Cancer Diagnosis
In Vitro Using
Monoclonal Antibodies

IMMUNOLOGY SERIES

Editor-in-Chief
NOEL R. ROSE
Professor and Chairman
Department of Immunology and
Infectious Diseases
The Johns Hopkins University
School of Hygiene and Public Health
Baltimore, Maryland

European Editor
ZDENEK TRNKA
Basel Institute for
Immunology
Basel, Switzerland

Additional Volumes in Preparation

Cancer Diagnosis In Vitro Using Monoclonal Antibodies

edited by

Herbert Z. Kupchik

*Boston University School of Medicine
and the Mallory Institute of Pathology
Boston, Massachusetts*

MARCEL DEKKER, Inc.   New York and Basel

Library of Congress Cataloging-in-Publication Data

Cancer diagnosis in vitro using monoclonal antibodies / edited by
  Herbert Z. Kupchik.
        p.   cm. -- (Immunology series ; 39)
    Includes index.
    ISBN 0-8247-7809-X
    1. Cancer--Diagnosis. 2. Antibodies, Monoclonal--Diagnostic use.
  I. Kupchik, Herbert Z. II. Series: Immunology series ;
  v. 39.
      [DNLM: 1. Antibodies, Monoclonal--diagnostic use. 2. Neoplasms-
  -diagnosis.   W1 IM53K v. 39 / QZ 241 C215]
  RC270.3.M65C36 1988
  616.99'40756--dc19
  DNLM/DLC
  for Library of Congress   88-27297
                                                    CIP

MARCEL DEKKER, INC.
270 Madison Avenue, New York, New York 10016

Current printing (last digit):
10 9 8 7 6 5 4 3 2 1

PRINTED IN THE UNITED STATES OF AMERICA

Dedicated to
Leona, Philip, and Aaron,
and in memory of
Mom

Series Introduction

Nothing has so challenged the imagination of the community of immunologists as tumor immunology. Clearly, antibodies are produced to any invading parasite or any injected foreign cell. Why not, then, to tumor cells? Surely, cancers act as the ultimate parasites, growing in an uncontrolled fashion and spreading through the body. They behave like foreign cells, but tumors fail to elicit an effective immune response. Protected by the physiological barriers that prevent responses to selfconstituents, they continue their unrestrained growth.

Immunization against tumors, then, has remained an unfulfilled dream of the immunologist. Still, immunology has made a useful contribution to oncology in another way. The specificity of the antibody and the sensitivity of serological reactions provide the most effective method for detection of unique structures of the cancer cells. Not cancer-specific in the classical sense, perhaps, but closely correlated with the malignancy, tumor markers have now been identified and put to good use for the diagnosis and monitoring of many cancers. The recent introduction of the hybridoma technique for the generation of large quantities of monoclonal antibodies of precise specificity has accelerated the development of new, more reliable tests.

In the present volume, Dr. Kupchik and his colleagues bring us up to date on this most rapidly expanding clinical application of fundamental immunological methodology.

Noel R. Rose
Professor and Chairman
Department of Immunology and
Infectious Diseases
The Johns Hopkins University
School of Hygiene and Public Health
Baltimore, Maryland

Foreword

"Once upon a time there were no tumor markers."

This might well be the line that the Brothers Grimm would have used for opening the story that unfolds in this volume dealing with monoclonal antibody assays for human cancers. Indeed, just over two decades ago, it was common wisdom that tumor markers, blood- or body-fluid-borne molecules that serve as "footprints of cancer," did not exist. This belief applied both to the biologic imperative of constituents required or generated with malignant transformation, as well as to the clinical situation wherein the measurement of certain constituents might be used in the diagnosis and management of cancer patients. The concept persisted despite the fact that Bence-Jones had described the first tumor marker in the urine of patients with multiple myeloma in 1846. Moreover, subsequent observations had led to descriptions of the ectopic production of hormones and enzymes by a number of tumors, most particularly bronchogenic cancers, sometimes giving rise to such conditions as the paraneoplastic syndromes. These demonstrations of what would now be termed "differentiation" or "phase-specific" tumor markers, depending upon the definitions being employed, still failed to excite further inquiry into the field of tumor markers, perhaps because such cases were described primarily as clinical curiosities.

The modern era of "tumor markerology," often called tumor immunology because of the techniques employed, is generally felt to have been ushered in by the description and definition of alpha$_1$-fetoprotein (AFP) and carcinoembryonic antigen (CEA). The paroxysms of optimism and pessimism that followed these reports are legion. It is only in the last few years that the lessons generated during the early, and rather chaotic, period of tumor markerology have been focused into the ever-more-aggressive search for increasingly sensitive and specific markers of tumor growth.

It has become clear that a substantial number of molecules found in body fluids may be of value to the clinician in the management of tumor patients. It has become equally clear that, for the moment, the major role to be played by assays for such materials is in the management of patients with established tumors before, during, and after therapy, but not in population screening. In the same vein, the data from populations cannot easily be applied to the individual patient and, hence, tumor marker assays must be used in conjunction with other available diagnostic tools for the tumor type being sought.

Conversely, tumor marker assays are important adjunctive diagnostic, and more importantly, prognostic aids and have important roles to play in the areas of immunohistology, immunocytology, and tumor localization by means of radioimmunoscintigraphy. At the present time, the role of tumor markers as targets for antibody-conjugated isotopes or drugs in "vectorial immunotherapy" remains to be more fully investigated, but the possibilities are very real.

The need for standardization of materials, methods, and study design in evaluating new and, indeed, old tumor marker assays is paramount. This has perhaps been the greatest single "sticking point" over the past two decades. Moreover, the semantic, and often philosophic, arguments about which molecule should be termed "tumor-specific" and which "tumor-associated" have, from a pragmatic standpoint, been largely resolved by appropriate definitions of where and when a marker is synthesized during embryologic development, specific periods of the cell cycle, or if it is produced exclusively during malignant transformation. In addition, a critically important distinction has been made between markers of clinical utility and cancer cell-specific molecules necessary for the integrity and invasive activities of tumor cells. Although the intellectual and scientific stimulation of such discussions is necessary, they should not be allowed to interfere with progress in the field but should, rather, speed the availability of carefully gathered data so that the marker in question may be assigned to its appropriate role in the field of tumor markers or dropped from the roster quickly.

From the foregoing, it should be underscored that the advent of monoclonal antibody technology, as applied to tumor markerology, has been a milestone event in this field where specificity, sensitivity, and molecular dissection are critical. Many chapters in this volume address state-of-the-art monoclonal antibody work as it applies to cancers of specific organ systems. These chapters were written by leading authorities on each of the tumor sites under consideration. Hence, this volume represents the present status of tumor markerology; a discipline at a turning point.

In reflecting on the contents of this book and future perspectives for tumor markers, including cellular microfluorometry, gene cloning of tumor markers, karyology in its broadest sense, and the increasing definitions of oncogenes and their products, one may begin to hope, again with the Brothers Grimm, that the closing statement in the field will be, "And they lived happily ever after."

Phil Gold, M.D., Ph.D.
Director
McGill University Medical Clinic
The Montreal General Hospital
Montreal, Quebec, Canada

Preface

The development of efficient (sensitive and specific) assays for the diagnosis of human cancer has been a high priority of cancer researchers for many years. With the advent of "the monoclonal antibody age," hopes and expectations were raised that the exquisite specificity afforded by such reagents would result in successful attainment of this goal. Numerous monoclonal antibodies that recognize a great variety of human tumor-associated macromolecules are described in this volume. Each contributor was challenged to discuss the state of knowledge of monoclonal antibodies related to his particular area of expertise and to evaluate the current and future benefits, limitations, and requirements of in vitro assay systems as applied to diagnosis and/or prognosis of nonhematopoietic human tumors.

Since cancer is not a single entity and can vary significantly among the different sites (organs) of the body (as well as within a particular organ), many of the antibodies are described within the context of tissue specificity. Nonetheless, the reader will note that several monoclonal antibodies are mentioned in more than one chapter since the tumor markers they recognize are found in different organs. The tumor markers CA 19-9, carcinoembryonic antigen, and placental alkaline phosphatase have been studied as discrete entities associated with a variety of malignant conditions. These were therefore afforded separate chapters. On the other hand, applications using monoclonal antibodies for the in vitro diagnosis of colonic carcinoma are derived from several studies and could not be confined to a single chapter. In a number of instances, monoclonal antibodies are described which may not be useful for assays of markers in body fluids. Many of these, however, can be used in immunocytochemical techniques for histopathologic identification and characterization. Several contributors have included studies of in vivo localization of radiolabeled monoclonal antibodies in human tumors grown in athymic mice. Such studies emphasize the importance of using all available means to identify those monoclonal antibodies that provide the greatest specificity and sensitivity for eventual diagnostic application. Finally, no volume describing monoclonal antibodies to human cancer would be complete without including a chapter describing the development of human antibodies to tumor markers since these may exhibit a different spectrum of reactivities than that seen with murine monoclonal antibodies.

I wish to extend my sincere appreciation to Mrs. Linda Stanger for her expert secretarial assistance and the contributors who responded to make this book as current as possible at the time of publication. It is hoped that the reader will appreciate the important contributions made to define the current role of monoclonal antibodies in the diagnosis of human cancer and that future investigations will benefit from the innovative studies described.

Herbert Z. Kupchik

Contents

Contents

Contributors

Miyako Abe, Ph.D. Dana Farber Cancer Institute, Harvard Medical School, Boston, Massachusetts

Robert C. Bast, Jr., M.D. Duke University Medical Center, Durham, North Carolina

Darell D. Bigner, M.D., Ph.D. Duke University Medical Center, Durham, North Carolina

Sandra H. Bigner, M.D. Duke University Medical Center, Durham, North Carolina

Michael J. Borowitz, M.D., Ph.D. Duke University Medical Center, Durham, North Carolina

T. Ming Chu, Ph.D. Roswell Park Memorial Institute, Buffalo, New York

Neil J. Finkler M.D. Brigham and Women's Hospital, Harvard Medical School, Boston, Massachusetts

Abraham Fuks, M.D. McGill Cancer Centre, McGil University, Montreal, Quebec, Canada

Victor E. Gould, M.D. Rush-Presbyterian-St. Luke's Medical Center, Chicago, Illinois

Michael G. Hanna, Jr., Ph.D. Bionetics Research, Inc., Rockville, Maryland

Martin V. Haspel, Ph.D. Bionetics Research, Inc., Rockville, Maryland

Daniel F. Hayes, M.D. Dana Farber Cancer Institute, Harvard Medical School, Boston, Massachusetts

Ingegerd Hellström, Ph.D., M.D. ONCOGEN, and University of Washington, Seattle, Washington

Karl Erik Hellström, Ph.D., M.D. ONCOGEN, and University of Washington, Seattle, Washington

Michael A. Hollingsworth, Ph.D. Duke University Medical Center, Durham, North Carolina

June Kan-Mitchell, Ph.D.   Kenneth Norris, Jr., Cancer Hospital and Research Institute, University of Southern California School of Medicine, Los Angeles, California

Carl S. Killian, Ph.D.   Roswell Park Memorial Institute, Buffalo, New York

Young Woo Kim, Ph.D.   Duke University Medical Center, Durham, North Carolina

Robert C. Knapp, M.D.   Brigham and Women's Hospital, Harvard Medical School, Boston, Massachusetts

Donald W. Kufe, M.D.   Dana Farber Cancer Institute, Harvard Medical School, Boston, Massachusetts

Herbert Z. Kupchik, Ph.D.   Boston University School of Medicine, and the Mallory Institute of Pathology, Boston, Massachusetts

Donald L. Lamm, M.D.   West Virginia Medical Center, Morgantown, West Virginia

Michael S. Lan, Ph.D.   Duke University Medical Center, Durham, North Carolina

Ching-Li Lee, Ph.D.   Roswell Park Memorial Institute, Buffalo, New York

Inchul Lee, M.D.   Rush-Presbyterian-St. Luke's Medical Center, Chicago, Illinois

Diane Logan, M.D.   McGill Cancer Centre, McGill University, Montreal, Quebec, Canada

Joel Lundy, M.D.   Winthrop Hospital, Mineola, and SUNY, Stony Brook, New York

Richard P. McCabe, Ph.D.   Bionetics Research, Inc., Rockville, Maryland

Roger E. McLendon, M.D. *   Duke University Medical Center, Durham, North Carolina

Richard S. Metzgar, Ph.D.   Duke University Medical Center, Durham, North Carolina

Malcolm S. Mitchell, M.D.   Kenneth Norris, Jr., Cancer Hosptial and Research Institute, University of Southern California School of Medicine, Los Angeles, California

Tsuneya Ohno, M.D., Ph.D.   Jikei University School of Medicine, Tokyo, Japan

---

Present affiliation: Tift General Hospital, Tifton, Georgia

Nicholas Pomato, Ph.D. Bionetics Research, Inc., Rockville, Maryland

James A. Radosevich, Ph.D. Northwestern University/VA Lakeside Medical Center, Chicago, Illinois

Steven T. Rosen, M.D. Northwestern University/VA Lakeside Medical Center, Chicago, Illinois

Jeffrey Schlom, Ph.D. National Cancer Institute, National Institutes of Health, Bethesda, Maryland

Derek F. Tucker, Ph.D. Imperial Cancer Research Fund, London, England

William W. Vick, M.D. Duke University Medical Center, Durham, North Carolina

Ming C. Wang, Ph.D. Roswell Park Memorial Institute, Buffalo, New York

Anthony Milford Ward, M.A., M.B., FRCPath. Royal Hallamshire Hospital, Sheffield, England

Vincent R. Zurawski, Jr., Ph.D. Centocor, Malvern, Pennsylvania, and Harvard Medical School, Boston, Massachusetts

Cancer Diagnosis
In Vitro Using
Monoclonal Antibodies

1
Monoclonal Antibodies in the Detection of Bladder Cancer

Richard P. McCabe, Martin V. Haspel, Nicholas Pomato, and Michael G. Hanna, Jr. / Bionetics Research, Inc., Rockville, Maryland

Donald L. Lamm / West Virginia Medical Center, Morgantown, West Virginia

INTRODUCTION

In 1986, there were an estimated 40,500 new cases of transitional cell carcinoma (TCC) of the bladder in the United States with an associated mortality of approximately 10,600. At one time, the incidence of TCC of the bladder was believed to be related to occupational exposure of workers to carcinogens, especially in the

1

rubber and dye industries, but the continued increase in disease incidence, even after safety measures have been taken to reduce the exposure to these workers, suggests that a broader range of environmental and dietary factors are involved (1).

Clinical detection of TCC is based primarily on examination of tumor cells in urine. However, this method of diagnosis (urinary cytology) is far from adequate. Of patients with well-differentiated (low-grade) tumors, often less than 30% will be identified (2), yet it is these patients who have the most favorable prognosis because low-grade tumors, when identified at an early stage, are more likely to respond to conservative treatment.

Once recognized as tumor cells, the grading of the cells as highly differentiated (grade I), intermediate (grade II), or poorly differentiated (grade III) becomes very important because the staging of the tumor and classifying the degree of differentiation are the principal factors considered in selecting a treatment regimen for the patient. Unfortunately, TCC is a highly heterogenous disease (3,4) with a variable histological appearance, which makes grading the cells a highly subjective procedure. Frequently, tumors scored as intermediate grade II are as aggressive as grade III tumors or behave like grade I tumors, which have a more favorable prognosis (5). Even with accurate information on grade and stage, the probability of recurrence can only be estimated; not withstanding, a substantial portion of tumors initially characterized as low-grade, early-stage tumors will recur (1,6). An adjunct to urinary cytological examination that would improve the detection of low-grade tumors and increase confidence in the prediction of which tumors are likely to recur would be an asset to the management of this disease.

Other characteristics of TCC cells, such as loss of blood group antigens (7-11), expression of T antigen (9, 12-14), and increased chromosomal number (5, 15, 16), correlate well with tumor grade and stage and, together with the grade and stage, may be helpful in predicting the malignancy of low-grade, early-stage cancer of the bladder (9). As promising as these markers are, however, individually they cannot be the determining factor for performing cystectomy. For example, although 90% of the tumors that test negative for blood group antigens will recur, nearly half of the tumors that test positive will also recur, so that testing for loss of blood group antigens has only limited value in predicting recurrence (10, 17), and if cystectomy were performed solely on this basis, many unnecessary operations would be performed (10, 17-18). Testing for blood group antigens is not a cut-and-dried procedure (19). The amount of antigen detected is influenced by subtle differences in methodology, and cutoffs for a positive test are subjective (19). A false-positive test result occurs with up to 30% of blood group 0 individuals, who represent 50% of the population (10). Subjectivity is especially important in laboratories where few tests are performed (19). The best use of blood group antigen detection is for estimating the probability of tumor invasion in a population at risk, rather than in an individual patient (10, 18). Evaluated together, however, blood group antigen deletion, T-antigen expression, and increased chromosomal number may be helpful for the individual patient. Additional study of these multiple markers and development of improved methodologies are needed.

Monoclonal antibody (MAb) technology provides the potential means of improving objectivity and accuracy in diagnosis, grading, and predicting recurrence of a tumor. Marker antigens identified with MAbs; in addition to blood group and T antigen, can be used to classify tumors for prospective determination of functional relationships among characteristics such as malignant behavior, structural abnormality, and marker expression. The same objectives may be realized whether the antibody-defined markers are detected by immuno-histochemistry with tumor cells or by immunoassay of antigens in urine, although the former approach has received the most attention. In addition, MAb technology offers many more new approaches in vivo tumor detection and tumor therapy than were possible to consider a few years ago.

IMMUNOHISTOCHEMISTRY WITH MONOCLONAL ANTIBODIES IN BLADDER CANCER

Although at least 26 MAbs reactive with TCC cells have been described (20-33), few have been characterized for the grade of tumor they recognize, and few have been found that specifically react with low-grade tumor cells (Table 1). Those antibodies that are reactive with low-grade tumors sometimes also react with normal urothelium, which limits their use in identifying tumor cells (34).

Fradat et al. (23) defined 11 distinct systems of cell surface antigens on normal and neoplastic bladder tissue with MAbs. Five of

Table 1 Monclonal Antibodies to Tumor Antigens Associated with Transitional Cell Carcinoma (TCC) of the Bladder

Antibody	Tissue/cell line reactivity	Ref.
A2	2/6 TCC cell lines	20
A80	4/6 TCC cell lines, normal kidney	
MAb 145	Normal bladder epithelium, lost in some TCC	21
D83.21	1/4 bladder tumor tissues	22
D6.2	3/4 bladder tumor tissues	
OM5	Low-grade bladder tumors, 50-60% normal urothelium	23
T23	6/46 bladder tumor tissue, no normal urothelial cell reactivity	23,34
T43	25/46 bladder tumor tissues, normal kidney, skin	23,34
T138	20/46 bladder tumor tissues, normal endothelium and kidney	23,34
JP165	2/10 bladder tumor tissues, no normal kidney reactivity	23
T101	4/10 bladder tumor tissues, some normal kidney reactivity	23
4B5	4/7 TCC cell lines, normal fibroblasts	24

S2C6	6/7 TCC cell lines, B lymphocyte	24
14B11	4/7 TCC cell lines, normal fibroblasts	24
HBA4	3/5 bladder tumor tissue, no normal tissue reactivity	25
HBE3	3/5 bladder tumor tissue, no normal tissue reactivity	25
HBE10	3/5 bladder tumor tissue, no normal tissue reactivity	25
9A7	5/15 TCC cell lines; low-, intermediate-, and high-grade bladder	26
2E1	tumor tissue, no normal tissue reactivity	
2A6		
3G2.C6	High-grade bladder tumors, no normal bladder reactivity	27
6F26.7.7	33/61 TCC cell lines, neutrophils (100%)	28
P7A5-4	7/8 bladder tumor tissues, no normal tissue reactivity	29
7E9	High-grade bladder tumors, no normal tissue reactivity	30
G4	High-grade bladder tumors and Ca in situ, 1/3 low-grade	31
E7	bladder tumors	

these systems defined antigens present on subsets of bladder tumors and absent from normal urothelium. A sixth system defined by MAb Om5 was the most restricted and was present only on low-grade tumors with a superficial papillary abnormality and on carcinomas in situ (23, 34). However, the Om5 antigen was expressed by 50-60% of normal urothelium samples (34). Overall, 16 of 19 superficial papillary tumors expressed Om5, as did six of eight carcinomas in situ (23, 34). Invasive tumors did not express Om5 (only three of 15 tested Om5-positive). Messing et al. (26) described three MAbs reactive with five cell lines and six primary transitional cell carcinomas tested. Primary tumors included four grade I and II tumors and two carcinomas in situ. No reactivity with normal tissue was detected. A study by Cordon-Cardo (35) provides further evidence that expression of antigens recognized by MAbs correlates with disease progression. In these experiments, about 80% of superficial papillary bladder tumors expressed URO-9 antigen but not URO-10 antigen. Conversely, about 90% of muscle-invasive or metastatic tumors expressed URO-10 but not URO-9 (35). Thus, these studies (23, 26, 34, 35) clearly establish that tumor cell-specific antigens exist on TCC cells and that MAbs to superficial tumors can be developed, although development of MAbs specifically reactive with low-grade tumors, and not reactive with normal tissue, may be difficult to achieve. A panel of MAbs, however, could be very useful in identifying tumors with the propensity to invade at an early stage when aggressive treatment would be successful. Additional work to characterize these antibodies and to develop additional antibodies with a focus on the potential clinical applications promises to be rewarding.

The strategy used in developing MAbs can greatly affect the nature of the antibodies produced. Most MAbs to TCC have been raised to bladder tumor cell lines. This approach has numerous advantages: Cell lines originating from a wide range of differentiation lineages in bladder cancer provide homogenous cell populations for immunization and serological and biochemical studies. However, there is no certainty that cell lines derived from grade I tumors have preserved the antigenic characteristics of low-grade tumors after years of subculture. Indeed, selection occurring during subculture commonly produces sublines that vary considerably from the originally isolated tumor cells. Fradet et al. (23), in describing their antibody to the Om5 antigen on superficial bladder tumor cells, reported the reactivity of the antibody with only four of 18 TCC cell lines but with strong reactivity with a high proportion of well-differentiated papillary bladder tumors. They concluded that raising antibodies to cell lines may not be the best approach to identifying antigens to low-grade TCC. It is a common finding that the use of cell lines produces few MAbs specifically reactive with low-grade tumors and, in many instances, MAbs isolated after immunization with cell lines have reacted less consistently with fresh tumor tissue than with other cell lines. The alternative to the use of cell lines is the use of fresh tumor tissue for immunization, an approach that seldom has been tried, although recognized as the better strategy. The fresh tissue approach seems better suited to the production of a broadly reactive reagent that recognizes low-grade tumor cells of most human TCC.

Metcalfe and Jamieson (36) recently found an unusual tumor marker, B5 antigen, present not on tumor cells but on the erythrocytes of patients with various types of malignancies, including TCC of the bladder. The marker is defined by an MAb. The antigen is not usually found on erythrocytes of normal individuals (18% of 249 people tested). Overall 80% of 98 bladder tumor patients expressed B5 on erythrocytes, as determined in MAb-based hemagglutination assay. More evaluation of this unusual marker is needed to establish its clinical value.

DETECTION OF SOLUBLE ANTIGENS IN URINE WITH MONOCLONAL ANTIBODIES

Clearly, urinary cytology and cell surface antigen expression alone are not yet sufficiently sensitive nor accurate for diagnosis of TCC, and cystoscopy, although quite effective in identifying lesions in the bladder, is not a completely benign procedure. Furthermore, once the primary tumor has been removed, patients must be monitored for years to ensure that they receive additional treatment at the earliest indication of tumor recurrence. A noninvasive, efficient, reliable, quantitative procedure that is useful both for detecting primary TCC and for monitoring patients after treatment is needed. An MAb-based radio-immunoassay (RIA) or enzyme-linked immunosorbent assay (ELISA) with sufficient sensitivity to detect small deviations from normal concentration levels of antigen would be ideally suited to automation and standardization as

required for a high-volume testing procedure. Several markers have
been evaluated (37-43). Most are of dubious value, lacking the
requisite sensitivity or specificity. Still others have not, as yet,
been fully evaluated. Currently, only carcinoembryonic antigen
(CEA) and urinary fibrin (ogen) degradation products (FDP) appear to have clinical value.

Soluble Antigen Excretion

Urinary CEA levels have been used by some workers as a means of
following responses to treatment or of assessing prognosis (44-45).
Pretreatment CEA levels of over 30 ng/ml are indicative of a poor
prognosis (45). Similar to serum assays used in the management of
many other types of cancer, decreasing urinary CEA levels after
treatment indicate a better prognosis than increasing levels. However, some bladder cancers produce little or no CEA and false-
positive results sometime occur because of infected urine or
urinary diversion (46). Consequently, other workers have concluded that urinary CEA is an unreliable marker of recurrence
(47-48), and thus, urinary CEA analysis has not become an accepted tool in the management of bladder cancer. This lack of acceptance is somewhat unjustified. Many workers are unaware of
appropriate applications of the CEA assay and have not evaluated
CEA in relation to other diagnostic or prognostic factors. When
combined with assessments of the stage and grade of the tumor
and with urinary cytological studies 4 months posttreatment, CEA
has proved to be most helpful in predicting a recurrence-free interval (44).

Analysis of FDP in urine also has been suggested as a reliable
indicator of bladder cancer (49-55), especially when used in conjunction with urinary cellular abnormalities (56-58). The FDP appear in urine when fibrin deposited in and around tumors or disseminated through the circulation in late-stage cancer is resolved
through the activity of plasmin (59). Plasmin degradation of fibrin
occurs with the sequential generation of well-defined fragments
of the entire molecule (Figure 1).

Analysis for FDP combined with urinary cytological studies
gave the correct diagnosis in 80% of the patients in one study (58)
and 86% of the patients in another study (56). In both of these
studies, the FDP assay methods were not quantitative and were

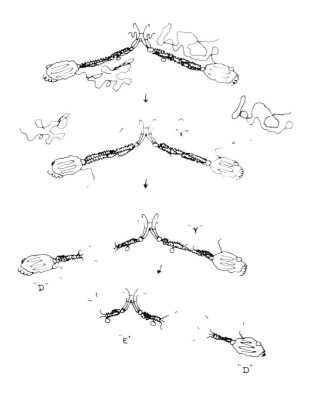

Figure 1 Schematic diagram depicting the plasmin-mediated generation of fibrin degradation products (FDP) from intact fibrinogen. Native fibrinogen is composed of three pairs of constituent chains in bilateral symmetry with a central "E" and two lateral "D" domains. The molecular weight is 340,000. The initial fragments released by plasmin are fragments of the carboxy-terminus of the A chain which extend as unfettered loops from the lateral D domains of the native fibrinogen. The looping portions are approximately 50,000-molecular weight and are degraded to smaller nonimmunogenic fragments not shown in the figure. The remaining fibrinogen fragment "X" is about 270,000. Plasmin acts on the trinodal remaining X portion to release one D region (85,000) generating fragment "Y" (170,000) consisting of the remaining D region attached to the central "E" domain. Finally, plasmin digests the Y fragment. Terminal digestion of native fibrinogen results in three fragments, two 85,000 D domains and one 55,000 E domain (*Source*: figure provided by R. F. Doolittle, University of California at San Diego.)

relatively insensitive (60). On the basis of these studies docu-
menting the clinical potential of determining FDP in the urine of
bladder cancer patients, we undertook development of an MAb-
based ELISA method for the rapid detection of urinary FDP. The
ELISA method was selected because of its many advantages over
RIA and hemagglutination inhibition (HAI) procedures. It is more
stable and convenient than RIA. Compared with HAI assays,
which are insufficiently sensitive for use as either a screen or a
monitor, the ELISA is much easier to perform, needs no prior
sample preparation or concentration, and can provide a quantitative analysis. The MAb enhances the specificity and reproducibility of the assay procedure.

Enzyme-Linked Immunosorbent Assay for Fibrin Degradation Products in the Urine of Bladder Cancer Patients

The MAb to the human urinary FDP was developed from spleen
cells of mice immunized with urine from a patient with bladder
cancer. Because the objective was to analyze a component of the
bladder tumor patient's urine, we decided to use this urine as the
immunogen, rather than the FDP generated in the laboratory,
which might be unrelated to the urinary FDP. The power of MAb
technology is that it allowed us to use the appropriate immunogen
without having to purify the material from its source.

The MAb developed (C-6) was an IgM with high apparent affinity for fibrinogen and was highly suitable as the capture moeity
in the solid-phase ELISA procedure. The specificity of C-6 was
determined to be directed to an epitope on terminal fibrin degradation product E by both indirect immonoprecipitation and
Western blot analysis. Figure 2 describes the evidence supporting
this specificity.

The solid-phase, capture-type ELISA was developed with the
MAb on polycarbonate-coated steel beads to capture urinary
fibronogen/ FDP. Polyclonal goat antihuman fibrinogen, conjugated with horseradish peroxidase (HRP), was used to detect the
captured fibrinogen or FDP. The assay was designed to detect
native fibrinogen as well as plasmin-digested fibrin (ogen) because
experiments, in which thrombin was added to patient urine to clot
intact fibrinogen, had shown that urinary fibrinogen was present
in both native and degraded forms (Table 2).

Table 2 Sensitivity of ELISA for Fibrinogen or FDP and Comparison with
the HAI Assay

	Titer or sensitivity	
Specimen	HAI method	ELISA
Highly positive urine from bladder tumor patient		
without thrombin	1:16	1:16
with thrombin	1:8	1:32
Fibrinogen standard	1250 ng/ml	39 ng/ml

Source: Ref. 55, reproduced with permission of the publisher.

The sensitivity of the ELISA was assessed by extinction titration of bladder cancer urine and a standard preparation of human fibrinogen. For reference purposes, the sensitivity of the ELISA was compared with that of the HAI method. Both tests indicated the same native fibrinogen/FDP ratio in tumor patient's urine (see Table 2). The ELISA assay was four times more sensitive than the HAI method in the urine assay and 32 times more sensitive than the HAI procedure in the fibrinogen standard assay (see Table 2).

Urine specimens from seven patients were assayed in triplicate in three consecutive ELISAs to determine the reliability of a single determination. Standard deviations ranged from 0.012 to 0.031 absorbance units.

The variance observed among specimens collected from the same patient was determined with tests on 14 collections from one patient assayed together in a single test (Figure 3). To determine daily variation in urinary FDP output, sequential determinations were performed on each voided specimen. The mean value was 0.705 ± 0.193 OD_{405} units. The large standard deviation reflected a single low value (0.198) obtained on the second collection day. A repeat analysis of the same specimens confirmed the validity of the assay result and of the aberrant single sample. At both day 1 and day 2, the lowest values were associated with the first-voided specimen. Except for the first specimen collection on day 2, the other collections were in agreement.

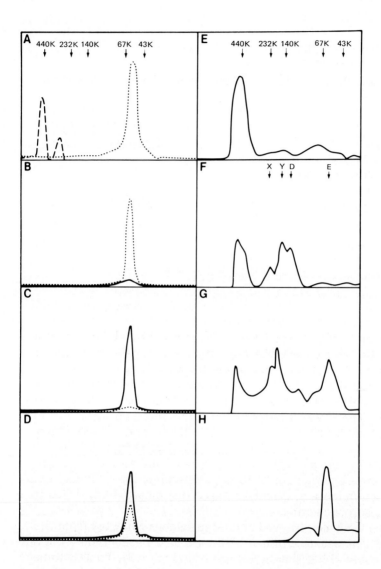

Figure 2

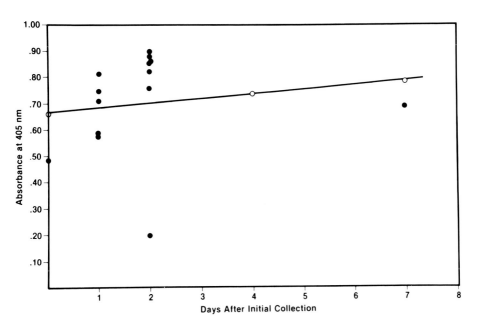

Figure 3   Results of ELISA (OD_{405nm}) of 14 urine specimens collected from one patient over a period of 7 days. Each closed circle is the mean of duplicate determinations. Open circles lie on the path of the best-fit regression line. Specimens were tested in the high-sensitivity ELISA procedure (*Source*: Ref. 55, reproduced with permission of the publisher.)

Figure 2   Specificity of C-6 MAb as demonstrated by immunoprecipitation (A-D) and Western immunoblot (E-H) of human fibrinogen and its plasmin degradation products reacted with C-6 MAb or rabbit antisera specific for degradation products D and E. Panel A, electrophoresis of ^{125}I-labeled fibrinogin before (dashed line) and after 8 hr digestion with 5 units human plasmin (dotted line). Panel B-D, electrophoresis of immunoprecipitated ^{125}I-labeled plasmin-digested fibrinogen (solid line) and of the supernatant remaining after immunoprecipitation (dotted line) with rabbit antisera to degradation product D (panel B), degradation product E (panel C), or C-6 MAb (panel D). Panel E-H, Western immunoblot of native human fibrinogen (panel E) and plasmin-digested fibrinogen (panels F-H) following electrophoresis and transfer to nitrocellulose. Immunoblots were developed with rabbit antisera to human fibrinogen (panel E), rabbit antiserum to degradation product D (panel F), rabbit antiserum to product E (panel G), or C-6 MAb (panel H). Electrophoresis was performed on 4 - 30% polyacrylamide gels using 37 µg protein in each lane. Top of each gel is at left margin of the panel. Each autoradiograph or Western immunoblot was scanned at 525 nm with a laser densitometer. Molecular weight markers were ferritin (440,000), catalase (232,000), lactate dehydrogenase (140,000), bovine serum albumin (67,000), and ovalbumin (43,000) (*Source*: Ref. 55 reproduced with permission of the publisher.)

Table 3   Analysis of Fibrinogen or FDP in Urine of Patients with Carcinoma of the Bladder. I. High-Sensitivity Assay[a]

Source of specimens (no. of patients)[b]	Assay result	No. of urine specimens (% total)	
		Uncertain values included	Uncertain values excluded[c]
BT+ patients (37)	Positive (TP)	92 (83)	90 (85)
	Negative (FN)[d]	19 (17)	16 (15)
	Uncertain		5
BT- patients (34)	Positive (FP)[e]	44 (34)	41 (33)
	Negative (TN)	87 (66)	82 (67)
	Uncertain		8

[a] The sensitivity of the assay was calculated by the formula (TP specimens/ Total specimens from BT+ patients) and was 83% (92/111), including uncertain values, and 85% (90/106), excluding uncertain values. Values within 0.05 OD units of the cutoff value were defined as uncertain. The accuracy of the assay was calculated by the formula (TP + TN specimens/ Total specimens) and was 74% (179/242), including uncertain values, and 75% (172/229), excluding uncertain values; TN, true negative; TP, true-positive.

[b] The total number of patients was 71. Each specimen was classified as BT+ or BT- depending upon whether or not the patient had clinically evident disease at the time of collection.

[c] Uncertain values were eliminated from each total for determination of the percentage.

[d] The false-negative (FN) rate for the assay was calculated by the formula (FN specimens/Total specimens) and was 8% (19/242), including uncertain values, and 7% (16/229), excluding uncertain values.

[e] The false-positive (FP) rate for the assay was calculated by the formula (FP specimens/Total specimens) and was 18% (44/242), including uncertain values, and 17% (41/229), excluding uncertain values. *Source*: Ref. 55, reproduced with permission of the publisher.

The occurrence of fibrinogen and FDP in the urine of bladder carcinoma patients, and the potential value of these determinations in the detection and management of this disease, were assessed with a coded panel of 412 randomly arranged specimens from 108 patients. The results are shown in Figure 4. In Tables 3 and 4, the results are broken down into patient categories for evaluation. The value of the assay is apparent in Figure 4, which shows that most specimens from tumor-bearing patients (BT+)

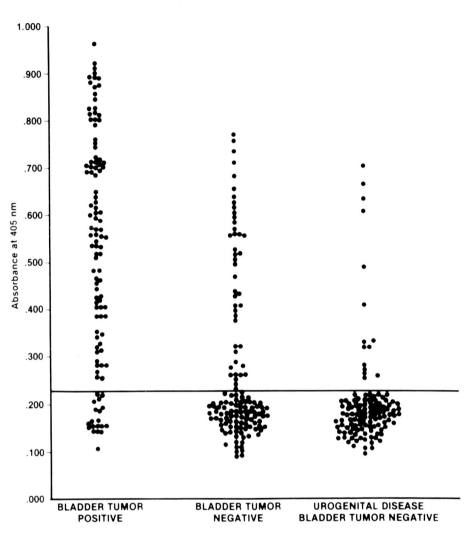

Figure 4   High-sensitivity ELISA. Scattergraph of individual specimen results
(OD405nm) grouped according to whether, at the time of specimen collection, the patients had clinically evident bladder carcinoma (bladder tumor-
positive), recent history of bladder carcinoma, but no current evidence of
disease (bladder tumor-negative), or urogenital tract inflammation or current
or prior evidence of prostatic or renal carcinoma (urogenital disease, bladder
tumor-negative), Each circle is the mean of duplicate determinations. Values
below the solid line were scored as negative, those above as positive (*Source*:
Ref. 55, reproduced with permission of the publisher.)

gave higher assay results than those from patients in the other groups. Given the standard deviations of 0.012 - 0.031 absorbance units for individual specimens, and as an aid in identifying positive and negative values, an uncertain zone within the assay extending 0.05 OD$_{405}$ units above and below the cutoff value was defined. Table 3 includes results presented and calculated both with and without inclusion of the uncertain values. However, exclusion of uncertain values had little impact on the overall evaluation because most specimens (229 of 242) did not fall within the uncertain zone. The high-sensitivity ELISA was 83-85% sensitive in detecting those patients with a clinically detectable tumor and 74-75% accurate in determining the current status of bladder carcinoma patients. The difference in overall accuracy compared with the sensitivity in detecting bladder cancer is a reflection of a 17-18% rate of false-positive values compared with 7-8% rate of false-negative values. In the analysis of specimens from patients with nonmalignant disease or tumors other than bladder carcinoma, the high-sensitivity ELISA showed 86% accuracy or specificity (see Table 4). It is important to emphasize that this group included

Table 4   Analysis of Fibrinogen or FDP in Urine of Patients with Non-Malignant Urogenital Disease or Tumors at Sites Other Than the Bladder. I. High-Sensitivity Assay[a]

Source of specimens (no. of patients)	Assay result	No. of negative specimens/ total specimens (%)
Patients with nonmalignant urogenital disease (32)	Negative (TN)	38/42 (90)
Patients with prostatic carcinoma (14)	Negative (TN)	43/48 (90)
Patients with renal carcinoma (4)	Negative (TN)	14/20 (70)

[a]The specificity of the assay was 86% (95/110) as calculated by the formula (Negative (TN) specimens/Total specimens). The rate of false-positive results of the assay was 14% (15/110 as calculated by the formula (Positive specimens/Total specimens). *Source*: Ref. 55, reproduced with permission of the publisher.

specimens from 29 patients with urinary tract infections. Eighty-six percent sensitivity exceeds the results that can be expected from other individual monitoring procedures. Furthermore, many other markers are nonspecifically elevated in patients with urinary tract infection or stones. The ability to differentially diagnose bladder cancer in these patients would be particularly useful.

Previous studies have reported elevated levels of urinary fibrinogen or FDP in upper, but not in lower, urinary tract infections (61). In our study, an elevated assay result was obtained in the high-sensitivity procedure for one patient with hematuria and in one with a renal stone; however, only one of 29 specimens from patients with urinary tract infection had an elevated assay value. Immunotherapy with bacille Calmette Guerin, which produces a marked inflammatory response in the bladder, was not associated with elevated assay values (D. Lamm, unpublished observations). Nevertheless, an elevated FDP value in association with an upper urinary tract infection would be interpreted with reservation pending more extensive clinical studies to establish this relationship.

The ELISA false-positive rate of 17% is low in comparison with that of other markers. The ELISA false-positive results appear to be caused by such factors as residual FDP excretion after tumor removal, irreversible kidney damage, or clinically undetected tumor recurrence. False-negative values can result from nonrepresentative urine collections (see Figure 3) or the presence of a tumor not associated with fibrinogen or FDP excretion. Long-term studies of individual patients and frequent sample collection will provide the data necessary to distinguish among these possibilities and will lessen the adverse effects of false assay values.

When designing the assay procedure, we selected sample volumes and reagent concentrations for maximum sensitivity, with the expectation that some values assigned as false-positive on the basis of a negative tumor status might, in actuality, be true-positive responses to a clinically undetected tumor. Whereas a false-positive value might subsequently be clinically proved to be a true-positive value, a false-negative value would be unlikely to change. However, this maximum level of sensitivity is not desirable in every application. Figure 5 and Tables 5 and 6 show the results obtained on the same panel with the assay redesigned to give a lower degree of sensitivity, but higher specificity, for bladder

Table 5 Analysis of Fibrinogen or FDP of Patients with Carcinoma of the Bladder. II. High-Specificity Assay[a]

Source of specimens (no. of patients)[b]	Assay result	No. of specimens %
BT[+] patients (38)		120
	Positive (TP)	60 (50)
	Negative (FN)[d]	60 (23)
BT[-] patients (36)		139
	Negative (TN)	123 (88)
	Positive (FP)[d]	16 (6)

[a]The sensitivity of the assay was calculated as described in Table 2 and was 50% (60/120). The accuracy of the assay was calculated as described in Table 3 and was 71% (183/259).
[b]Total number of patients was 74. Specimens from individual patients were classified as either BT[+] or BT[-] according to the presence of clinically evident disease at the time of collection.
[c]The rate of false-negative (FN) results was 23% (60/259) as calculated by the formula described in Table 3.
[d]The rate of false-positive (FP) results was 6% (16/259) as calculated by the formula described in Table 3. *Source*: Ref. 55 reproduced with permission of the publisher.

Table 6 Analysis of Fibronogen or FDP in Urine of Patients with Non-malignant Urogenital Disease or Tumors at Sites other Than the Bladder. II. High-Specificity Assay[a]

Source of specimens (no. of patients)	Assay result	No. of negative specimens/ total specimens (%)
Patients with nonmalignant urogenital disease (33)	Negative (TN)	41/42 (98)
Patients with prostatic carcinoma (15)	Negative (TN)	47/49 (96)
Patients with renal carcinoma (4)	Negative (TN)	21/22 (95)

[a]The specificity of the assay was 96% (109/113) as calculated as described in Table 4. The rate of false-positive results was 4% (4/113) as calculated by the formula described in Table 4. *Source*: Ref. 55, reproduced with permission of the publisher.

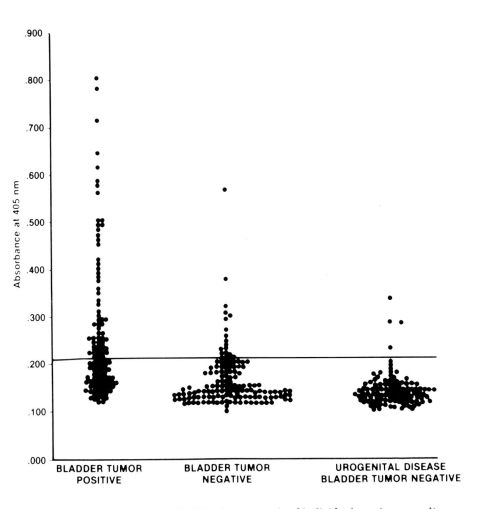

Figure 5 High-specificity ELISA. Scattergraph of individual specimen results (OD_{405nm}) grouped according to whether, at the time of specimen collection, the patients had clinically evident bladder carcinoma (bladder tumor-positive), recent history of bladder carcinoma but no current evidence of disease (bladder tumor-negative), or urogenital tract inflammation or current or prior evidence of prostatic or renal carcinoma (urogenital disease, bladder tumor-negative). Each circle is the mean of duplicate determinations. Values below the solid line were scored as negative, those above as positives. (*Source*: Ref. 55, reproduced with permission of the publisher.)

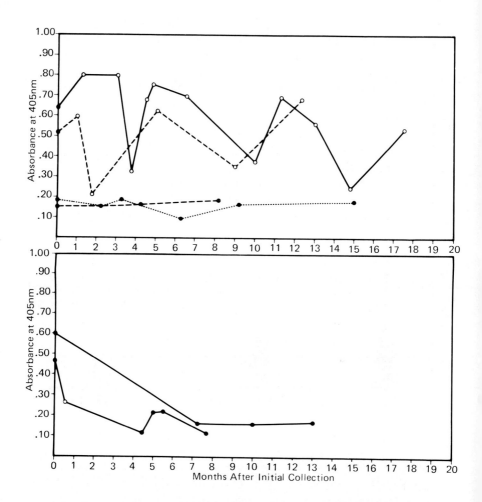

Figure 6 Top frame: ELISA results (OD_{405nm}) with urine specimens from four patients collected over periods of up to 17.5 weeks. Open circles represent results on specimens from two patients with clinically evident bladder tumor (BT^+) throughout the monitoring period. Closed circles represent results from two patients with a prior bladder tumor, but no clinical evidence of disease (BT^-) throughout the monitoring period.

      Bottom frame: ELISA results (OD_{405nm}) with urine specimens from two patients. Both patients had clinically evident bladder tumors (BT^+) (open circles) at the beginning of the monitoring period and after treatment became (BT^-) (closed circles). (*Source*: Ref. 55 reproduced with permission of the publisher.)

cancer. In the patients with bladder cancer, the false-positive rate fell to 6% of the total (see Table 5) and in the patients with non-malignant urogenital disease, the false-positive rate fell to 4% (see Table 6). Table 7 compares the two assay procedures. The high-sensitivity procedure appears better for predicting tumor status in patients with bladder cancer; however, its specificity for bladder carcinoma (76%) is not as high as that of the high-specificity procedure (92%). Clearly, the choice of procedure will be dictated by the intended use of the assay. For screening, specificity is extremely important, and a lower level of sensitivity may be acceptable; for monitoring tumor status in patients known to have bladder cancer, higher sensitivity to the recurrence of tumor is more important, and a lower level of specificity may be acceptable.

The monitoring of treatment efficacy requires frequent specimen analysis. The more frequent the analysis, the less significant are false-positive or false-negative results because the pattern of assay values rather than individual results form the basis of interpretation. Any marked change in assay results would be readily confirmed in a subsequent assay. Figure 6 illustrates this point with data from several patients from whom urine specimens were collected over a period of several weeks. The data in Figure 6 (top) are typical of most patients. Assay results were consistently within the positive or negative range, although wide fluctuations were apparent, and a drop to the negative range or rise to positive value on a single specimen collection was not indicative of a change in tumor status. In addition, the ELISA was sensitive to changes in tumor burden as reflected in Figure 6 (bottom); two patients with no detectable disease after surgery produced assay values that fell after treatment and remained in the negative range on subsequent assays. Decreasing assay values after tumor removal were expected. Occasionally, the assay value did not become negative immediately after surgery but was persistently and decreasingly positive for several weeks before eventually becoming and remaining negative.

Finally, it was important to consider whether the analysis of urinary fibrinogen or FDP was equivalent to, or superior to, a simple protein assay in predicting tumor status. When the results of the high-sensitivity assay were compared with the protein concentrations of each sample, many discrepancies between protein content and assay result were apparant, and no overall correlation

Table 7 Compilation of Assay Results

Evaluation variable	Formula	% from high-sensitivity assay	% from high-sensitivity assay
Sensitivity	No. of TP[a] specimens / Total no. of specimens from BT+ patients	83 (92/111)	50 (60/120)
Accuracy	No. of TP specimens + TN specimens / Total no. of specimens	78 (274/352)	78 (292/372)
Specificity	No. of TN specimens (exluding specimens from BT- patients) / nonmalignant urogenital disease or cancer at sites other than the bladder	86 (95/110)	96 (109/113)
Overall specificity	No. of TN specimens / No. of specimens from BT- patients and specimens from patients with nonmalignant urogenital disease or cancer at sites other than the bladder	76 (182/241)	92 (232/252)
False-negative	No. of FN specimens / Total no. of specimens	5 (19/352)	16 (60/372)
False-positive	No. of FP specimens / Total no. of specimens	17 (59/352)	5 (20/372)

[a] TP, true-positive; TN, true-negative; FP, false-positive. Source: Ref. 55, reproduced with permission of the publisher.

of assay value with protein concentration was found. This supports the belief that the FDP in the urine are arising from the activation of plasminogen and degradation of fibrin in the tumor and are not the result of leakage of serum proteins through damaged renal glomeruli.

FUTURE PROSPECTS

The ability to detect and treat urinary bladder carcinomas in vivo using radiolabeled antibodies will be among the most important contributions of MAb technology to the overall management of this disease. The ability to specifically concentrate themselves in tumor tissue along with the radionuclide or therapeutic agent attached to them is the basic premise of antibody-mediated in vivo tumor detection and therapy. Monoclonal antibodies labeled with radioactive isotopes have been shown to be useful for the clinical identification of tumor sites in patients with various types of malignances (62-66), but no clinical studies in bladder cancer have been reported. However, experimental studies have established the feasibility of the concept in bladder cancer. Gross et al. (67), using their A2 MAb produced to RT4 bladder carcinoma cells, have demonstrated specific localizations of the radiolabeled A2 antibodies in RT 4-nude mouse xenografts and the capacity to readily detect the tumor tissue by external gamma scintigraphy. Bubenik et al. (30) have reported similar results in tumor detection by radio-immunoscintigraphy using their 7E9 MAb to T-24 bladder carcinoma cells xenografted to nude mice.

Techniques for applying MAbs to in vivo detection and therapy are being evaluated in clinical trials. Antibody-drug and antibody-toxin conjugates are now being developed in the clinic. However there are problems that, although not preventing limited in vivo use of MAbs, may very well prevent the clinical realization of the full potential of this technology. These problems include cross-reactivity with normal tissues (65,66,68,69), low avidity of fragmented antibody (70-71), and effects of specific antigens in the circulation (72). These problems may be circumvented by careful selection of antibodies and are, therefore, not conceptual limitations; however, the fact that all murine antibodies and antibody fragments are immunogenic in patients with functioning immune systems (73-79) is a general and potentially serious limitation.

Human antimouse antibody responses develop in most patients after one administration of whole-mouse immunoglobulin and in approximately 50% of patients after three or more injections of murine F (ab')$_2$ or Fab' fragments (74). Antimurine antibody can abrogate the effectivenss of the MAb (75) and could result in immune complex-mediated serum sickness. Human antibodies are of great interest for this reason. Toxicity to foreign proteins (urticaria, fever, nausea, anaphylaxis) should not be a problem with human antibodies, and repeated doses of the same antibody could potentially be administered without eliciting human antibody responses that would interfere with therapy or tumor detection. Anti-idiotypic responses that develop would be antibody-specific and circumvented by use of a second or third antibody of different specificity. Unlike the immune response to murine antibodies, an immune response to one human antibody should not have any effect on the use of other human antibodies in the same patient. Human antibodies can potentially be applied in the same patient over periods of several months to years to detect tumor, specifically concentrate toxic agents in tumor tissue, and monitor the results of the therapy regimen.

In 1985 we reported the development of over 20 human MAbs from the peripheral blood lymphocytes of patients with colon cancer (76). Recently, we reported on the pharmacokinetics of two of these human MAbs in nude mice and on their tumor-specific localization in human colon tumor xenografts and on their external detection by radioimmunoscintigraphy (77). A current diagnostic-therapeutic clinical trial with colon carcinoma patients has established the absence of systemic toxicity with up to 100 mg of these antibodies. There is no evidence of reactivity to the antibodies,and metastatic tumor lesions have been identified in liver, lung, bone, and tissue in five of six patients now being studied (R. Steis, unpublished).

The human MAbs were developed with the lymphocytes of patients participating in an active specific immunotherapy trial for colon cancer (78). Current research is focused on producing more human MAbs using cells from patients in other clinical immunotherapy trials. Immunotherapy of bladder cancer using intravesicular bacille Calmette Guérin is now the most effective treatment for superficial bladder cancer (79-80). In the patients so treated, an active immune response to the tumor is apparently induced. Lymphocytes from these patients can be used to develop human MAbs to bladder cancer in the same manner as was used to develop the MAbs from the lymphocytes of colon cancer patients. Such MAbs may be useful in identifying secondary tumor sites, monitoring the progress of systemic therapy, and monitoring the delivery of therapeutic agents to metastatic tumor. In addition, because it can be expected that antibodies developed from patients immunized to their own tumor tissue will recognize a more restricted range of antigens, and possibly an entirely different class of antigens, then those recognized by mice immunized with human bladder carcinoma cells from cell culture, human MAbs may identify antigens useful in the in vitro identification of low-grade tumor cells for primary diagnosis by urinary ELISA or staining of exfoliated cells.

SUMMARY

Monoclonal antibody technology has the potential of providing reagents to reliably and consistently detect cell surface markers and soluble urinary antigens associated with bladder tumors and correlated with the aggressive potential of the disease. The heterogeneity of tumors makes it unlikely that any single MAb will be useful with all tumors. As an initial step in the use of MAbs to detect recurrence of bladder tumor, the FDP assay is encouraging. The high-specificity procedure is extremely accurate (92-95%) with a low rate of false-positive results (5%), a level of accuracy that is important in screening individuals at increased occupational or environmental risk of developing bladder cancer. In addition to causing needless concern to the patient, falsely elevated assays necessitate further clinical examination, which ultimately would include cystoscopic examination, the mainstay of the diagnosis of bladder cancer, but a procedure that is neither innocuous nor inexpensive.

Urinary cytological studies, the current noninvasive standard for the detection of bladder cancer, is notoriously inaccurate in low-grade tumors. In contrast, urinary ELISA appears to accurately detect both high-grade and low-grade lesions. The ELISA procedure also offers important technical and practical advantages over cytological examination. It is a semi automated procedure that can be used by a relatively unskilled technician to screen 200-300 urine specimens in a few hours. Thus, it is much less expensive and time-consuming than microscopic examination of urine. Furthermore, internal controls and standards included with each 96-well assay plate could provide a quick and accurate means of evaluating the reliability of the assay and of scoring assay results.

In the future, human MAbs developed from bladder cancer patients undergoing bacille Calmette Guérin immunotherapy will be used to identify tumor lesions outside the bladder and to specifically deliver cytotoxic agents to the metastic bladder tumor tissue.

REFERENCES

1. R. S. Weinstein, in *AUA Monographs: Bladder Cancer* (W. W. Bonney and G. R. Prout, Jr., eds.), William & Wilkins, Baltimore (1982), p. 3.
2. G. Koss, M. R. Malamed, and R. E. Kelly, *J. Natl Cancer Inst. 43*:233 (1969).
3. G. R. Prout, Jr., in *AUA Monographs: Bladder Cancer* (W. W. Bonney and G. R. Prout, Jr., eds.), Williams & Wilkins, Baltimore (1982), p. 149.
4. M. N. El-Boklainy, *J. Urol. 124*:20 (1980).
5. B. Czerniak and L. G. Koss, *Cancer 55*:2380 (1985).
6. A. A. Narayana, S. A. Leoning, D. J. Slyman, and D. A. Culp, *J. Urol. 130*:56 (1983).
7. J. M. DeCenzo, P. Howard, and C. E. Irish, *J. Urol. 114*:874 (1975).
8. J. D. Johnson and D. L. Lamm, *J. Urol. 123*:25 (1980).
9. N. Javadpour, *Urol. Clin. N. Am. 11*:609 (1984).
10. R. P. Huben, *Urology*, 23(Suppl. 3):10 (1984).
11. T. J. Stephenson, J. L. Williams, and K. Gelsthorpe, *Br. J. Urol. 57*:148 (1985).
12. J. L. Summers, J. S. Coon, R. M. Ward, W. H. Falor, A. W. Miller, and R. S. Weinstein, *Cancer Res. 43*:934 (1983).
13. J. A. Vafier, N. Javadpour, G. F. Worsham, and K. J. O'Connell, *Urology 23*:348 (1984).
14. R. S. Weinstein, A. W. Miller, and J. S. Coon, *Prog. Clin. Biol. Res. 153*: 249 (1984).
15. W. H. Falor and R. M. Ward, *Acta Cytol. 20*:270 (1976).
16. S. D. Fossa, O. Kaalhus, and O. Scott-Knudson, *Eur. J. Cancer 13*:1155 (1977).
17. W. J. Catalona, *Urology 18*:113 (1981).

18. K. B. Cummings, *Cancer 45*:1849 (1980).
19. C. Limas, J. Coon, P. H. Lange, and R. S. Weinstein, in *AUA Monographs: Bladder Cancer* (W. W. Bonney and G. R. Prout, Jr., eds.), Vol. 1, Williams & Wilkins, Baltimore (1982), p. 69.
20. H. B. Grossman, *J.Urol. 130*:610 (1983).
21. A. Rearden, D. A. Nachtscheim, D. M. Frisman, P. Chiu, D. A. Elmajian, and S. M. Baird, *J. Immunol. 131*:3073 (1983).
22. G. L. Wright, Jr., M. L. Beckett, J. J. Starling, P. F. Schellhammer, S. M. Sieg, L. E. Ladaga, and S. Poleskic, *Cancer Res. 43*:5509 (1983).
23. Y. Fradet, C. Cordon-Cardo, T. Thompson, M. E. Daly, W. F. Whitmore, Jr., K. O. Lloyd, M. R. Melamed, and L. J. Old, *Proc. Natl. Acad. Sci. USA 81*:224 (1984).
24. H. Koho, S. Paulie, H. Ben-Aissa, I. Jonsdottir, Y. Hansson, M. L. Lundblad, and P. Perlmann, *Cancer Immunol. Immunother. 17*:165 (1984).
25. T. Masuko, H. Yagita, and Y. Hashimoto, *J. Natl. Cancer Inst. 72*:523 (1984).
26. E. M. Messing, J. E. Bubbers, K. E. Whitmore, J. B. deKernion, M. S. Nestor, and J. L. Fahey, *J. Urol. 132*:167 (1984).
27. D. A. Young, G. R. Prout, Jr., and C. W. Lin, *Cancer Res. 45*:4439 (1984).
28. O. R. Baricordi, A. Sensi, C. DeVinci, L. Melchiorri, G. Fabris, E. Marchetti, F. Corrado, P. L. Muttiuz, and G. Pizza, *Int. J. Cancer 35*:781 (1985).
29. H. Ben-Aissa, S. Paulie, H. Koho, P. Biberfield, Y. Hansson, M. L. Lundblad, H. Gustafson, I. Jansdottir, and P. Perlmann, *Br. J. Cancer 52*:65 (1985).
30. J. Bubenik, J. Kieler, P. Perlmann, S. Paulie, H. Koho, B. Christensen, Z. Dienstbier, H. Koprivova, J. Pospisil, and P. Pouckova, *Eur. J. Cancer Clin. Oncol. 21*:701 (1985).
31. D. K. Chopin, J. B. deKernion, D. L. Rosenthal, and J. L. Fahey, *J. Urol. 134*:260 (1985).
32. I. C. Summerhayes, R. A. McIlhinney, B. A. Ponder, R. J. Shearer, and R. D. Pocock, *J. Natl. Cancer Inst. 75*:1025 (1985).
33. L. K. Trejdosiewicz, J. Southgate, J. A. Donald, J. R. Masters, P. J. Hepburn, and G. M. Hodgers, *J. Urol. 133*:533 (1985).
34. Y. Fradet, C. Cordon-Cardo, W. F. Whitmore, Jr., M. R. Melamed, and L. J. Old, *Cancer Res. 46*:5183 (1983).
35. C. Cordon-Cardo, *Cancer Res.* (in press).
36. S. M. Metcalfe and N. V. Jamieson, *Ann. R. Coll Surg. Engl. 66*:399 (1984).
37. A. P. Monaco, J. J. Gozzo, R. M. Schlesinger, and S. D. Codish, *Ann. Surg. 182*:325 (1975).

38. E. J. Sanford, J. R. Drago, T. J. Rohner, G. F. Kessler, L. Sheehan, and A. Lipton, *J. Urol. 113*:218 (1975).
39. R. K. Chawla, A. D. Wadsworth, and D. Rudman, *J. Immunol. 121*:1636 (1978).
40. N. S. Rote, R. K. Gupta, and D. L. Morton, *Int. J. Cancer 26*:203 (1980).
41. S. Kumar, C. B. Costello, R. W. Glashan, and B. Bjorklund, *Br. J. Urol. 53*:578 (1981).
42. S. R. DeFazio, J. J. Gozzo, and A. P. Monaco, *Cancer Res. 42*:2913 (1982).
43. S. Kubota, M. Okada, K. Imahori, and N. Ohsawa, *Cancer Res. 43*:2363 (1983).
44. B. Wahren and F. Edsmyr, *Urol. Res. 6*:221 (1978).
45. B. Wahren, B. O. Nilsson, and R. Zimmerman, *Cancer 50:139* (1982).
46. J. A. Lessing, *J. Urol 120*:1 (1978).
47. V. Betkerur, R. Rao, V. Hlaing, H. Rhee, G. Baumgartner, and P. Guinan, *Urology 16*:16 (1980).
48. R. W. Glashan, E. Higgins, and A. M. Neville, *Eur. Urol. 6*:344 (1980).
49. M. Ohtaki, *Jpn. J. Urol. 68*:1172 (1977).
50. J. A. Martinez-Pineiro, C. Pertuse, E. Masanto, V. G. Zancajo, M. Massallon, G. Losada, and F. Ortesa, *Eur. Urol. 4*:348 (1978).
51. S. Ueda, H. Hirayama, M. Arita, and K. Ikesami, *Jpn. J. Urol. 69*:1241 (1978).
52. E. A. Alsabti, *Eur. Surg. Res. 11*:185 (1979).
53. T. Tanahashi, *Nippon Hinyokika Gakkai Zasshi 70*:553 (1979).
54. T. Tanahashi, *Nippon Hinyokika Gakkai Zasshi 71*:1047 (1980).
55. R. P. McCabe, D. L. Lamm, M. V. Haspel, N. Pomato, K. O. Smith, E. Thompson, and M. G. Hanna, Jr., *Cancer Res. 44*:5886 (1984).
56. T. Tanahashi, Y. Matsumara, H. Ohmori, and T. Tanaka, *Acta Med. Okayama 32*:139 (1978).
57. K. Uemura, J. Tanaka, N. Yoshitake, S. Noda, and K. Etoh, *Nishinippon Hinyokika 41*:497 (1979).
58. Z. Wajsman, P. D. Williams, J. Greco, and G. P. Murphy, *Urology 12*:659 (1978).
59. R. P. McCabe and J. H. Evans, *Surv. Synth. Pathol. Res. 2*:1 (1983).
60. C. Merskey, G. J. Kleiner, and A. J. Johnson, *Blood 28*:1 (1966).
61. J. A. Whitworth, K. F. Fairley, and M. A. McIvor, *Lancet 1*:234 (1973).
62. D. M. Goldenberg, F. H. Deland, and E. Kim, *N. Engl. J. Med. 298*:1384 (1978).
63. A. A. Epenetos, K. E. Briton, J. Mather, J. Shepherd, M. Granowska, J. Taylor-Papadimitriou, C. C. Nimnon, H. Durbin, L. R. Hawkins, and J. S. Malpas, *Lancet 2*:999 (1982).

64. J.-P. Mach, J.-F. Chatal, J. D. Lumbroso, F. Buchegger, M. Forni, J. Ritschard, C. Berche, J.-Y. Douillard, S. Carrel, M. Herlyn, Z. Steplewski, and H. Koprowski, *Cancer Res. 43*:5593 (1983).
65. N. C. Armitage, A. C. Perkins, M. V. Pimm, P. A. Farrands, R. W. Baldwin, and J. D. Hardcastle, *Br. J. Surg. 74*:407 (1984).
66. M. D. Gross, R. W. Skinner, and H. B. Grossman, *Invest. Radiol. 19*:530 (1984).
67. J. A. Carrasquillo, K. A. Krohn, P. Beaumier, R. W. McGuffin, J. P. Brown, K. E. Hellstrom, I. Hellstrom, and S. M. Larson, *Cancer Treat. Rep. 68*:317 (1984).
68. S. M. Larson, J. P. Brown, P. W. Wright, J. A. Carrasquillo, I. Hellstrom, and K. E. Hellstrom, *J. Nucl. Med. 24*:123 (1983).
69. P. J. Moldofsky, J. Powe, C. B. Mulherne, U. Hammond, H. F. Sears, P. A. Gatenby, S. Steplewsky, and H. Koprowski, *Radiology 149*:549 (1983).
70. T. Maillet, A. C. Roche, F. Therain, and M. Monsigny, *Cancer Immol. Immunother. 19*:177 (1975).
71. B. Ballou, J. M. Reiland, G. Levine, R. J. Taylor, W.-C Shen, H. J.-P. Reyser, D. Solter, and T. R. Hakala, *J. Surg. Oncol. 31*:1 (1986).
72. C. Berche, J.-P. Mach, J.-D., Lumbroso, C. Langlais, F. Aubry, F. Buchegger, S. Carrel, P. Rougier, C. Parmentos, and M. Tubiana, *Br. Med. J. 285*:1447 (1982).
73. R. Levy and R. A. Miller, *Fed. Proc. 42*:2650 (1983).
74. J. C. Reynolds, J. A. Carrasquillo, A. M. Keenan, M. E. Lora, P. Sugarbaker, P. Abrams, K. Foon, J. L. Mulshine, J. Roth, D. Colcher, J. Schlom, and S. M. Larson, *J. Nucl. Med. 27*:1022 (1986).
75. D. Hyams, J. C. Reynolds, J. A. Carasquillo, P. Perentesis, S. M. Larson, M. Morin, D. Simpson, J. Schlom, and D. Colcher, *J. Nucl. Med. 27*:922 (1986).
76. M. V. Haspel, R. P. McCabe, N. Pomato, N. J. Janesch, J. V. Knowlton, L. C. Peters, H. C. Hoover, Jr., and M. G. Hanna, Jr., *Cancer Res. 45*: 3951 (1985).
77. R. P. McCabe, L. C. Peters, M. V. Haspel, N. Pomato, and M. G. Hanna, Jr., *Cancer Res.* (submitted for publication).
78. H. C. Hoover, Jr., M. G. Surdyke, R. B. Dangel, L. C. Peters, and M. G. Hanna, Jr., *Cancer Res. 55*:1236 (1985).
79. D. L. Lamm, D. E. Thor, and W. D. Winters, *Cancer 48*:82 (1981).
80. H. W. Herr, *Uremia Inves. 8*:257 (1984-1985).

2
Monoclonal Antibodies and Diagnosis of Brain Neoplasms

Roger E. McLendon, * William W. Vick, Sandra H. Bigner, and
Darell D. Bigner/ Duke University Medical Center, Durham, North Carolina

INTRODUCTION

The application of immunological techniques to histogical sections offers the possibility of phenotypic characterization of the morphologically heterogeneous central nervous system tumors. Mono-

---

*Present affiliation : Tift General Hospital, Tifton, Georgia

specific polyvalent antisera have been difficult to generate for neuropathological applications because few biochemical antigens of diagnostic utility in the brain have been purified. These problems have arisen because of the difficulty in the biochemical purification of neural antigens, because of the cross-reactivity of the various neural antigens, and because of the subsequent loss of these antigenic markers in neoplasia. Monoclonal technology allows the use of impure antigen, thus overcoming a number of the problems inherent in polyvalent antisera including antigen identification, antibody supply, and antibody specificity to produce continuous clones of antibody-producing cells. Although the initial time consumed in generating and characterizing a monoclonal antibody (MAb) is longer than that for an equivalent polyvalent antiserum, once established the purified supernatant requires only minimal testing.

Although a number of MAbs have been produced against neural antigens, no comprehensive reviews exist that examine their specificity as provided by the characterization data published on these MAbs. As there are no standardized means of testing MAb specificity, several techniques have been applied for this purpose. To judge each MAb, the relative utility of each technique used to determine specificity must be known. Radioimmunoassay (RIA), immunoblot electrophoresis, and immunohistochemistry are the most commonly used methods for measuring different aspects of MAb specificity. The RIA method with cell cultures is a rapid means of screening secreting clones to determine if the supernatant reacts with a culture line that expresses the target antigen. The specificity of the RIA-positive clonal supernatants can be tested by immunoblot electrophoresis, a sensitive means of testing MAb specificity against a homogeneous antigen preparation separated according to electrophoretic mobilities, transferred, or "blotted," onto nitrocellulose paper, upon which the MAb is applied, using indirect peroxidase localization techniques.

These clones may then be tested by immunohistochemistry to determine the cellular distribution of the antigen. Although this technique is, in some ways, the most sensitive means of determining specificity, immunohistochemistry will not always differentiate between two antigens that coexist in a cell, such as the myelin-associated antigens. Thus, immunohistochemistry alone is not sufficient to verify the specificity of a MAb.

For categorization purposes, the MAbs that are now available can be separated into two groups: MAbs against antigens identified by biochemical means, and MAbs against antigens identified initially by the MAb itself. The first category of neural antigens includes S-100, the intermediate filaments, neuron-specific enolase, glutamine synthetase, and a_2 glycoprotein. The second category is so extensive that all MAbs cannot be covered here. Rather, this discussion is focused on a small group of MAbs representative of this category, including those described by Wikstrand, Bourdon, and others from Bigner's laboratory, by Kemshead, Coakham, and collaborators in England, among others. Although experience with MAbs against CNS tumor-associated antigens is limited, these efforts have permitted the elucidation of some principles, goals, and pitfalls in the characterization of monoclonally defined neural neoplastic-associated antigens.

BIOCHEMICALLY DEFINED ANTIGENS

S-100

In 1965, Moore (1) described a protein that he believed was unique to the nervous system. He named this protein S-100 because it was soluble in neutral pH, 100% ammonium sulfate. The exact function of the protein has not been determined, but studies have defined a calcium-binding role (2). Biochemically, the protein is dimeric, being composed of combinations of a-subunits and β-subunits. Subunit S-100ao is, therefore, composed of an a-a combination, S-100a is a-β, and S-100b is β-β. Subunit S-100ao is preponderantly confined to tissues of macrophage-monocyte origin (3), where as S-100a and S-100b, although not confined to the central nervous system (CNS), have a restricted distribution among tissues of neuroectodermal, ectodermal, and mesodermal origin (4-6).

Early immunochemical studies utilizing polyvalent antisera produced conflicting results, partially because of technical problems in purifying the antisera and partially because of poor tissue fixation allowing the water-soluble, low-molecular-weight (21,000) S-100 dimers to diffuse. Recent studies, in which these artifacts were strictly controlled, have found S-100 reactivity in the normal CNS confined to astrocytes and the Bergman glial cells and in the peripheral nervous system (PNS) to the Schwann cells and the satellite cells found in peripheral ganglia. Furthermore, nonneural immunoreactivity has been found in melanocytes and Langerhans cells of skin, in the interdigitating reticular cells of lymph nodes, in chondrocytes of both neural crest and mesodermal origin, in ductular myoepithelial cells, and in T lymphocytes. Neither normal neurons nor ependymal cells have been found to contain any S-100 protein, whereas recent evidence suggests that normal oligodendrocytes are also negative for the protein (reviewed in 7, 8) (Table 1).

The early studies on S-100 reactivity have used absorbent-purified polyvalent antisera and have shown that the immunolocalization of S-100 has its greatest value in the differential diagnosis of spindle cell neoplasms (4). Neoplasms of Schwann cells, melanocytes, smooth muscle, striate muscle, fibroblasts, or meninges may be difficult to distinguish from one another in the routine hematoxylin-eosin-stained sections. In studies with polyvalent antisera, only the tumors of Schwann cell, astrocytic, and melanocytic origin, including neurofibromas, acoustic neuromas, traumatic neuromas, granular cell tumors, neurilemmomas, some malignant nerve sheath sarcomas, astrocytomas of all grades, and malignant melanomas, express S-100 (4, 5, 8-10). Spindle cell tumors that produce negative reactions for S-100 include leiomyomas, leiomyosarcomas, rhabdomyosarcomas, fibrosarcomas, malignant fibrous histiocytomas, alveolar soft-part sarcomas, Ewing's sarcoma, and meningiomas (4,7,10), although conflicting results on meningiomas exist (4, 11).

Nonspindle-cell tumors that exhibit S-100 positivity include chordomas, histiocytosis X (eosinophilic granuloma), pleomorphic adenomas of salivary glands, cartilaginous tumors, lipomas, liposarcomas, and some osteogenic sarcomas (correlating with the cartilaginous portion of the tumor((4,5). Nakajima et al. (6) have reported an infiltrating ductal carcinoma of the breast to be S-100-positive. Although S-100 reactivity has been described in T lymphocytes, no hematological malignancies have been described that express S-100. No oat cell carcinoma, Merkel cell tumor, or medullary carcinoma of the thyroid has yet been reported to express S-100 (10).

In the central nervous system, most primary neoplasms give positive reactions of S-100, including gliomas, schwannomas, and some pituitary adenomas, pinealomas, and medulloblastomas. Meningiomas, in most studies, have been negative. Controversy surrounds the S-100 content of the oligodendroglioma. Although histological studies (11) have ruled out the presence of S-100 in normal oligodendroglia, in studies of snap-frozen, fresh non-reactive brain, using polyvalent antisera, positivity in the oligo-dendroglioma has been observed (5,6).

These reports, using polyvalent antisera, emphasize the desirability of a standard anti-S-100 MAb reactive with formalin-fixed tissues. Several S-100 MAbs have been reported (12-16). The MAb 15E2E2 of Gillespie and Golden (Figure 1), which reacts with both S-100 and S-100a, has been extensively tested on formalin-fixed tissues and exhibits a staining intensity and pattern on both CNS and peripheral neoplasms comparable with that of polyvalent antisera (8). The MAb of Haan et al. (11) also reacts with both S-100a and S-100b by immunoblot electrophoresis and reacts specifically in the normal rat CNS with astrocytes as defined by double-labeling studies with the glial fibrillary acidic protein. Marks et al. (14) have produced an MAb that, by plate-binding radioimmunoassay, by immunoprecipitation sodium dodecyl sulfate-polyacrylamide gel electrophoresis (SDS-PAGE) studies, and by positive immunoperoxidase reactivity with the C-6 glioma line, was considered to be specific for S-100. This MAb's re-activity in tissue sections was not reported in the original study. Van Eldik et al. (15) have reported two MAbs (1A1 and 404) specific for the β-specificity which produce significantly different results from the other MAbs and the cross-reactive polyvalent antisera now commonly in use.

Vanstapel et al. (16) have reported the production and charac-terization of three MAbs that by immunoblot studies react with an epitope common the the a-subunit and β-subunit of S-100. In a follow-up study on both normal and neoplastic tissues, these authors (17) compared the immunoreactivity of their MAbs with an S-100 polyvalent antiserum from a commercial source and found markedly different staining. Their MAbs stained both normal and neoplastic liver; adenocarcinomas of gastric, colonic, and gallbladder origin; and histiocytes. Furthermore, no staining was present in sections of two of five Schwann cell sections. These unusual histological reactivities require further studies before this MAb may be applied in diagnostic situations.

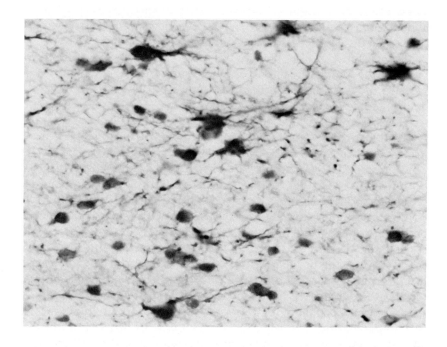

Figure 1   Anti-S100 MAb 15 E2E2 of Gillespie stains both the reactive astrocytes and the oligodendroglia in this formalin-fixed, paraffin-embedded non-
neoplastic brain section (X 540).

Intermediate Filament Proteins

Intermediate filaments are a major constituent of many cells both
in vivo and in vitro. Along with the larger-diameter microtubules
(23 nm) and the smaller-diameter microfilaments (6 nm), intermediate filaments (8-10 nm diameter) compose the cytoskeletal
architecture of higher eukaryotic cells. Although each intermediate filament is comprised of one to three smaller repetitive
subunits, these polypeptides are encoded by a large multigene pool
and are expressed differentially in various tissues. Given the subunit structure, five classes of intermediate filaments are recognized: (1) glial fibrillary acidic protein, detected in astrocytes; (2)
neurofilaments, characteristic of neurons; (3) cytokeratins, specific for cells of epithelial origin; (4) desmin, found preponderantly

in smooth, skeletal, and cardiac muscle cells; and (5) vimentin, the nonspecific filament that can be found in cells of ectodermal, mesodermal, endodermal, and neuroectodermal origin (18,19).

Glial Fibrillary Acidic Protein

The intermediate filament, glial fibrillary acidic protein (GFAP), has proved to be an important marker of glial cells in diagnostic neuropathology. This protein was first independently isolated by two groups, Mori et al. (20) using brains from patients with Tay-Sachs disease and Eng et al. (21) using brains from patients with multiple sclerosis. Subsequent studies have found these two proteins to be identical (reviewed in 20). Although GFAP was originally purified from pathologically altered brains, bovine spinal cord has become the source most commonly employed for the production of the purified protein used in the induction of both antisera and MAbs (22,23).

Biochemical studies have shown that GFAP may exist in two forms, a water-soluble form and a water-insoluble form (21,24). Both forms have identical molecular weights (51,000) (25) and amino acid contents (21,25), and both forms can repolymerize into filaments under specific in vitro conditions (27). The biochemical and physiological role of each form is uncertain, as a number of factors including postmortem autolysis (28) have been found to alter their distribution; however, the soluble form is believed to represent an actual physiologic state and is thought to explain the GFAP immunoreactivity found in certain neoplasms that lack ultrastructurally demonstrable intermediate filaments, such as the astroblastoma (24).

The distribution of GFAP in the central nervous system has been well documented in studies using highly specific antisera (22). The most intensely staining cells of the nonreactive, non-neoplastic central nervous system are the fibrillary astrocytes of the cerebrum (30). Protoplasmic astrocytes also exhibit GFAP reactivity, as do the Bergman glia of the cerebellum (31) and rare ependymal cells, which some investigators believe to be tanycytes (32). The GFAP reactivity has also been described in pituicytes of the posterior lobe (22,23), the supportive cells of the pineal gland (34,35), and in the Müller cells of the retina (36). After injury, fibrillary astrocytes, ependymal cells, Bergman radial glia, and retinal Müller cells all become strongly immunoreactive (22).

Outside of the central nervous system, GFAP immunoreactivity has been described in both the sciatic nerve and small unmyelinated nerves, which might represent Schwann cell reactivity (37-39), in the enteric glia (40), in the lens epithelium of the eye (41), and in the metaplastic cartilage of a mixed salivary gland tumor (42). Although the antisera used to identify these antigens may have been recognizing a cross-reactive, or shared, epitope on an unrelated protein, immunoblot studies have found the immunoreactive protein in the lens epithelium to be a 51-kd protein that comigrates with GFAP and reacts with a well-characterized MAb to GFAP in immunoblot studies (41). Preliminary studies using three well-characterized MAbs to GFAP did not identify any reactivity in four schwannomas (43).

The distribution of GFAP in CNS neoplasms has been well described in a number of reviews using both MAbs and polyvalent antisera (29,30,32,44-47). Astrocytomas of all grades exhibit GFAP reactivity with the well-differentiated neoplasms exhibiting virtually 100% reactivity of the cells. Most studies have found GFAP immunoreactivity to decrease with increasing anaplasia. Our experience with these tumors suggests that anaplastic astrocytomas and low-grade, or well-differentiated, astrocytomas are both strongly positive. In glioblastoma, however, the immunoreactivity varies markedly from the tumors preponderantly composed of small anaplastic cells that exhibit a low percentage of positive cells, to the tumors composed of large bizarre cells that have a high percentage of positive cells (43).

The presence of GFAP reactivity in oligodendrogliomas and ependymomas has been well documented (45,46). Several authors have suggested that GFAP immunoreactivity in these neoplasms might reflect the stages in development of both the oligodendrocyte and the ependymal cell in which GFAP production is manifest (48). In contrast to the oligodendrocyte, however, the ependymal cell may exhibit GFAP positivity in reactive processes, such as ventriculitis and obstructive hydrocephalous (49). An occasional choroid plexus papilloma may also be positive for GFAP (44, 50, 51). Because normal choroid plexus epithelium lacks intermediate filaments, Rubinstein and Brucher (52) have suggested that this phenomenon represents focal ependymal differentiation in this tumor.

A neoplasm in which GFAP immunoreactivity has been of help in classification has been the so-called intracranial fibrous xanthoma that is found in pediatric patients. The finding of GFAP positivity in these tumors led to the ultrastructural recognition of intermediate filaments and the reclassification of a subgroup of these neoplasms as xanthoastrocytomas (53).

Monoclonal antibodies to GFAP have been described. Collins (54) has described MAb C9, which exhibits GFAP specificity by immunoblot studies and by immunohistochemistry on both fresh-frozen and formalin-fixed, frozen tissues. This MAb has been of use in the cytological recognition of glial cells in smear preparations of CNS tissues (55). Its reactivity is lost in paraffin-embedded tissues, however, suggesting that the epitope recognized by the MAb is sensitive either to the effects of processing or to reagents in the paraffin itself (55). Albrechtsen et al. (56) have described an MAb (GFAP-3) that was monospecific for GFAP by indirect immunoprecipitation, by immunoblot analysis, and by immunohistochemistry on frozen tissues. Like the MAb of Collins, this MAb exhibits weak and inconsistent reactivity on formalin-fixed, paraffin-embedded tissues. Lee et al. (57) have described four MAbs ($2.2B_{10}$, $2.1B_{12}$, $1.1A_2$, $3.1E_{12}$) that were monospecific to GFAP by enzyme-linked immunosorbent assay (ELISA), immunoblot studies, and by immunohistochemistry on sections from fresh-frozen and mercuric chloride-fixed, paraffin-embedded tissues. Trojanowski et al. (58) have further studied the diagnostic utility of these MAbs on 100 Zenker's or Bouin's-fixed CNS and PNS neoplasms and found the MAbs to be specific for glial elements. Debus et al. (58) have described the production of 10 MAbs that are monospecific for GFAP by immunoblot analysis and by immunohistochemistry on frozen sections of astrocytomas fixed in either formalin or alcohol. The application of these MAbs on formalin-fixed, paraffin-embedded tissues has not been reported.

From Bigner's laboratory, Pegram, in collaboration with Eng, produced three MAbs that were monospecific for GFAP by RIA, immunoblot analysis, and immunohistochemistry of both fresh-frozen and formalin-fixed, paraffin-embedded tissues (23). On competitive inhibition analyses, these MAbs were found to identify either the same, or spatially close, epitopes. Further studies on these MAbs found that a "cocktail" composed of equal concen-

trations of each MAb resulted in the immunohistochemical localization of GFAP comparable with that of a high-titer, monospecific
polyvalent antisera on 71 intracranial and intraspinal neoplasms
that had been fixed in formalin and embedded in paraffin (Figure
2) (43). Absorption analyses carried out on brain homogenates on
11 different species demonstrated that these MAbs identified
phylogentically conserved epitopes (23). Immunohistochemical
studies on dog, cat, rat, and human brains have further supported
these findings. This study additionally reported the characterization of another eight MAbs that, although reacting with GFAP,
also reacted with vimentin or one of the neurofilament subunits
(23). This cross-reactivity with epitopes also present on the other
intermediate filaments is a well-recognized problem in the production of monospecific MAbs to these proteins (59-62).

Neurofilaments

Hoffman and Lasek (63) were the first to propose that the components of slow axonal transport recognized as neurofilaments
consisted of triplets, now identified as 68-kD, 160-kD, and 212-kD
proteins (64,65).

In early studies, polyvalent antisera raised to each of the
triplet proteins cross-reacted with the other two subunits (36,65-
67), suggesting a homologous substructure shared by the subunits.
Further studies, however, have found that the subunits are trans-
lated from distinct mRNAs, thus confirming the triplet proteins
as distinctive entities (67). Homologous regions have been identified between the neurofilaments and other intermediate filaments:
a 40% homology in amino acid sequence has been demonstrated
between an isolated fragment of the porcine neurofilament 68-kD
subunits and portions of desmin and vimentin from the same
species (68). In experiments using highly specific polyvalent antisera on neurofilament-rich neuronal cytoskeletons, antisera against
the 68-kD and 145-kD proteins produced a continuous decoration
of the ultrastructural filament, whereas the 200-kD protein antisera produced discontinuous labeling (66,69). These studies suggest that while each neurofilament is composed of all three subunits, the 68-kD, and probably the 145-kD, proteins are localized
to the filament backbone, whereas the 200-kD subunit appears to
be involved with side-arm appendage structure.

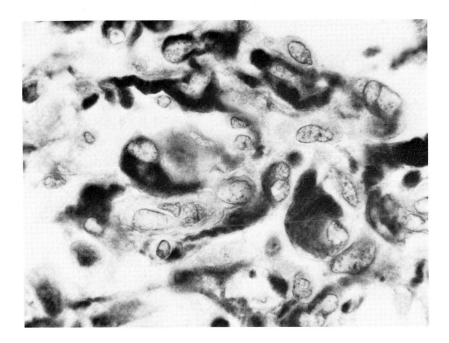

Figure 2   Anti-GFAP monoclonal cocktail composed of a mixture of three anti-GFAP MAbs produces intense cytoplasmic reactivity in this glioblastoma multiforme (X 1000).

Neurofilaments are characteristic of most (70), but not all (69), neurons. Immunohistochemical studies have shown that the individual neurofilament proteins vary in the different neuronal populations; thus, while most axons exhibit all three proteins in comparatively large amounts, only small amounts of the 200-kD protein are detected in certain brain stem neurons or in the dendrites and cell bodies of cerebral pyramidal cells (58,71). Cerebellar granule cells apparently lack neurofilaments (71). Developing neurons exhibit a differential expression of neurofilament, with the 68-kD and the 145-kD subunits the first to appear followed by the 212-kD protein (72,73).

Lee et al. (74) have reported MAbs specific for each individual neurofilament protein, as determined by immunoblot electrophoresis and immunohistochemistry. MAb 4.3F9, which recognizes both the 145-kD and the 212-kD proteins in $HgCl_2$ formalin-fixed, paraffin-embedded tissues was used by Trojanowski et al. (44,58,75,76), who found neurofilament reactivity in 2 of 3 carotid body tumors, 4 of 4 gangliogliomas, 2 of 2 ganglioneuroblastomas, 3 of 3 ganglioneuromas, 1 of 6 neuroblastomas, 4 of 6 pheochromocytomas, and 1 of 1 ovarian teratoma. No neurofilament reactivity was found in any gliomas, carcinoids, or other nonneuronal tumors. Trojanowski et al. have also reported the localization of the 68-kD protein in esthesioneuroblastomas (77). Interestingly, no staining was identified in any of 10 medulloblastomas or in one pineoblastoma. These findings suggested to these investigators that neurofilament reactivity may, in addition to labeling a cell as neuronal, provide information about the degree of cellular differentiation.

In addition to the antineurofilament MAb studied by Lee and associates, Debus et al. (58) have reported two MAbs (NF1 and NEI 4) for the 200-kD protein, one MAb for the 145-kD protein (NN18), and one MAb for the 68-kD protein (NR4) that were monospecific by immunoblot electrophoresis and immunohistochemistry on both cell cultures and fresh-frozen rat brain. The NR4 MAb when applied to 24 neuroblastomas and was variably reactive with 18 of the neoplasms. Wood and Anderton (78) have also reported an MAb that specifically binds neurofilament in fresh-frozen tissue sections. Neither its protein subunit specificity nor its application to neoplasms, has, however, been reported.

Vimentin

Vimentin lacks the cytological specificity of the other intermediate filaments, as it has been identified in cells of ectodermal, mesodermal, endodermal, and neuroectodermal origin (19). In the neuroectoderm, vimentin is coexpressed with neurofilaments in developing neurons and with glial fibrillary acidic protein in both developing glia and mature astrocytes, including Bergman glia and fibrous astrocytes (38,79). Furthermore, mature ependymal cells, tanycytes, meningothelial cells, mesenchymal cells of the choroid plexus, and vascular smooth muscle may express vimentin (19). The practical application of vimentin reactivity appears to be limited in the diagnosis of CNS neoplasms. Although meningiomas express vimentin as their only intermediate filament (80,81), this information has been of little practical use in differentiating these neoplasms or in subclassifying them.

Cytokeratins

Keratin is the most complex of the five types of intermediate filaments. There have been at least 19 types of cytokeratins identified, all varying in mass (range 40-67 kD) and isoelectric point. Previous investigations have demonstrated that the overall type of cytoskeleton is not changed after malignant transformation, which means that neoplasms with epithelial differentiation may still express its original cytokeratin spectrum. With the increasing development of antikeratin MAbs, the potential exists of ultimately "fingerprinting" various types of epithelia and carcinomas to establish diagnoses in poorly differentiated neoplasms (82). Central nervous system neoplasms that express cytokeratin include the choroid plexus neoplasms, the chordoma (83) and the colloid cyst (84).

This marker has been used to differentiate the chordoma from the cytokeratin-negative cartilaginous sarcomas. The application of cytokeratin-specific MAbs to CNS neoplasms may also be useful in confirming the diagnosis of metastatic carcinomas (84).

Desmin

Desmin is highly restricted in its expression and is characteristic of smooth, skeletal, and cardiac muscle in normal adult tissues. Although the distribution of the protein has not been demonstrated in the CNS, it probably resides in vascular smooth muscle cells. Antibodies against desmin have been used to identify spindle cell sarcomas of muscle cell origin and is, thus, potentially useful in the diagnosis of primary and metastatic rhabdomyosarcoma and metastatic leiomyosarcoma in the central nervous system.

Myelin-Related Antigens

Myelin-Associated Glycoprotein

Myelin-associated glycoprotein (MAG), originally described by Quarles et al. (85), is distributed throughout the myelin lamellar structure. It is concentrated in the periaxonal region of both the PNS and CNS myelin sheath, although biochemical studies suggest that the CNS and the PNS proteins are not biochemically identical

(86). As MAG has been investigated primarily for its role in the pathogenesis of autoimmune demyelinating diseases, its application to the diagnosis of brain tumors is not well documented. The MAb HNK-1 (Leu-7), however, which was primarily described for its recognition of human natural killer (NK) lymphocytes, recognizes an MAG epitope (87,88). Perentes and Rubinstein (89, 90) have found Leu-7 reactivity in most peripheral neurogenic tumors and oligodendrogliomas. In these studies, moderate to weak reactivity was also noted in the majority of astrocytic gliomas, as well as 4 of 10 ependymomas, 3 of 7 choroid plexus papillomas, 7 of 14 medulloblastomas, 3 of 5 esthesioneuroblastomas, and in 1 pineocytoma. These investigators did not identify Leu-7 reactivity in any of 4 pineoblastomas. Caillaud et al. (91) found HNK-1 staining in 2 meningiomas, 1 medulloblastoma, 11 neuroblastomas, 3 neuroepitheliomas, 5 esthesioneuroblastomas, and 3 retinoblastomas, as well as in 4 of 16 Ewing's sarcomas, 2 of 6 nephroblastomas, 1 of 2 chrondrosarcomas, and 1 of 7 melanomas. No staining was identified in any of the embryonal sarcomas, fibrosarcomas, tenosynovial sarcomas, osteosarcomas, hematopoietic malignancies, carcinomas, or adenomas tested. The restricted distribution of this antigen, therefore, makes the reactivity of this MAb useful in the diagnosis of the peripheral spindle cell tumor in which the schwannoma is a consideration.

Myelin Basic Protein

The 18.5-kD myelin basic protein (MBP), also known as the P_1 protein, composes 30-40% of the protein content of myelin (86). The MBP is present in all mammalian species, including man, in both CNS and PNS myelin. Monoclonal antibodies to MBP have been reported by Sires et al. (92), Hickey et al. (76), Fritz and Chou (93), and Carnegie et al. (94). The biochemical epitopes recognized by a number of these MAbs have been characterized by Hruby et al. (95). All of these MAbs react with formalin-fixed, paraffin-embedded brain tissues, staining myelin specifically. One anti-MBP MAb (C12-225-6) of Hickey has been found to produce staining in $HgCl_2$-fixed tissues of comparable intensity to that of an anti-MBP polyvalent antisera. Another MBP MAb has been reported by Mogallon et al. (96); the biochemical specificity of which has not been reported to date.

P_0 and P_2 Proteins

Two antigenic proteins of potential utility in diagnostic pathology are the P_0 and the P_2 proteins (97,98). The P_0 protein constitutes approximately half the total protein content of peripheral nerve myelin. This basic glycoprotein (28-30 kD) is found throughout the multiple layers of the myelin sheath by immunohistochemistry, being present in both in the Schwann cell cytoplasm and membrane (86). To date, no MAbs to the P_0 protein have been reported. The P_2 protein, also a basic protein, is primarily confined to the Schmidt-Lantermann clefts of peripheral nerve myelin (99) and apparently is not a component of all peripheral myelinated nerves (100). Franko et al. (101) have produced an MAb specific for the P_2 protein by solid-phase RIA, by immunohistochemistry on fresh-frozen tissue sections, and by complement activation studies on both the native protein in peripheral nervous system myelin and in an artificial bilayer. There are no reports yet on the application of this MAb to human neurogenic tumors.

Galactocerebroside C

An additional myelin-associated antigen is the immunogenic glycolipid, galactocerebroside (GalC) (102). The major experience with this antigen has been gained from tissue culture studies, from which it is known that GalC is a developmentally expressed antigen in both nonneoplastic Schwann cells and oligodendroglia (103). Two MAbs to GalC have been described. The MAb of Ranscht et al. (103) is monospecific for GalC by ELISA studies, as well as antibody absorption analyses using cholesterol micelles both with and without incorporated galactosphyngolipid. The MAb of Rostami et al. (102). is monospecific for GalC by RIA on microtiter GalC-coated plates, by immunofluorescence of cultured cell lines, and by complement-mediated cytotoxicity assays of oligodendroglial cultures. There have been no reported application of either of these MAbs on neoplastic tissues.

Carbonic Anhydrase

Carbonic anhydrase II (CA II) (30 kD) has been purported to be a marker for oligodendroglia by both enzyme histochemistry and by immunohistochemistry (reviewed in 103; 20). Ghandour et al. (104) have used MAbs to CA I and CA II and have determined, by both electron immunohistochemistry and by CA II-GFAP double-labeling studies that CA II is specific for oligodendroglia in the normal rat cerebellum. These studies demonstrated that CA II is preponderantly a membrane-bound antigen localized to the oligodendroglial cell body, with little CA II found in the myelin sheath and only a small fraction of CA II soluble in the oligodendroglial cell cytoplasm. This MAb to CA II has not yet been applied to any human tumors, thus, it remains to be determined whether or not this marker maintains its oligodendroglial specificity in neoplasia.

Neuron-Specific Enolase

Enolase, an enzyme in the glycolytic pathway that catalyzes the interconversion of 2-phosphoglycerate and phosphoenolpyruvate, exists as multiple isoenzyme dimers formed from three subunits (a, β, and γ). The γ subunit of enolase is present in disproportionately large amounts in nervous tissue; indeed, the γ-γ isoenzyme, initially referred to as the 14-3-2 protein by Moore, was originally isolated and studied as a "brain-specific" protein (104). Many investigators, using highly specific antisera, observed γ-reactivity confined to neurons in normal central and peripheral nervous tissue (105-110). Hence, the term neuron-specific enolase (NSE) was applied to the γ-γ dimer, replacing the original 14-3-2 designation (108). The current consensus on γ-activity is that, within the CNS, neuronal enolase activity is due to the γ-subunit while a-subunit activity is largely confined to glial cells (111).

The distribution of γ-activity within normal tissues was later expanded beyond the neuronal localization to encompass central and peripheral neuroendocrine cells, which remains consistent with their recognized relation to neuronal tissue. Consequently, γ-activity has been reported in pinealocytes, pituitary cells, thyroid parafollicular cells, adrenal medullary chromaffin cells, and islet of Langerhans cells (112,113). The quantity of the γ-subunit varies widely within these neuronal and nonneuronal cell populations, and certain neuroendocrine cells (e.g., pinealocytes) contain considerably more enzyme than other neuronal cells (e.g. dorsal root ganglion neurons) (113). γ-Subunit activity has been localized in reactive astrocytes, although normal astrocytes appear to be without this isoenzyme. In addition, a wide variety of unrelated normal cell types have been shown to contain small amounts of the γ-subunit of NSE; these are blood and bone marrow cells, various smooth muscle cells, and certain kidney cells. Nonneuronal, nonneuroendocrine cells contain signficantly smaller quantities of the γ-subunit, expressing primarily the a-γ enzyme with very little of the γ-γ form.

Because of the small quantities of γ-isomer present in the cell types mentioned earlier, the enzyme must be considered as only operationally specific for eurons and neuroendocrine cells in normal tissues. Even this operational specificity is lost in neoplastic tissues. In addition to astrocytomas, glioblastomas, and oligodendrogliomas, CNS tumors found to contain significant amounts of γ immunoreactivity include ependymomas, meningiomas, pineoblastomas, pituitary adenomas, choroid plexus tumors, medulloblastomas, and chordomas. Neoplasms of the PNS found to contain NSE include neuroblastomas, ganglioneuromas, paragangliomas, and schwannomas. Fibroadenoma of the breast, mammary carcinoma, ovarian carcinoma, renal cell carcinoma, nodular goiter, and giant cell tumor of the tendon sheath, are also positive (114-116). Therefore, because of the heterogeneous tumor population that may express NSE, the usefulness of its localization is currently restricted. The quantitation of the amount of enzyme present within the tissue may prove much more helpful than the detection of its presence in neoplastic tissues (112).

Monoclonal antibodies specific for NSE have been difficult to generate because of resulting cross-reactivity with non-neuronal enolase (NNE). Seshi and Bell (118) described a method of obtaining purified NSE and subsequent generation of murine MAbs using a hybridoma technique. Two MAbs (8304EB11.6A19 and 8304CF5.4L7) were found to react only with NSE and not with NNE, based on solid-phase RIA. Immunohistochemistry on formalin-fixed, paraffin-embedded tissues have shown these MAbs to specifically label pyramidal cells, nerve fibers, and small-cell carcinomas; no reactivity was observed with liver, a source rich in NNE.

Glutamine Synthetase

Glutamine synthetase (GS) is a key enzyme in the detoxification of ammonia in the brain as well as the metabolism of γ-aminobutyric acid and γ-glutamic acid. Immunohistochemical studies on

Table 1 Cellular Distribution of Antigens

Antigen	Neural nonneoplastic	Somatic nonneoplastic	Neoplastic neural
S-100	Astrocytes	Melanocyte	Schwannoma
	Bergman glia	Langerhans cell of skin	Melanoma
	Schwann cell	Reticular cell of lymph node	Astrocytoma
	Satellite cell	Chondrocyte	Oligodendroglioma (?)
		Myoepithelial cell of ducts	Neuroma
		T lymphoctye	
			Granular cell tumor
			Chordoma
			Eosinophil granuloma
			Pleomorphic adenoma
			Chondroma
			Lipoma
			Liposarcoma
			Pituitary adenoma
			Pinealoma
			Medulloblastoma
			Meningioma (?)

GFAP	Astrocyte Bergman glia Pitucyte Tanycyte (?) Muller cell of retina Schwann cell (?) Pineal supportive cell Enteric glia Lens epithelium	Astrocytoma Ependymoma Choroid plexus Papilloma (?) Oligodendroglioma Ganglioglioma Xanthoastrocytoma
Neurofilaments	Neurons	Carotid body tumor Ganglioglioma Ganglioneuroblastoma Ganglioneuroma Neuroblastoma Pheochromocytoma Ovarian teratoma Esthesioneuroblastoma
Vimentin	Meningothelial cell Tanycyte Ependymal cell Mesenchymal cell of choroid plexus Vascular smooth muscle Cells of nonepithelial origin	Of limited use in intracranial neoplasms

Table 1 (Continued)

Antigen	Neural nonneoplastic	Somatic nonneoplastic	Neoplastic neural
Cytokeratin	Notochord Choroid plexus	Epithelial cell	Chordoma Colloid cyst Craniopharyngioma
Desmin	Vascular smooth muscle	Smooth muscle Striate muscle Cardiac muscle	Metastatic neoplasms of muscular origin
Myelin-associated glycoprotein	Oligodendroglia Schwann cell	Unknown	Astrocytoma[a] Ependymoma Choroid plexus papilloma Medulloblastoma Esthesioneuroblastoma Pineocytoma Meningioma Neuroblastoma Retinoblastoma
Neuron-specific enolase	Neuron Pinealocytes Pituitary cell	Parafollicular cell Adrenal medullary	Astrocytoma Oligodendroglioma Ependymoma

chromaffin cell
dorsal root ganglia

Islet of Langerhans cell

Meningioma
Medulloblastoma
Pineoblastoma
Pituitary adenoma
Choroid plexus
neoplasms
Chordoma
Neuroblastoma
Ganglioneuroma
Paraganglioma
Schwannoma
Fibroadenoma of breast
Mammary carcinoma
Ovarian carcinoma
Renal cell carcinoma
Nodular goiter
Giant-cell tumor of
tendon sheath

aDetermined by Leu-7 MAb.

normal brain tissue has shown that GS is restricted to astrocytes (119). Glutamine synthetase is not restricted to astrocytes in the human body; liver also contains this enzyme. In the CNS, however, GS appears to be cell-type restricted. By utilizing polyvalent antisera to GS, Pilkington and Lantos (119) have reviewed the immunoreactivity of 20 intracranial neoplasms and compared it with that obtained with an anti-GFAP antisera. Here, the immunological reactivity for GS coincided with that for GFAP. Furthermore, GS reactivity correlated with the degree of anaplasia, with the better-differentiated gliomas being strongly reactive. In one case, however, a discrepancy arose between the results of the GFAP and GS antisera, a poorly differentiated, probably metastatic, neoplasm was negative for GFAP and positive for GS. These results indicate that further work is necessary to determine the GS reactivity in both primary and metastatic CNS neoplasms. Although the enzyme is not cell-type specific, if its presence in neoplastic cells is restricted, its utility as a confirmatory test for astrocytic lineage will be enhanced.

a_2-Glycoprotein

a_2-Glycoprotein was first described by Warecka and Bauer in 1967 as a brain-specific protein that migrated in the a_2-range in immunoelectrophoresis. Although much empirical data suggested a glial origin, histochemical proof of glial-specificity was not determined until 1982 (121). Subsequent immunohistochemical studies have not been performed on gliomas to determine if this specificity is conserved in neoplasia; however, biochemical studies on human tumors have detected the presence of a_2-glycoprotein in both astrocytomas and mixed astrocytic-oligodendroglial neoplasms. Furthermore, this study did not find a_2-glycoprotein in any of 11 glioblastomas, 4 medulloblastomas, 2 ependymomas, 2 spongioblastomas, 1 oligodendroglioma, 3 meningiomas, or in 3 adenocarcinomas metastatic to CNS (121). Additional histochemical studies on this antigen, especially in neoplasms, seem to be warranted. No MAb to this antigen is now available.

Gangliosides

Gangliosides are sialic acid-containing glycosphingolipids. These amphipathic molecules derive their antigenic identity from their carbohydrate hydrophilic portions that project outward into the extracellular matrix from the cell membrane where they are anchored by their hydrophobic ceramide portions. Gangliosides are important molecules in the CNS, having been implicated in receptor functions and cellular interactions. Gangliosides are the receptor molecules for tetanus toxin and cholera toxin, both of which bind neuronal cells in histologic sections as well as in cell culture. A developmentally regulated ganglioside has been found to be expressed in 6- to 13-day-old rat fetuses and is quantitatively and qualitatively regulated in embryogenesis (122,123). Willinger and Schachner (122) have found the expression of ganglioside GM1, the cholera toxin receptor, is developmentally regulated and is restricted in the cerebellum to the post mitotic granule cells in the embryonic rat. Importantly, however, myelin also contains a large amount of GM1 and represents a source of cross-reactivity. The initial experience with gangliosides as tumor marks has come from MAbs generated by immunization with cell preparations derived from either human melanoma or spontaneous rat brain tumors. An example of the former is the MAb 4.2 of Yeh et al. (124) which recognizes a ganglioside structurally similar to GD3. An example of the latter is the MAb D1.1 generated against the rat-derived B49 cell line which recognizes an O-acetylated sialic acid-containing ganglioside migrating between GM1 and GM2 on one-dimensional gel electrophoresis (125). Some of these melanoma MAbs also cross-react with gliomas. Among these MAbs are the anti-OFA-I-1 MAb that recognizes GM2 and the anti-OFA-I-1 MAb that recognizes GD2, both described by Irie and coworkers (126-128).

One MAb to a ganglioside-related antigen that has received considerable attention is the A2B5 MAb, a murine MAb raised against chick retinal cells (129). It was initially considered to be neuron-specific but, subsequently, has been found to react broadly with cells of neuroectodermal derivation and with stratified squamous epithelium. The MAb demonstrates a potential problem in the generation of ganglioside MAbs in that Fredman et al. (130) have shown that it reacts not with one specific ganglioside but with an epitope shared on many ganglioside fractions. In neoplastic tissue, the reactivity of the MAb reflects the broad distribution of its epitope, binding to malignant gliomas, meningiomas, schwannomas, medulloblastomas, neuroblastomas, and metastatic carcinomas; no binding has been noted on choroid plexus tumors or lymphomas (131).

Recent studies have shown that human glioma biopsies contain a marked increase of the gangliosides GM3 and GD3, with a concomitantly significant reduction in the major normal brain gangliosides GM1, GD1a, GD1b, and GT1b (132). These studies also identified several gangliosides whose migration patterns in thin-layer chromatography were distinct from any of the previously described gangliosides. By utilizing large amounts of cultured human glioma cells that were free from brain contaminants, Fredman et al. (133) found that GM2 and GD2 were also expressed in substantial quantities, again with little or no of the major normal gangliosides. Mansson et al., (134) using the Duke malignant glioma cell line, D-54 MG, isolated a previously undescribed, structurally unique ganglioside exhibiting a lactotetraosylceramide configuration. This finding, although important, was not unexpected because several epithelial and neuroectodermal neoplasms have been found to express tumor-associated glycospingolipids (135-140). Although the functional implication of these qualitative and quantitative alterations in ganglioside expression are not known, the diagnostic importance of these alterations lies in the ability of monospecific MAbs developed against these molecules to specifically react with tumor cells.

MONOCLONALLY DEFINED NEURAL ANTIGENS

The identification and purification of antigens has also been approached by the immunization of laboratory animals with fetal brain preparations or with neoplastic cell culture preparations from which hybridomas are produced and from which clones secreting antibodies reacting with antigens of neuroectodermal interest are identified (141). The characterization of the specificity of these MAbs is almost entirely by RIA on short-term cultures and cell lines and by immunohistochemistry on human brain biopsy specimens. In some instances, partial purification and characterization of these MAb-defined antigens has been done. It is important, that extensive experience be gained with these MAbs in the diagnostic setting for which they are intended before any recommendations concerning their diagnostic utility can be rendered. The most extensive experience with diagnostic application of any of these MAbs has been in the laboratories of Kemshead, Coakham, and collaborators, and Bigner and collaborators.

Coakham et al. (142-145), Garson et al. (146), and Vick et al. (147) have employed panels of well-characterized MAbs as an adjunct to conventional histological techniques in the diagnosis of CNS tumors. They have found that on the basis of characteristic MAb reactivity profiles, it is possible to distinguish between gliomas, medulloblastomas, neuroblastomas, schwannomas, meningiomas, and choroid plexus tumors, as well as metastatic carcinomas and lymphomas. The investigators have used primarily three MAbs, specific for certain primary CNS elements, in an antibody panel approach to the identification of the neoplasms.

UJ13A

Monoclonal antibody UJ13A, an IgG1 MAb raised against 16-week-old human fetal brain, is specific for most cells of neuroectodermal origin based on indirect immunofluorescence on frozen sections of a wide variety of normal fetal, pediatric, and adult tissues (148). In addition to recognizing CNS tissues and peripheral nerves, other cell types derived from the neuroectoderm (adrenal medulla, sympathetic chain, arachnoid granulations, thymic epithelium, and nerve fiber plexi in the gastrointestinal tract) are also recognized. Rare cross-reactivity with antigens outside of the neuroectoderm has been noted, with staining of thyroid epithelial cell luminal borders being the only known example in adult tissues. In addition to the binding pattern observed in the adult, the antibody stains certain kidney tubule cells and a subset of thymic cells in fetal tissues. In neoplastic tissue, MAb UJ13A recognizes gliobastomas, astrocytomas, oligodendrogliomas, ganglogliomas, ependymomas, meningiomas, schwannomas, medulloblastomas, neuroblastomas, retinoblastomas, thymomas, and oat-cell carcinomas; choroid plexus tumors do not stain (144, 148). Malignant melanomas, which are also of neuroectodermal origin, have been consistently negative with this antibody. Malignancies of nonneuroectodermal derivation that stain with MAb UJ13A are Wilms' tumor and rhabdomyosarcoma (148). Monoclonal antibody UJ13A does not react with lymphomas or carcinomas (with the exception of oat-cell carcinoma), and thus has been shown to be a useful agent for distinguishing primary CNS tumors from lymphoma and metastatic carcinomas (142-144, 146, 148).

UJ127.11

Monoclonal antibody UJ127.11, an IgG1 immunoglobulin also generated against 16-week-old human fetal brain, recognizes a 220-240-kd glycoprotein, which is not fibronectin, associated with the plasma membrane (149). Studies using indirect immunofluorescence on normal fetal and adult tissues have shown that this antigen is restricted in its expression to adult cells of neuronal origin as well as to fetal brain of 14- and 27-weeks gestation, adult cerebellum and temporal lobe, nerve fiber plexi in the esophagus and colon, and adrenal medullary cells. By immunofluorescence and modified RIA, MAb UJ127.11 has been shown to bind five neurobastoma cell lines and one melanoma cell line. The screening of a wide variety of normal nonneuroectodermally derived tissues revealed reactivity in occasional renal tubules. In one major study, MAb UJ127.11 reacted with 5 of 7 neuroblastomas, 38 of 54 neuroblastomas metastatic to bone marrow, 3 of 3 retinoblastomas, 1 of 1 cerebral neuroblastoma, 1 of 1 medulloblastoma, and 1 of 1 ganglioglioma; no reactivity was demonstrated in glioblastomas, meningiomas, schwannomas, choroid plexus papillomas, or various malignancies of nonneuroectodermal origin (149). Although 15 ependymomas exhibited weak reactivity, this reactivity was confined to cells with astrocytic characteristics; further studies by Coakham et al. (144) have not found any additional ependymomas to react with this MAb. Subsequent work with UJ127.11 has supported these findings, as well as finding reactivity in schwannomas. Therefore, MAb UJ127.11 appears useful in the diagnosis of neuronal malignancies, schwannomas, and melanomas.

UJ181.4

Monoclonal antibody UJ181.4 also an IgG1 immunoglobulin raised in the same fusion against 16-week-old human fetal brain tissue as the previous MAbs, reacts with a cell membrane antigen present in fetal brain but not expressed in normal adult tissues (146). In neoplastic tissues, strong reactivity is found in neuroblastic neoplasms including the medulloblastomas and neuroblastomas (142, 143, 145, 146). Weak staining has also been found in 5 of 31 high-grade gliomas, 3 of 6 oligodendrogliomas, and 1 of 41 metastatic carcinomas with no staining seen in any astrocytomas, ependymomas, meningiomas, schwannomas, choroid plexus tumors, or lymphomas (144).

Antiglioma Monoclonal Antibodies

Wikstrand et al. (151,152) have described the development of four antihuman fetal brain MAbs whose reactivity in normal adult tissues is restricted to lymphoid tissues and to malignant neuroecto-dermal neoplasms among neoplastic tissues. Monoclonal antibody 4D2, as tested on various cultured cell lines, bound to 5 of 14 glioblastomas, 1 of 2 melanomas, 1 of 3 neuroblastomas, and 1 of 5 fetal fibroblast cell lines in cell surface radioimmunoassay (C5-RIA), and to one neuroblastoma, fetal brain and liver, and adult spleen in an immunoperoxidase histochemistry assay. The MAb 7H10 bound to cell lines of 13 of 14 glioblastomas, 1 of 3 neuroblastomas, and 1 medulloblastoma by CS-RIA and to 13 of 13 glioblastomas, 1 neuroblastoma, and to fetal brain, liver, spleen, thymus, and adult spleen by immunoperoxidase histochemistry. Neither of these MAbs bound to any of six carcinoma cell lines or to five sarcoma cell lines by CS-RIA. However, MAb 7H10 was absorbed by Hodgkins' lymphoma tissue, whereas MAb 4D2 was not. The MAbs 1H8-2 and 1H8-3 (152) were also recognized epitopes present on human neuroectodermal neoplasms as well as fetal tissues. The MAb 1H8-3 reacted with 9 of 14 glioblastomas, 2 of 3 neuroblastomas, 1 of 2 melanomas, and 1 medulloblastoma by radioimmunoassay on these cultured cell lines. Monoclonal antibody 1H8-2 had a more restricted reactivity pattern as determined by positive RIA on the cell lines of 7 of 14 glioblastomas, 2 of 3 neuroblastomas, 1 medulloblastoma, and 2 of 3 fetal skin fibroblast lines. Neither of these MAbs bound either the non-neuroectodermal neoplasms or normal adult tissues including brain, thymus, lymph node, liver, kidney, lung, skin, and pancreas.

Monoclonal antibodies 2F3, 4C7, and 5B7 (153) were the result of innoculation of mice with the malignant glioma cell line D-54 MG. The MAb 2F3 recognizes a highly restricted epitope, as evidenced by its reactivity with 5 of 12 glioblastoma cell lines and of 1 of 4 fetal skin lines by CS-RIA and with 9 of 11 human glioblastomas in tissue section by immunoperoxidase histochemistry;

this MAb did not react with any of the melanomas, neuroblastomas, meningiomas, or control noncentral nervous system tumors
tested, nor with any of the fetal tissues tested. The MAbs 4C7 and
5B7 react with neuroectodermally conserved epitopes as evidenced
by MAb 4C7 reactivity with 1 of 6 melanoma, 2 of 3 neuroblastoma, and 4 of 12 glioblastoma cell lines by CS-RIA and by MAb
5B7 reactivity with 1 of 6 melanoma cell lines. In addition, MAbs
4C7 and 5B7 also reacted with normal fetal skin cell lines by CS-
RIA and with fetal brain and thymus in tissue sections.

Bourdon and co-workers (154) used the malignant glioma cell
line U-251 MG as the immunogen to produce the MAb 81C6 that
recognizes a glioma-mesenchymal extracellular matrix (GMEM)
antigen. Antibody 81C6 recognized the GMEM antigen in 14 of 16
gliomas, 1 of 3 neuroblastomas, 1 of 7 melanomas, 2 of 6 sarcoma
cell lines, and 8 of 9 fibroblast cell lines. Differential expression in
neoplasia was exhibited by both the 81C6 antigen and the pre-
veiously mentioned 1H8-2 antigen (155). The 81C6 antigen was
detected in 5 of 8 glioblastomas but in only 1 of 6 astrocytomas,
whereas the 1H8 antigen was detected in 6 of 7 glioblastomas and
1 of 6 astrocytomas (distinct from the 91C6-positive astro-
cytoma). The 81C6 antigen has not been detected in normal adult
or fetal brain. Furthermore, this antigen was not detected in any
of the carcinoma or myeloid-lymphoid cell lines examined. The
GMEM antigen was distinct from previously described forms of
fibronectin, laminin, collagen types I - V, hyaluronic acid, chon-
droitin sulfate, and heparin by absorption analysis and immunohistology.

The MAbs C12 and D12 (156), also produced from the innoculation of mice with D-54 MG cells, also recognize highly restricted tumor-associated epitopes. By indirect CS-RIA, the two
MAbs exhibited distinct reactivity patterns, with C12 binding 9 of
17 gliomas and D12, 8 of 17 gliomas. Both MAbs reacted with the
same 1 of 3 medulloblastoma cell lines, 1 of 2 melanoma cell lines,
and cell lines derived from 12- and 16-week gestation fetal brain in
immunoperoxidase histochemistry performed on a panel consisting of both fresh-frozen and formalin-fixed, paraffin-embedded
tissues. On this panel C12 reacted with 6 of 7 glioblastomas,
whereas D12 reacted with 2 of 7. Morphologically, C12 reacted
with an antigen that was consistently confined to the cell membrane and cytoplasm, whereas D12 recognized an antigen found in

the cytoplasm, cell membrane, and in some gliomas, the extracellular matrix.

CONCLUSION

The future of MAbs in diagnostic neuropathology extends in several directions. As diagnostic pathology incorporates the techniques of cell culture to understand the in vitro characteristics of neoplasms, especially in relation to chemotherapeutic sensitivity, MAbs will be useful in identifying if molecular mechanisms of resistance are present. These molecules include such enzymes as O-6-alkylguanine DNA transferase, implicated in correcting DNA cross-linking induced by alkylating agents (157). As pathology incorporates the techniques of molecular genetics, MAbs will be used to detect oncogene products, such as the epidermal growth factor produced by the *c-erb b* oncogene, which is increased in gliomas (158,159). Monoclonal antibodies will continue to be powerful descriminatory agents in identifying cellular antigens. The use of whole-cell preparations derived from cell culture lines of CNS neoplasms has proved its usefulness in selecting tumor-associated antigens (141). The development of monospecific MAbs reactive against cell-type-specific and tumor-associated neural antiens will continue to progress as improved methods in the identification and purification of neural antigens are developed. In turn, the MAbs will contribute substantially to the understanding of not only the cellular distribution of these antigens in the CNS but also the functional significance of these antigens.

Although this volume is confined to the applications of MAbs to the in vitro diagnosis of CNS neoplasms, the future of these reagens also includes in vivo diagnosis and therapy. The role of the pathologist will be to bridge the gap between in vitro diagnosis and in vivo application. One recent study demonstrated a correlation between MAbs that react with antigens located in the extracellular matrix and the ability of that antibody, when radiolabeled, to localize neoplastic tissues in an athymic mouse-human glioma xenograft model (160,161). Although confined to an athymic mouse-xenograft model, this study suggests that the interpretation of morphological reactivity patterns will be an important consideration in screening MAbs for in vivo localization and therapy. Thus, the advent of these reagents will require not only expert histological interpretation but also experience in interpreting reactivity patterns.

REFERENCES

1. B. W. Moore, *Biochem. Bioplys. Res. Commun. 19*:739 (1965).
2. M. V. Starostina, T. K. Malup, and S. M. Sviridov, *J. Neurochem. 36*: 1904 (1981).
3. T. Akagi, K. Takahashi, and Y. Ohtsuki, *J. Leuk. Biol. 36*:131 (1984). (abstr.)
4. S. W. Weiss, J. M. Langloss, and F. M. Enzinger, *Lab. Invest. 49*:299 (1983).
5. H. J. Kahn, A. Marks, H. Thom, and R. Baumal, *Am. J. Clin. Pathol. 79*:341 (1983).
6. T. Nakajima, S. Watanabe, Y. Sato, T. Kameya, T. Hirota, and Y. Shimosato, *Am. J. Surg. Pathol. 6*:715 (1982).
7. P. S. Golden and G. Y. Gillespie (submitted for publication).
8. S. C. Loeffel, G. Y. Gillespie, S. A. Mirmiran, E. W. Miller, P. Golden, F. B. Askin, and Siegal GP, *Arch. Pathol. Lab. Med. 109*:117 (1985).
9. C. M. Jacque, M. Kujas, A. Poreau, M. Raoul, P. Collier, J. Racadot, and N. Baumann, *J. Natl. Cancer Inst. 62*:479 (1979).
10. K. Stefansson, R. Wollman, and M. Jerkovic, *Am. J. Pathol. 106*:261 (1982).
11. E. A. Haan, B. D. Boss, and M. Cowan, *Proc. Natl. Acad. Sci. USA 79*: 7585 (1982).
12. P. S. Golden, G. Y. Gillespie, and J. M. Bynum (submitted for publication).
13. G. Y. Gillespie and P. S. Golden (submitted for publication).
14. A. Marks, J. Law, J. B. Mahoney, and R. Baumal, *J. Neurochem. 41*: 107 (1983).
15. Van Eldik, B. Ehrenfried, and R. A. Jensen, *Proc. Natl. Acad. Sci. USA 81*:6034 (1984).
16. M.-J. Vanstapel, B. Peeters, J. Cordell, W. Heyns, C. De Wolf-Peters, V. Desmet, and D. Mason, *Lab. Invest. 52*:232 (1985).
17. M.-J. Vanstapel, K. C. Gatter, C. D. W-Peeters, D.Y. Mason, V.D. Desmet, *Am. J. Clin. Pathol. 85*:160 (1986).
18. E. Lazarides. *Ann. Rev. Biochem. 51*:219 (1982).
19. M. Osborn and K. Weber, *Lab. Invest. 48*:372 (1983).
20. T. Jones and D. D. Bigner, in *Human Cancer Markers* (S. Sell and B. Wahren, eds), Humana Press, Clifton, N.J. (1982), p. 381.
21. L. F. Eng, *Brain Res. 28*:351 (1971).
22. L. F. Eng and S. DeArmond, in *Progress in Neuropathology* (H. M. Zimmerman, ed.), Vol. 5, Raven Press (1983), New York p. 19.

23. C. N. Pegram, L. F. Eng, C. J. Wikstrand, R. D. McComb, Y. Lee and D. Bigner, *Neurochem. Pathol. 3*:119 (1980).
24. S. J. DeArmond, L. F. Eng, and L. J. Rubinstein, *Pathol. Res. Pract. 168*:374 (1980).
25. L. F. Eng, J. Vanderhaeghen, A. Bignami, and B. Gerstl, *Brain Res. 28*: 351 (1971).
26. G. H. DeVries, W. T. Norton, and C. S. Raines, *Science 172*:1370 (1972).
27. Lucas, *Neurochem. Res. 5*:247 (1980).
28. S. J. DeArmond, M. Fajardo, S. A. Naughton, and L. F. Eng: *Brain Res. 262*:275 (1983).
29. L. F. Eng and L. J. Rubinstein, *J. Histochem. Cytochem. 26*:513 (2978).
30. S. J. DeArmond and L. F. Eng, *Prog. Exp. Tumor Res. 27*:92 (1984).
31. P. E. Duffy, L. Graft, Y.-Y. Huang, and M. M. Rapport, *J. Neurol. Sci. 40*:133 (1976).
32. J. H. N. Deck, L. F. Eng, J. Bigbee, and S. M. Woodcock, *Acta Neuropathol. 42*:183 (1978).
33. U. Suess and V. Pliska, *Brain Res. 221*:27 (1981).
34. H. R. Highely, J. A. McNulty, and G. Rowden, *Brain Res. 304*:117 (1984).
35. S. C. Papasozomenos, *J. Neuropathol. Exp. Neurol. 42*:391 (1983).
36. R. G. Dixon and L. F. Eng, *J. Comp. Neurol. 195*:305 (1981).
37. D. Dahl, N. Chi, L. Miles, B. Nguyen, and A. Bignami, *J. Histochem Cytochem. 30*:912 (1982).
38. S.-H. Yen and K. Fields, *J. Cell Biol. 88*:115 (1981).
39. K. L. Fields and S.-H. Yen, *J. Neuroimmunol. 8*:311 (1985).
40. K. R. Jessen and R. Mirsky, *J. Neuroimmunol. 8*:377 (1985).
41. J. S. Hatfield, R. P. Skoff, H. Maisel, L. F. Eng, and D. D. Bigner, *J. Neuroimmunol. 8*:347 (1985).
42. Y. Nakazato, J. Ighizeki, K. Takahashi, H. Yamaguchi, T. Kamei, and T. Mori, *Lab. Invest. 48*:621 (1982).
43. R. E. McLendon, P. C. Burger, C. N. Pegram, L. F. Eng, and D. D. Bigner, *J. Neuropathol. Exp. Neurol.* (in press) (1986).
44. J. Q. Trojanowski, V. Lee, and W. W. Schlaepfer, *Hum. Pathol. 15*:248 (1984).
45. N. A. Tascos, J. Parr, and N. K. Gonatas, *Hum. Pathol. 13*:454 (1982).
46. J. D. M. Van der Muellen, H. J. Houthoff, and E. J. Ebels, *Neuropathol. Exp. Neurobiol. 4*:177 (1978).
47. M. E. Velasco, D. Dahl, U. Roessman, P. and Gambetti, *Cancer 45*:484 (1980).
48. B. H. Choi and R. C. Kim, *Science 223*:407 (1984).
49. U. Roessman, M. E. Velasco, S. D. Singely, and P. Gambetti, *Brain Res. 200*:13 (1980).

50. A. L. Taratuto, H. Molina, and J. Monges, *Acta Neuropathol. 59*:304 (1983).
51. C. Jacque, C. Vinner, M. Kujas, M. Faoul, J. Racadot, and N. Baumann, *J. Neurol. Sci. 35*:147 (1978).
52. L. J. Rubinstein and J. M. Brucher, *Acta Neuropathol. 53*:29 (1981).
53. J. J. Kepes, L. J. Rubinstein, and L. F. Eng, *Cancer 44*:1839 (1979).
54. V. P. Collins, *Acta Pathol. Microbiol. Immunol. Scand. 91*:269 (1983).
55. V. P. Collins, *Acta Cytol. 28*:401 (1984).
56. M. Albrechtsen, A. C. von Gerstenburg, and E. Bock, *J. Neurochem. 42*:86 (1984).
57. V. M.-Y. Lee, C. D. Page, H.-L. Wu, W. W. Schlaepfer, *J. Neurochem. 42*:25 (1984).
58. E. Debus, G. Flugge, K. Weber, and M. Osborn, *EMBO J. 1*:41. (1982).
59. R. M. Pruss, R. Mirsky, M. C. Raff, R. Thorpe, A. J. Dowding, and B. H. Anderton, *Cell 27*:419 (1981).
60. A. M. Gown and A. M. Vogel, *J. Cell. Biol. 95*:414 (1982).
61. S. K. R. Pixley, Y. Kobayashi, and J. deVellis, *J. Neurosci Res. 12*:525 (1984).
62. D. Dahl, M. Grossi, and A. Bignami, *Histochemistry 81*:525 (1984).
63. P. Hoffman and R. Lasek, *J. Cell Biol. 66*:351 (1975).
64. W. W. Schlaepfer and L. Freeman, *J. Cell Biol. 78*:653 (1978).
65. R. Liem, S.-H. Yen, G. Saloman, and M. Shelanski, *J. Cell Biol. 79*:637 (1978).
66. M. Willard and C. Simon, *J. Cell Biol. 89*:198 (1981).
67. H. Czosnek, D. Soifer, and H. Wisniewski, *J. Cell Biol. 85*:726 (1980).
68. D. Dahl, *FEBS Lett. 111*:152 (1980).
69. N. Geisler, U. Plessmann, and K. Weber, *Nature 296* (1982).
70. G. Sharp, G. Shaw, and K. Weber, *Exp. Cell Res. 137*:403 (1982).
71. R. Leim, C. Keith, J. Leterrier, E. Trenkner, and M. Shelanski, *Cold Spring Harbor Symp. Quant. Biol. 46*:341 (1982).
72. G. Shaw, M. Osborn, and K. Weber, *Eur. J. Cell Biol. 26*:68 (1981).
73. G. Shaw and K. Weber, *Nature 298*:277 (1982).
74. E. Debus, K. Weber, and M. Osborn, *Differentiation 25*:193 (1983).
75. V. M.-Y. Lee, H. Wu, and W. W. Schlaepfer, *Proc. Natl. Acad. Sci. USA 79*:6089 (1982).
76. J. Q. Trojanowski, M. A. Obrocka, and V. M.-Y. Lee, *J. Histochem Cytochem. 31*:1217 (1983).
77. W. F. Hickey, V. M.-Y. Lee, L. J. McMillan, T. J. McKean, J. Gonatas, and N. K. Gonatas, *J. Histochem. Cytochem. 31*:1126 (1983).
78. J. Q. Trojanowski, V. M.-Y. Lee, N. Pillsbury, and S. Lee, *N. Engl. J. Med. 307*:159 (1982).
79. J. Wood and B. Anderton, *Biosci. Rep. 1*:263 (1981).
80. A. Bignami, T. Raju, and D. Dahl, *Dev. Biol. 91*:186 (1982).

81. W. C. Halliday, H. Yeger, G. F. Duwe, and M. J. Phillips, *J. Neuropathol. Exp. Neurol. 44*:617 (1985).
82. K. Schweichheimer, J. Kartenbeck, R. Moll, and W. Franke, *Lab. Invest. 51*:584 (1984).
83. D. Cooper, A. Schermer, and T.-T. Sun, *Lab. Invest. 52*:243 (1985).
84. C. M. Coffin, M. R. Wick, J. T. Braun, and L. P. Dehner, *Am. J. Surg. Pathol. 10*:394 (1986).
85. P. C. Burger, M. Makek, and P. Kleihues, *Acta Neuropathol.* (in press) (1986).
86. R. H. Quarles, J. L. Everly, and R. O. Brady, *J. Neurochem. 21*:1177 (1973).
87. M. R. Lees and S. W. Brostow, in *Myelin* (P. Morell, ed.), Plenum Press, New York (1984).
88. S. Schuller-Petrovic, W. Gebhart, H. Lassmann, H. Rumpold, and D. Kraft, *Nature 306*:179 (1983).
89. G. Stoll, G. Schwendemann, K. Heininger, A. J. Steck, and K. V. Toyka, *J. Neurol. Neurosurg. Psychiatry 48*:635 (1985).
90. E. Perentes and L. J. Rubinstein, *Acta Neuropathol.* (in press) (1986).
91. E. Perentes and L. J. Rubinstein, *Acta Neuropathol. 68*:319 (1985).
92. J.-M. Caillaud, S. Benjelloun, J. Bosq, K. Braham, and M. Lipinski, *Cancer Res. 44*:4432 (1984).
93. L. R. Sires, S. Hruby, E. C. Alvord Jr, I. Hellstrom, K. E. Hellstrom, M. W. Kies, R. Martenson, G. E. Deibler, E. D. Beckman, and J. E. Casnellie, *Science 214*:87 (1981).
94. R. B. Fritz and C.-H. J. Chou, *J. Immunol. 130*:2180 (1983).
95. J. A. Carnegie, M. E. McCully, and H. A. Robertson, *J. Histochem. Cytochem. 28*:308 (1980).
96. S. Hruby, E. C. Albord Jr, R. E. Martenson, G. E. Deibler, W. F. Hickey, and N. K. Gonatas, *J. Neurochem. 44*:637 (1985).
97. R. Mogollon, N. Penneys, J. A. Saavedra, and M. Nadji, *Cancer 53*:1190 (1984)
98. M. Mukai, *Am. J. Pathol. 112*:139 (1983).
99. H. B. Clark, H. Minesky, D. Agrawal, and H. C. Agrawal, *Am. J. Pathol. 121*:96 (1985).
100. B. D. Trapp, L. J. McIntyre, R. H. Quarles, N. H. Sternberger, and H. deF. Webster, *Proc. Natl. Acad. Sci. USA 76*:3552 (1979).
101. S. J. DeArmond, G. E. Deibler, M. Bacon, M. E. Kies, and L. F. Eng, *J. Histochem. Cytochem. 28*:1275 (1980).
102. M. C. Franko, C. L. Koski, C. J. Gibbs, D. E. McFarlin, and D. C. Gajdusek, *Proc. Natl. Acad. Sci. USA 79*:3618 (1982).
103. A. Rostami, P. A. Eccleston, D. H. Silberberg, M. Hirayama, R. P. Lisak, D. E. Pleasure, and S. M. Phillips, *Brain Res. 298*:203 (1984).

104. B. Ranscht, P. A. Clapshaw, J. Price, M. Noble, and W. Seifert, *Proc. Natl. Acad. Sci, USA 79*:2709 (1982).
105. M. S. Ghandour, O. K. Langley, G. Vincendon, G. Gombos, D. Fillippi, N. Limozin, C. Dalmasso, and G. Laurent, *Neuroscience 5*:559 (1980).
104. B. Ranscht, P. A. Clapshaw, J. Price, M. Noble, and W. Seifert, *Proc. Natl. Acad. Sci. USA 79*:2709 (1982).
105. M. S. Ghandour, O. K. Langley, G. Vincendon, G. Gombos, D. Fillippi, N. Limozin, C. Dalmasso, and G. Laurent, *Neuroscience 5*:559 (1980).
106. B. Moore and D. McGregor, *J. Biol. Chem. 240*:1647 (1965).
107. M. S. Ghandour, O. K. Langley, G. Labourdette, G. Vincendon, and G. Gombos, *Dev. Neurosci. 4*:66 (1981).
108. D. Schmechel, M. Brightman, and P. Marangos, *Brain Res. 190*:195 (1980).
109. D. Schmechel, P. Marangos, A. Zis, M. Brightman, and F. Goodwin, *Science 199*:313 (1978).
110. J. Royds, M. Parson, C. Taylor, and W. Timperley, *J. Pathol. 137*:37 (1982).
111. V. Pickel, D. Reis, P. Marangos, and C. Zomzely-Neurath, *Brain Res. 105*:184 (1976).
112. D. Schmechel, *Lab. Invest. 52*:239 (1985).
113. D. Schmechel, P. Marangos, and M. Brightman, *Nature 276*:834 (1976).
114. P. Marangos, D. Schmechel, A. Parma, R. Clark, and F. Goodwin, *J. Neurochem. 33*:319 (1979).
115. S. Vinores, J. Bonnin, L. J. Rubinstein, and P. Marangos, *Arch. Pathol. Lab. Med. 108*:536 (1984).
116. K. Haglid, C. Carlsson, and D. Stavrou, *Acta Neuropathol. 24*:187 (1973).
117. M. Wick, B. Scheithauer, and K. Kovacs, *Am. J. Clin. Pathol. 29*:703 (1983).
118. B. Seshi and E. Bell, *Hybridoma 4*:13 (1985).
119. M. D. Norenberg and H. M. Hernandez, *Brain Res. 161*:303 (1979).
120. G. J. Pilkington and P. L. Lantos, *Neuropathol. Appl. Neurobiol. 8*: 227 (1982).
121. M. S. Ghandour, O. K. Langley, G. Gombos, G. Vincedon, and K. Warecka, *Neuroscience 7*:231 (1982).
122. K. Warecka, *J. Neurol. Sci. 26*:511 (1975).
123. R. Mirsky, L. M. B. Wendon, P. Balck, C. Stolkin, and D. Bray, *Brain Res. 148*:251 (1978).
124. M. Willinger and M. Schachner, *Develop. Biol. 74*:101 (1980).
125. M.-I. Yeh, I. Hellstrom, K. Abe, S.-I. Hakomori, K. E. Hellstrom, *Int. J. Cancer 29*:269 (1982).
126. D. A. Cheresh, A. P. Varki, N. M. Varki, W. B. Stallcup, J. Levine, and R. A. Reisfeld, *J. Biol. Chem. 259*:7453 (1984).

127. R. F. Irie, A. G. Giuliano, and D. L. Morton, *J. Natl. Acad. Sci. 80*: 367 (1979).
128. M. Katano, N. Sidell, and R. F. Irie. *Ann. N.Y. Acad. Sci. 47*:426 (1983).
129. T. Tai, J. C. Paulson, L. D. Cahan, and R. Irie, *Proc. Natl. Acad. Sci. 80*:5392 (1983).
130. G. S. Eisenbarth, F. S. Walsh, and M. Nirenberg, *Proc. Natl. Acad. Sci. USA 76*:4913 (1979).
131. P. Fredman, J. L. Magnani, M. Nirenberg, and V. Ginsburg, *Arch. Biochem. Biophys. 223*:661 (1984).
132. H. Coakham, J. Garson, B. Brownell, P. Allan, E. Harper, and J. Kemshead, *S. Afr. J. Surg. 22*:13 (1984).
133. P. Fredman, H. von Holst, V. P. Collins, A. Ammar, B. Kellheden, L. Granholm, and L. Svennerholm, *Neurol. Res. 8*:123 (1986).
134. P. Fredman, L. Svennerholm, C. J. Lewis, S. H. Bigner, J. Mark, and D. D. Bigner (submitted for publication).
135. J.-E. Mansson, P. Fredman, D. D. Bigner, K. Mollin, B. Rosengreen, H. S. Friedman, and L. Svennerholm, *FEBS Lett. 201*:109 (1986).
136. J.-E. Mansson, P. Fredman, O. Nilsson, L. Lindholm, J. Holmgren, and L. Svennerholm, *Biochim. Biophys. Acta 834*:110 (1985).
137. C. S. Pukel, K. O. Lloyd, R. Travassos, W. G. Dippold, H. F. Oettgen, and L. J. Old, *J. Exp. Med. 155*:1133 (1982).
138. H. Koprowski, Z. Steplewski, K. Mitchell, M. Herlyn, and P. Fuhrer, *Somatic Cell Genet. 5*:957 (1979).
139. E. Nudelman, S.-I. Hakomori, R. Kannagi, S. Levery, M.-Y. Yeh, K. E. Hellstrom, and I. Hellstrom, *J. Biol. Chem. 257*:12752 (1982).
140. S.-I. Hakomori and R. Kannagi, *J. Natl. Cancer Inst. 71*:231 (1983).
141. J. L. Magnani, M. Brockhaus, D. F. Smith, V. Ginsburg, M. Blaszcyk, K. F. Mitchell, Z. Steplewski, and H. Koprowski, *Science 212*:55 (1981).
142. C. J. Wikstrand and D. D. Bigner, in *Monoclonal Antibodies in Cancer* (S. Sell and R. A. Reisfeld, eds.), Humana Press, Clifton, N.J. (1985), p. 365.
143. H. Coakham, B. Brownell, E. Harper, J. Garson, P. Alan, and E. Lane, *Lancet 1*:1095 (1984).
144. H. Coakham, J. Garson, B. Brownell, and J. Kemshead, *Prog. Exp. Tumor Res. 29*:57 (1985).
145. H. Coakham, J. Garson, P. Allan, E. Harper, B. Brownell, J. Kemshead, and E. Lane, *J. Clin. Pathol. 38*:165 (1985).
146. J. Kemshead and H. Coakham, *J. Pathol. 141*:249 (1983).
147. J. Garson, H. Coakham, P. Allan, E. Harper, B. Brownell, J. Kemshead, B. Lane, and P. Beverley, in *Protides of the Biological Fluids*; 31st Colloq. (H. Peeters, ed.), Pergamon, Oxford (1983), p. 853.
148. W. W. Vick, S. H. Bigner, C. J. Wikstrand, D. E. Bullard, J. T. Kem-

shead, H. Coakham, J. Schlom, W. W. Johnston, and D. D. Bigner (submitted for publication).

149. P. Allan, J. Garson, E. Harper, U. Asser, H. Coakham, B. Brownell, J. Kemshead, *Int. J. Cancer 31*:591 (1983).

150. C. J. Wikstrand, M. A. Bourdon, C. N. Pegram, and D. D. Bigner, *J. Neuroimmunol. 3*:43 (1982).

151. J. Kemshead, J. Fritschy, J. Garson, P. Allan, H. Coakham, S. Brown, and U. Asser, *Int. J. Cancer 31*:187 (1983).

152. C. J. Wikstrand and D. D. Bigner, *Cancer Res. 42*:267 (1982).

153. C. J. Wikstrand, M. A. Bourdon, C. N. Pegram, and D. D. Bigner, *J. Neuroimmunol. 3*:42 (1982).

154. C. J. Wikstrand, S. H. Bigner, and D. D. Bigner, *J. Neuroimmunol. 6*: 169 (1984).

155. M. A. Bourdon, C. J. Wikstrand, H. Furthmayr, T. J. Matthews, and D. D. Bigner *Cancer Res. 43*:2796 (1983).

156. C. J. Wikstrand and D. D. Bigner, in *Diseases of the Nervous System* (A. K. Asbury, G. M. McKhann, and W. I. McDonald, eds.), Ardmore Medical Books, W. B. Saunders, Philadelphia (1985), (in press).

157. C. J. Wikstrand, R. E. McLendon, D. E. Bullard, P. Fredman, L. Svennerholm, and D. D. Bigner. (submitted for publication).

158. W. J. Bodell, R. Cheitlin, T. Aida, M. S. Berger, and M. R. Rosenblum, Sixth International Conference on Brain Tumor Research And Therapy, Asheville, N.C. (1985).

159. T. A. Liberman, H. R. Nusbaum, N. Razon, R. Kris, I. Lax, H. Soreq, N. Whittle, M. D. Waerfield, A. Ullrich, and J. Schlessinger, *Nature 313*: 144 (1985).

160. T. A. Liberman, N. Razon, A. D. Bartal, Y. Yarden, J. Schlessinger, and H. Soreq, *Cancer Res. 44*:753 (1984).

161. C. J. Wikstrand, R. E. McLendon, S. Carrel, J. T. Kemshead, J.-P. Mach, H. B. Coakham, N. de Tribolet, D. E. Bullard, M. R. Zalutsky, and D. D. Bigner, (submitted for publication) (1986).

162. R. E. McLendon, C. J. Wikstrand, M. A. Bourdon, and D. D. Bigner, *J. Neuropath. Exp. Neurol. 45*:318 (1986).

3
Monoclonal Antibody Assays for Breast Cancer

Donald W. Kufe, Daniel F. Hayes, Miyako Abe / Dana Farber Cancer Institute, Harvard Medical School, Boston, Massachusetts

Tsuneya Ohno / Jikei University School of Medicine, Tokyo, Japan

Joel Lundy / Winthrop Hospital, Mineola, and SUNY, Stony Brook, New York

Jeffrey Schlom / National Cancer Institute, National Institutes of Health, Bethesda, Maryland

INTRODUCTION

Breast cancer is a major cause of morbidity and mortality in
this country; one woman in 11 will ultimately develop this disease.
Initial surgical approaches with the use of radical mastectomy
markedly improved the survival rate; however, there has been
little further improvement (1). Although the local tumor can be
controlled with surgery and radiotherapy, residual systemic micrometastases result in high recurrence rates with a 10-year disease-
free survival in less than 50% of the patients. Metastatic spread to
the axillary nodes can be evaluated by surgical sampling at the
time of mastectomy. However, the detection of disease in the
internal mammary nodes or at distal sites has been more difficult.
Adjuvant chemotherapy directed at these undetectable metastases
has resulted in a slight increase in absolute survival at 5 years for
premenopausal women with involved nodes (2). However, metastatic disease still develops in a substantial number of patients for
whom no curative therapy is currently available. Thus, the development of more effective diagnostic and therapeutic approaches are clearly needed for control of this disease.

More effective diagnostic approaches may be achieved by the
use of antibodies specifically reactive with breast cancer cells.
Tumor cells in both animals and humans have been shown to express distinct cell-surface antigens that distinguish them from normal tissues. These tumor-associated antigens (TAA) are of biological and clinical interest. However, the definition of a TAA is difficult, because it is nearly impossible to prove that an antigen is
absent from normal tissues at all stages of embryonic development and subsequent cellular differentiation. Nonetheless, initial
efforts to identify human mammary tumor-associated antigens were
successful using polyclonal antisera. However, these studies were
hampered by the heterogeneity of the antibody populations and
the amount of available immunoglobulin. More recently, a variety
of monoclonal antibodies (MAbs) have been produced which react
with distinct antigens expressed by human mammary tissues. This
chapter will review some of the characteristics of these MAbs and
focus on their use in in vitro diagnostic assays.

MONOCLONAL ANTIBODIES REACTIVE WITH
HUMAN BREAST TUMORS

Monoclonal antibodies have been generated against human breast tissues using the following immunogens: (1) human milk-fat globule membranes; (2) human mammary tumor cell lines; and (3) extracts of human breast tumors.

Several groups have generated MAbs against human milk-fat globule membranes (3-8). These antibodies react strongly with lactating breast tissues and to a lesser extent with the normal resting breast. A characterization of the cell-surface antigens defined by these MAbs has revealed molecules with molecular weights of 46,000, 70,000, and 400,000 (5,8). The higher-molecular-weight antigen is a mucinlike glycoprotein with a high sugar content (8).

Human mammary tumor cell lines have also been used as immunogens by several laboratories (9-11). The MAb generated against the ZR-75-1 cell line reacts with approximately half of malignant tumors and with more than 80% of benign mammary lesions (11). The MCF-7 and SK-BR-3 breast carcinoma cell lines have been employed as immunogen in the generation of MAbs F36/22 and M7/105 (12). The MAb F36/22 reacts with normal mammary epithelial membranes and milk-fat globule membranes, whereas MAb M7/105 reacts only with membranes of malignant cells (12). The expression of F36/22 antigen also correlates with the breast tumor estrogen receptor level (13). This antigen is expressed on other adenocarcinomas and has a molecular weight of over 400,000. The MCF-7 cell line has also been used as immunogen in the production of MAb 10-3D2 (14) and MAb MBr1 (15, 16). The MAb 10-3D2 binds to all breast carcinoma cell lines tested, as well as to a number of other human carcinomas by solid-phase radioimmunoassay (SP-RIA) (14). This antibody precipitates a 126,000-molecular weight protein and does not bind to normal mammary epithelium. In contrast, MAb MBr1 reacts with both normal and malignant breast epithelium (15,16).

Other investigators have utilized membrane-enriched extracts of human metastatic mammary tumor cells as immunogens to generate and characterize MAbs reactive with determinants that would be maintained on metastatic, as well as primary, human mammary carcinoma cells. Assays using tumor cell extracts, tissue sections, and live cells in culture have been employed to reveal the diversity of the MAbs generated (17-21). Several MAbs are reactive with up to 80% of primary breast carcinomas but are unreactive with a variety of normal human tissues. These antibodies show limited cross-reactivity with certain other carcinomas, but they are uniformly unreactive with tumors of mesenchymal origin. The most specific member of this group is MAb B72.3, which reacts with a 220,000-400,000 high-molecular-weight glycoprotein complex found in 50% of human mammary carcinomas and 80% of human colon carcinomas. Another MAb, designated DF3, was prepared against a membrane-enriched extract of a human breast carcinoma metastatic to the liver (22). This MAb reacts with a 300,000-400,000-molecular weight breast tumor-associated glycoprotein that is detectable on the cell surface of human breast carcinoma cells.

The generation of MAbs against breast carcinoma-associated antigens may provide useful diagnostic reagents in (1) immunoperoxidase-staining studies of primary or metastatic breast tumors, (2) monitoring for mammary epithelial antigens in plasma or serum, and (3) radioimmunodetection studies. Because this chapter focuses on the in vitro diagnosis of human breast carcinomas, we will limit our attention to immunoperoxidase studies and assays that monitor circulating antigen. The MAb DF3 serves as an example of a reagent useful in both of these areas. Thus, the remainder of this chapter will review studies with MAb DF3, as space limitations preclude a more comprehensive analysis of each MAb already listed as reactive with breast carcinomas.

IMMUNOPEROXIDASE STUDIES WITH MONOCLONAL ANTIBODY DF3

Reactivity with Malignant Mammary Carcinomas

Initial characterization of MAb DF3 was directed toward defining expression of the reactive antigen in breast cancers. Several histological types of human malignant mammary carcinomas were examined for reactivity with MAb DF3 using the ABC immunoperoxidase method and 5-μm sections of formalin-fixed tissues.

Monoclonal antibody DF3 was reactive with 78% of 32 infiltrating ductal carcinomas (IDC) (22). As shown in Figure 1, the proportion of tumor cells staining within each of the 25 IDCs ranged from a few to over 90%. Furthermore, the staining pattern for these carcinomas was primarily cytoplasmic (Figures 2A and 2B). A similar staining pattern was observed for mammary carci-

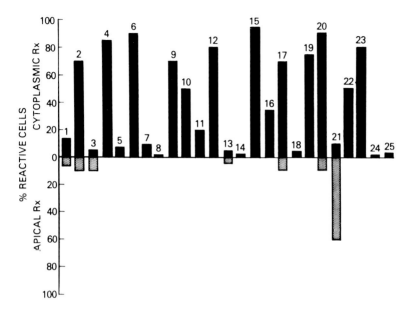

Figure 1   Reactivity of MAb DF3 with infiltrating duct carcinoma. Each bar represents a different patient. The dark areas represent the percentage of tumor cells with a cytoplasmic reaction: the striped areas represent the percentage of tumor cells displaying MAb DF3 reactivity on apical borders.

nomas containing both infiltrating ductal and intraductal elements.

The reactivity with infiltrating elements was compared in nine separate breast cancer specimens (22). The percentage of reactive cells varied for individual tumors, and the infiltrating elements of each tumor displayed a higher degree of cytoplasmic reactivity than the intraductal component. Similar staining patterns were observed with in situ, medullary, and infiltrating lobular carcinomas (22). The three infiltrating locular carcinomas and one medullary carcinoma showed only cytoplasmic staining. In contrast, the in situ carcinomas had various degrees of cytoplasmic and apical border reactivity.

Reactivity with Benign Breast Lesions

In contrast to the cytoplasmic reactivity observed with the malignant breast tissues, MAb DF3 showed reactivity with only the

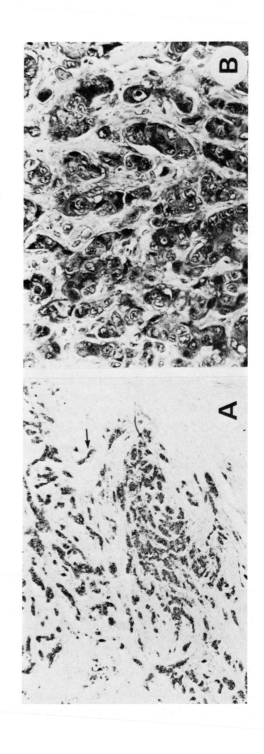

72

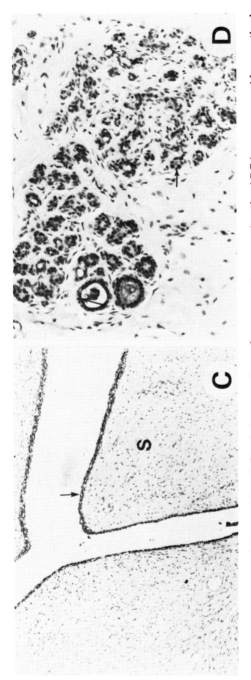

Figure 2 Reactivity of MAb DF3 with fixed tissue sections of mammary tumors using the ABC immunoperoxidase method: (A) infiltrating ductal carcinoma with strong cytoplasmic reactivity (54×); (B) higher magnification of (A) (330×); (C) fibroadenoma showing MAb DF3 reactivity on apical borders of cell (arrow), S is stroma; (D) fibrocystic disease showing apical staining of the cell lining of the cyst (large arrow) and normal gland (small arrow) (130×).

73

apical borders of all benign breast lesions. Figures 2C and 2D
show the apical reactivity of MAb DF3 in fibroadenomas and
fibrocystic disease, respectively. A similar pattern of reactivity
was observed with a lactating breast tissue. Approximately 10-
20% of normal ducts from breast tumor patients also showed a
slight apical staining. However, none of five fibroadenomas, only
one of eight fibrocystic disease specimens, and no normal duct
cells showed any evidence of cytoplasmic MAb DF3 reactive antigen.

Table 1 summarizes reactivities on the basis of cytoplasmic
staining alone. From this criteria, 78% of malignant lesions were
positive, whereas only one of 13 benign lesions displayed this pattern of reactivity.

Antigen Distribution in Primary and Metastatic Lesions

Primary and metastatic breast carcinomas from three patients
were also examined for reactivity with MAb DF3. As detailed in
Table 2, all metastatic disease to axillary lymph nodes and distal
sites was positive. The pattern of reactivity for distal metastatic
disease was uniformly cytoplasmic as observed with the primary
breast carcinomas. One exception was the lung metastasis ob-

Table 1   Cytoplasmic Reactivity of MAb DF3 with Human Mammary
Tumors[a]

Tissue	Total no. tested	No. reactive with MAb DF3 (%)	
Malignant			
infiltrating ductal	32	25	(78)
infiltrating and intraductal	12	9	(75)
other	7	6	(86)
Total	51	40	(78)
Benign			
fibroadenomas	5	0	
fibrocystic disease	8	1	(13)
Total	13	1	(8)

[a]By immunoperoxidase staining.
Source: Modified from Ref. 22, with permission.

Table 2 MAb DF3 Antigen Distribution in Primary and Metastatic Mammary Carcinoma Lesions[a]

	% Reactive cells in tumor		
Site of tumor	Patient 1	Patient 2	Patient 3
Primary	60	70,100,60,80[b]	50
Metastases			
axillary node	40	60	70,80[b]
distant			
bone	55	90	
brain			50
kidney		5	
liver	40		
lung	40	60,10[b]	90
meninges		45	
ovary		95	

[a]By immunoperoxidase staining.
[b]Different lesions.
Source: Ref. 22, reproduced with permission.

tained from patient 1, which also revealed some degree of apical staining. The reactivity of breast tumor metastases with MAb DF3 is demonstrated in Figure 3. Figure 3A shows the strongly staining breast carcinoma cells metastatic to the ovary (see Table 2, patient 2). Figure 3B reveals strongly reactive metastatic disease in the bone marrow of the same patient.

Reactivity with Nonbreast Tissues

Numerous tissues were examined for cells reactive with MAb DF3. All cell types of normal adult spleen, colon, bone marrow, heart, stomach, duodenum, skin, and adrenal cortex were negative. Epithelial cells of several organs reacted with MAb DF3. This reactivity was, in general, on the apical borders (Table 3). The highest percentage of stained cells were seen in the collecting and distal tubules of the kidney and in the epithelial and glandular cells of the uterus and endocervix (see Table 3).

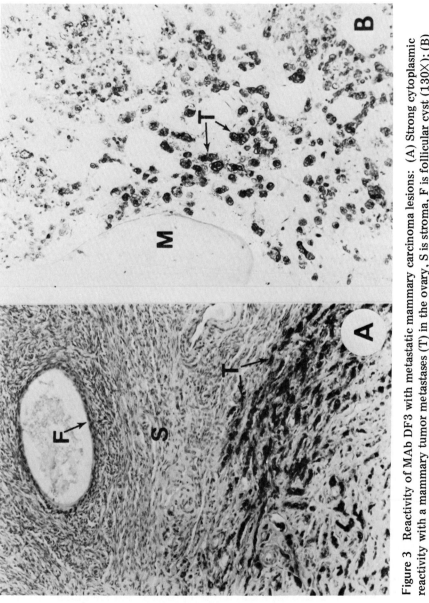

Figure 3   Reactivity of MAb DF3 with metastatic mammary carcinoma lesions: (A) Strong cytoplasmic reactivity with a mammary tumor metastases (T) in the ovary, S is stroma, F is follicular cyst (130×); (B) Positive metastatic tumor cells (T) in the bone marrow (M) (× 220).

Table 3 Reactivity of MAb DF3 with Normal Human Tissues[a]

Tissue	Total No. tested	No. reactive with MAb DF3 (% reactive cells)	Type of cell reactive with MAbDF3
Stomach	2	1 (5)	Gastric glands
Duodenum	1	0	
Colon	3	0	
Liver	4	2 (10-25)	Epithelial cells along bile ducts
Fetal liver	1	0	
Gallbladder	3	2 (5-80)	Epithelial cells
Spleen	2	0	
Lung	7	3 (5-25)	Alveolar and bronchiolar cells
Heart	1	0	
Kidney	7	5 (15-100)	Convoluted distal and collecting tubules
Bladder	1	1 (10-30)	Transitional epithelial cells
Testis	1	1 (5)	Epithelial cells along seminiferous ducts
Uterus	1	1 (100)	Epithelial cells, cells of glands
Endocervix	2	2 (100)	Mucus-secreting glandular epithelial cells
Exocervix	3	0	
Skin	1	0	
Sebaceous gland	3	3 (50-70)	Alveolar cells
Sweat gland	3	3 (10-80)	Secretory tubule cells
Adrenal cortex	1	0	
Thyroid	1	1 (10)	Folicular cells
Bone marrow	2	0	

[a]By immunoperoxidase staining.

Forty-six nonmammary carcinomas of various sites were analyzed for reactivity with MAb DF3 (Table 4). Various degrees of antigen expression were observed for these specimens. There was no detectable reactivity of MAb DF3 with colon carcinomas, thus clearly distinguishing this antibody from F36/22 which reacts with these tumors (13). In contrast, MAb DF3 reactivity was observed with a variety of other adenocarcinomas. Pancreatic and uterine adenocarcinomas had the highest percentage of tumor cells with cytoplasmic reactivity. The intensity and pattern of staining was generally lower for other carcinomas. There was no detectable reactivity with a panel of tumors of mesenchymal origin.

Table 4   Reactivity of MAb DF3 with Nonmammary Carcinomas

Tumors	No. tested	% Reactive tumor cells
Colon adenocarcinomas	14	0,0,0,0,(5)[a],0,(1), 0,0,0,(5),0,(5),(1)
Transitional cell carcinomas of the bladder	9	10(5),(1),20(5),20, 0,10,50,(5),(5)
Ovarian adenocarcinomas	2	(25),80(30)
Carcinoma in situ of the cervix	2	20,20[b]
Pancreatic adenocarcinomas	3	60,70,70,(50)
Prostatic adenocarcinomas	9	0,0,60,(30),15,5,1,0,0
Adenocarcinomas of the uterus	7	(70),90,(40),70,(65), (25),70,(60),80, (75),100,(20)
Metastatic carcinoid	1	0

[a]Number given are total percentage of reactive tumor cells (cytoplasmic and apical), numbers in parenthesis are the percentage of reactive tumor cells with apical concentration of antigen only.
[b]Here, 5% of the normal cells were positive, with cytoplastic staining.

Monoclonal Antibody DF3 Reactivity and Degree of
Breast Carcinoma Differentiation

Potential applications of immunoperoxidase staining with MAb
DF3 would be to (1) define the degree of breast tumor differentiation and (2) to predict the prognosis after primary breast
therapy. For example, MAbs produced from milk-fat globule
membranes react more strongly with well-differentiated as compared with undifferentiated breast tumors (3). There is no available MAb, however, that histopathologically defines prognosis,
as does, for example, nodal status. The availability of an MAb
that is predictive of disease-free survival on the basis of immunoperoxidase-staining patterns might obviate the need for axillary
dissection, an essential, but nontherapeutic and potentially mor-
bid step in determining the need for adjuvant chemotherapy.

Human mammary tumors were thus evaluated for the level
of DF3 antigen as a correlate to clinicopathologic factors related
to the degree of tumor differentiation: nuclear grade (NG),
histological grade (HG), and estrogen receptor (ER) status (23).
Carcinomas with NG 1 and 2 contained significantly more DF3
antigen compared with tumors with NG 3 (p = .002) (23). A
similar relationship was obtained between percentage of DF3-
positive tumors and histological grade. Seventeen of 19 tumors
with HG 1 and 2 scored positive for reactivity with MAb DF3
(23). In contrast, only 11 of 27 tumors with HG 3 scored positive (p = .001). These findings suggested that reactivity with
MAb DF3 is significantly associated with the degree of differentiation as determined by both nuclear and histological grade.

The previously reported (24-28) correlation between hormone receptor content and histological grade prompted a further
examination of the relationship between MAb DF3 reactivity and
ER status. Only one of 23 ER-positive tumors had less than 10%
MAb DF3-reactive cells. In contrast, only six of 23 ER-negative
tumors had 10% or more cells positive for reactivity with MAb
DF3 (23). These results were significantly different (p < .001).
Because 20 of 23 tumors were ER-progesterone receptor (PgR)-
positive, no statement can be made related to correlation with ER-
positive, PgR-negative tumors. In addition, because only four
patients were premenopausal, no attempt was made to analyze
this group independently.

All of the 15 HG 1 and 2 tumors that were ER-positive were also positive for MAb DF3 reactivity. Seven of eight HG 3 tumors that were ER-positive were also reactive with MAb DF3 (23). Similarly, 17 of 18 NG 1 and 2, ER-positive tumors were reactive with MAb DF3. Finally, each of the five NG 3, ER-positive tumors were reactive with MAb DF3, while only two of 15 NG 3, ER-negative tumors demonstrated this reactivity (p = .001) (23).

These studies, thus, demonstrate that reactivity of primary breast tumors with MAb DF3 correlates significantly with at least three (NG, HG, ER status) important factors associated with risk of recurrence in lymph node-negative patients. The use of MAb DF3 reactivity in conjunction with other clinicopathological factors may, therefore, provide additional prognostic information that would further define the biological course of individual patients with breast cancer. Additional prognostic indicators would be particularly useful in the lymph node-negative patient group. Another group at risk are those patients selected for excision of the primary tumor (i.e., lumpectomy) and subsequent radiation therapy. A high NG, extensive intraductal involvement, and high mitotic activity have resulted in local recurrence rates approaching 40% in this group of patients (29). The significant correlation between MAb DF3 reactivity and HG may, for example, further define patients at risk in this group. Although this study has not explored the relationship between MAb DF3 reactivity and prognosis, the results should provide the basis for extending the use of this MAb as an adjunct to ER status in defining the biological behavior of individual breast carcinomas.

Other MAbs have been evaluated in similar studies. The MAbs generated against purified human milk-fat globule membranes (Mam-3, HMFG 1, and HMFG 2) were reacted with sections of 100 primary breast carcinomas (30). A tendency toward a greater proportion of tumors binding the antibodies was observed among the highly differentiated tumors when compared with the less-differentiated carcinomas. However, no apparent relationship was observed between the presence of antigen and menopausal status, lymph node status, or ER status. Tumors lacking PgR (eight of nine) also lacked reactivity to Mam-3 (30). Other studies with Mam-3 have indicated a better survival for patients with tumors positive for this antigen (31). Another study using HMFG 1 identified 22 of 175 patients with reactive tumors and a good prognosis, while 13 patients not reactive with the MAb had early recurrence (32). The good-prognosis group had tumors with a low HG and a high degree of tubule formation. However, subsequent studies with MAbs HMFG 1 and HMFG 2 found no correlation between staining and either tumor differentiation or prognosis (33). Finally, patients whose tumors exhibited intense staining with MAb NCRC 11 had an improved survival compared with those with less intensely staining tumors (34). The MAb NCRC 11 recognizes an antigen that has a distribution similar to that of antibodies prepared against milk-fat globule membrane (4,5). These studies, however, are limited by their retrospective design. A prospective trial of patients undergoing adjuvant therapy is currently underway.

DETECTION OF BREAST CANCER METASTASES IN BODY FLUIDS AND BONE MARROW USING MONOCLONAL ANTIBODIES

The cytopathological diagnosis of cells in serious effusions has certain limitations. Malignant cells are often difficult to differentiate from reactive mesothelial cells. Furthermore, even when malignant cells are recognized, there may be difficulty in determining the tissue of origin. The development of MAb technology, however, has enhanced the diagnostic potential of breast cancer cytopathology.

Several MAbs have been used to study malignant effusions. The Ca1 antibody has been reported to distinguish malignant from nonmalignant cells in 21 of 25 malignant effusions (35). More recent studies, however, have indicated some cross-reactivity of this MAb with mesothelial cells (36). The MAb HMFG 2 has similarly been reported to be reactive with cancer cells but not with mesothelial or endothelial cells (37). Furthermore, MAbs MBr1 and Mov2, which react with distinct antigens expressed on both breast and ovarian carcinomas, have been used to demonstrate malignant cells in pleural and peritoneal effusion in eight of 21 (38%) patients with metastatic breast cancer and previously negative cytological examinations (38).

We have also monitored patterns of immunocytochemical staining of malignant and benign cells in effusions using MAbs DF3 and B72.3 (39). The MAb B72.3 showed positive staining with 36 of 39 (92%) adenocarcinomas versus staining in only one

of 12 (8%) other neoplasms. In contrast to staining of adenocarcinomas, MAb B72.3 stained no mesothelial cells in 68 specimens. The MAb DF3 showed a reaction pattern to adenocarcinomas similar to that of MAb B72.3, although this antibody also
had reactivity with mesothelial cells. Thus, MAb B72.3, but not
MAb DF3, is highly selective in distinguishing adenocarcinoma
cells from mesothelial cells. More selective antibodies, however,
are required to determine if tumor cells in effusions originated
in breast tissue.

Monoclonal antibodies have also been used to identify malignant cells in the cerebrospinal fluid. The MAB LE61, directed
against epithelial cytokeratin, and MAb AUAI, directed against
an epithelial "proliferation" antigen, were used to diagnose and
characterize carcinomatous meningitis in five of six cases (40).
A routine cytological examination was nondiagnostic in three of
these patients.

Another potential application of MAbs is in the evaluation
of breast cyst fluid. The use of MAb Ca1, however, did not reliably differentiate between benign and malignant breast epithelial
cells (41). Similar studies with other antibodies have yet to be
reported.

Monoclonal and polyclonal antibodies have been used to
screen bone marrows from patients with breast cancer. Antisera against epithelial membrane antigen (EMA) has been reported
to detect tumor cells in 31 of 110 (28%) patients with nonmetastatic primary breast cancer (42). More recently, a panel of
MAbs, including LE61, HMFG 2, and E29 (anti-EMA) detected
bone marrow metastases in two patients with breast cancer (44).
Results of routine cytological examination were negative in one
of these patients.

Finally, the use of high-dose chemotherapy, with autologous
bone marrow transplantation in patients with breast cancer, has
been under investigation (45). The ability to detect occult bone
marrow involvement by metastatic breast cancer could have an
impact on the success of this approach. Monoclonal antibodies
directed against breast carcinomas would be useful both in determining bone marrow involvement and as potential reagents to
eliminate these cells. There are, however, no published reports
that examine the role of MAbs in "purging" bone marrows from
patients with breast cancer.

CHARACTERIZATION OF DF3 ANTIGEN

Expression of DF3 antigen has, thus, been shown to correlate with the degree of human breast tumor differentiation and estrogen receptor status (23). Furthermore, DF3 antigen is detectable in human milk (46). These findings have suggested that MAb DF3 reacts with a milk-related antigen that might be useful as a biochemical marker of differentiated mammary epithelial cells. The suggestion that MAb DF3 reacts with a differentiation antigen has also been supported by the demonstration of enhanced DF3 antigen expression after treatment of breast carcinoma cells with butyric acid or phorbol ester (46,47), known inducers of differentiation.

In view of the possible role of DF3 antigen in differentiated functions of mammary epithelium, we have developed an approach to purify the cross-reactive species by using gel filtration and antibody affinity chromatography (48). The affinity-column-purified DF3 antigen was absorbed by wheat germ agglutinin and peanut agglutinin but not by concanavalin A or lentil lectin. In contrast, wheat germ agglutinin inhibited MAb DF3 reactivity with the purified antigen, whereas little, if any, inhibition occurred with peanut agglutinin. These findings are, thus, consistent with the involvement of terminal N-acetyl-d-neuraminic acid, or N-acetylglucosamine residues, or both, in the antigenic site. The DF3 antigenicity was also sensitive to neuraminidase but not to chondroitinase ABC, chondroitinase AC, chondroitin-4-sulfatase, or hyaluronidase. Furthermore, DF3 antigen was sensitive to Pronase, subtilisin BPN', and α-chymotrypsin. The presence of O-glycosidic linkages between carbohydrate and protein in the DF3 antigenic site was further supported by the presence of $NaBH_4$-sensitive sites. Together, these results suggest that sialyl oligosaccharides present on a peptide backbone are required for maintaining DF3 antigenicity. Similar findings have been demonstrated for DF3 antigen purified from both human milk and breast cancer effusions. However, the DF3 antigen in human milk consisted of a single high-molecular-weight species, whereas the tumor-associated antigen consisted of at least two distinct glycoproteins with molecular weights of 330,000 and 450,000. These findings are relevant to the demonstration that distinct high-molecular-weight DF3 antigens are elevated in the circulation of patients with breast carcinoma.

DETECTION OF CIRCULATING DF3 ANTIGEN
IN PATIENTS WITH BREAST CANCER

Another diagnostic approach using MAbs reactive with human breast carcinomas could involve monitoring for circulating human mammary epithelial antigens. Breast tissue markers, such as casein (49), α-lactalbumin (50), glycosyltransferases (51), glycolipids (52), phospholipids (53), gross cystic disease protein, and carcinoembryonic antigen (CEA) (54), have been detected in the circulation by a variety of techniques. With the exception of CEA, none has gained acceptance as a breast cancer marker. Although of some clinical value, CEA levels have proved to be too nonspecific and insensitive to be generally applicable in the serological detection and evaluation of human breast carcinoma (55).

Human mammary epithelial antigens detected by MAbs prepared against human milk-fat globule have been shown to be elevated in sera of patients with disseminated cancer of the breast and other organs (56). Similarly, a breast epithelium antigen (100 kd) defined by MAb 24-17.2 has been detected in increased amounts in the sera of patients with breast cancer (57). Although both assays appear promising, neither has been applied to monitor the clinical course. More recently, double-determinant assays have been used to detect elevated circulating F36/22 (58) and Mam-6 (59) antigen levels in patients with metastatic breast cancer. We have also developed a radioimmunoassay (RIA) and an enzyme-linked immunoassay (EIA) with MAb DF3 to monitor circulating DF3 antigen levels in patients with breast cancer (60). These assays will be described in some detail.

DF3-DF3 Double-Determinant Assays

Figure 4 illustrates representative profiles using the EIA. The DF3 antigen was detectable in the plasmas from three patients with breast cancer and from three control subjects. However, DF3 antigen levels were undetectable at a 1:125 dilution of plasmas from all three normal females, whereas significant amount of peroxidated MAb DF3 bound at similar dilutions of plasmas from the three patients. The EIA profiles were similar to those obtained by RIA. Thus, the level of DF3 antigen was higher in patients than in controls. Plasma or serum samples yielded identical results.

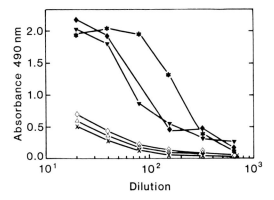

Figure 4 Effect of plasma dilution on binding of peroxidated MAb DF3.
Plasma samples from patients with metastatic breast cancer (closed diamond,
triangle, asterisk) and from normal women (open diamond, triangle, asterisk)
were diluted serially and assayed for DF3 antigen in the sequential double-
determinant EIA.

The detection of circulating DF3 antigen prompted further
analysis using transblot techniques to determine the molecular
weight of the reactive species. Figure 5 shows the results obtained from plasmas from breast cancer patients and normal subjects. Antigenic heterogeneity was observed in both patients and
controls. The MAb DF3 reactivity was preponderantly found with
antigens of three different molecular weights ranging from
300,000 to approximately 400,000. Although similar patterns
were observed in breast cancer patients and controls, the extent
of reactivity was clearly greater with plasmas obtained from breast
cancer patients. These findings by transblot analysis are, thus, in
concert with the RIA and EIA results. Further, the transblot
approach yields additional information regarding the molecular
weight of the cross-reactive antigens.

The RIA, EIA, and transblot assays have been used to monitor
circulating DF3 antigen levels in a larger series of breast cancer
patients and normal subjects. Figure 6 summarizes the EIA
assay results of samples from 58 patients with metastatic breast
cancer and 111 apparently normal females. The EIA DF3 antigen
units were determined after comparison with a frozen primary ref-

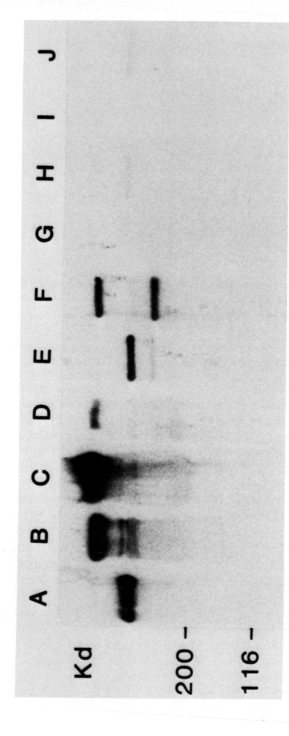

Figure 5 Reactivity of MAb DF3 with a metastatic breast carcinoma and plasma samples: (A) membrane-enriched fraction of a breast carcinoma metastatic to liver (0.5 μg); (B-F) plasma samples from patients with metastatic breast cancer (1 μl); (G-J) plasma samples from normal women (1 μl). The antigen preparations were subjected to electrophoresis on a 3-15% SDS-polyacrylamide gel, transferred to nitrocellulose paper, and analyzed for reactivity with MAb DF3.

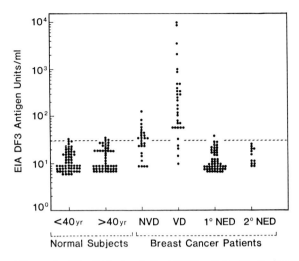

Figure 6   The EIA circulating DF3 antigen levels in normal women, patients with metastatic breast cancer, and patients with breast cancer free of detectable disease. Samples from 111 normal women, 58 patients with metastatic breast cancer (NVD, 26 patients; VD, 32 patients), and 65 patients with a prior history of breast cancer ($1°$ or primary disease; $2°$ or metastatic disease), but who were free of detectable disease (NED) at the time of sampling were assayed for EIA DF3 antigen level. Relative EIA DF3 antigen units per milliliter were determined at an absorbance of 0.75 (490 nm) and by reference to the frozen breast tumor standard. The dotted line represents an arbitrary level to distinguish elevated values.

erence standard. By use of this approach, only six of 111 normal subjects had EIA DF3 antigen levels $\geqslant$ 30 U/ml (mean $\pm$ SD 13 $\pm$ 88). Furthermore, similar results were obtained with normal women younger or older than 40 years. In contrast, 42 of 58 patients (72%) with breast cancer had EIA DF3 antigen levels $\geqslant$ 30 U/ml (mean $\pm$ SD 545 $\pm$ 1781). The difference between all breast cancer patients and all normal subjects was significant ($p <$ .001). Twenty-eight of 32 patients (88%) with visceral disease (VD) had EIA DF3 antigen levels $\geqslant$ 30 U/ml, whereas 14 of 26 patients (54%) with nonvisceral disease (NVD) had EIA DF3 antigen value above this level. The EIA DF3 antigen levels in patients with visceral disease (mean $\pm$ SD 973 $\pm$ 2350) were significantly different from those patients with nonvisceral disease (mean $\pm$ SD 37 $\pm$ 27) ($p <$

.001). Furthermore, the difference between EIA DF3 antigen levels obtained with NVD patients and all normal subjects was significant ($p < .001$). Finally, 50 of 52 patients with primary and 13 of 13 patients with metastatic breast cancer who were free of detectable disease at the time of sampling had EIA antigen levels that were < 30 U/ml.

It was of further interest to determine if serial measurements of circulating DF3 antigen levels would vary with the clinical course. Therefore, we monitored DF3 antigen levels in patients with metastatic breast cancer who were subsequently treated with chemotherapy. A representative profile obtained by RIA is illustrated in Figure 7A. This patient had an RIA DF3 antigen level of 700 U/ml just before beginning chemotherapy. Clinical response was obtained after 1 month of therapy, and at that time, the RIA DF3 antigen level had declined to 20 U/ml. The RIA DF3 antigen levels ranged between 15 and 70 U/ml while the patient received chemotherapy and remained in clinical remission. A similar example of a patient monitored for EIA DF3 antigen levels is illustrated in Figure 7B. This patient initially presented with an EIA DF3 antigen level of 80 U/ml. After achieving a complete response with chemotherapy, the EIA DF3 antigen level decreased to below 30 U/ml. The EIA DF3 antigen level, however, increased while this patient remained off chemotherapy, predating clinical detection of recurrent disease (32 months). Hepatic and pulmonary metastasis were eventually detected at 48 months and an unsuccessful attempt at retreatment with chemotherapy was associated with persistently elevated levels of EIA DF3 antigen. These serial findings have been confirmed by transblot analysis. Finally, serial EIA DF3 antigen levels were monitored in five patietns with progressive breast cancer, and in each one there was an increase in DF3 antigen level. Three of these patients were subsequently treated with hormonal therapy or chemotherapy, and the declines in EIA DF3 antigen levels paralleled partial and complete clinical responses.

We also monitored circulating DF3 antigen levels in patients with other benign and malignant disease. For this, serum EIA DF3 antigen levels were determined for 17 patients with benign breast diseases (60). None of these patients had EIA DF3 antigen levels ≥ 30 U/ml (mean $\pm$ SD 14.8 $\pm$ 17.3). There was also no detectable elevation of circulating DF3 antigen in 71 patients with

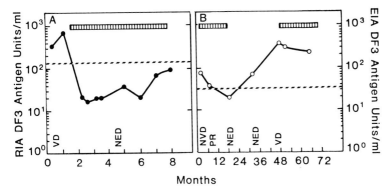

Figure 7 Circulating DF3 antigen levels and clinical course. (A) Serial samples froma patient with metastatic breast cancer assayed for RIA DF3 antigen levels; (B) serial samples from another patient with metastatic breast cancer assayed for EIA DF3 antigen levels. The dotted line represents arbitrary levels to distinguish elevated values in the RIA (150 U/ml) or EIA (30 U/ml). Hatched areas represent treatment with chemotherapy.

esophageal, gastric, or colorectal carcinomas. Of the 48 patients with colorectal tumors, 25 had liver involvement, which suggests that hepatic metastases per se did not cause elevations in circulating DF3 antigen. Furthermore, only two of 58 patients with pancreatic malignancies and one of 11 patients with lung cancer had DF3 levels > 30 U/ml. Elevated DF3 antigen levels were, however, detected in 27% of patients with hepatoma and 47% of patients with ovarian cancer. Finally, 10 of 66 patients with benign liver disease had DF3 antigen levels > 30 U/ml (60).

CA15-3 Assay

We have further monitored circulating DF3 antigen in patients with breast cancer using a bideterminant immunoradiometric assay (IRMA), designated CA15-3 (61). The CA15-3 IRMA combines MAb 115D8 (6) in the solid phase and radiolabeled MAb DF3 as tracer.

Distribution of Circulating CA15-3 Levels in Normal Women and Patients with Breast Cancer

The percentage of 1050 normal control subjects, for whom CA15-3 levels are elevated above reference values, is listed in Table 5. The CA15-3 levels were > 22 U/ml in 99 subjects (9.4%) and > 25 U/ml in 58 (5.5%) subjects. Furthermore, only 14 (1.3%) of these subjects had CA15-3 levels > 30 U/ml, and only five (0.5%) and one (0.09%) had levels > 35 U/ml and 40 U/ml, respectively. In contrast, 31 patients with primary breast cancer had a mean CA15-3 antigen level of 26.9 ± 30 U/ml. Nine of these patients (29%) had CA15-3 levels > 22 U/ml, seven (23%) had CA15-3 levels > 25 U/ml, and only two (7%) had CA15-3 levels > 40 U/ml.

The CA15-3 levels were > 22 U/ml in 73% of 158 patients with metastatic breast cancer (mean ± SD 175.4 ± 520 U/ml) (see Table 5). Additionally, 52% of these patients had levels > 40 U/ml. Of 26 patients with local recurrence, 13 (50%) had levels > 22 U/ml, and six (23%) had values > 40 U/ml (mean ± SD of 34.4 ± 44 U/ml). These data for patients with only local recurrence are not significantly different from those obtained from patients with advanced stage IV primary carcinomas of the breast (see Table 5). In contrast, patients, with bone metastases only had significantly higher CA15-3 levels (mean ± SD of 104.0 ± 137 U/ml) than did those with local recurrence ($p < .001$). Similarly, patients with hepatic metastases, with or without other sites of disease, had even higher CA15-3 levels (mean ± SD of 544.9 ± 1163 U/ml).

Comparison of Circulating CA15-3 and Carcinoembryonic Antigen in Patients with Breast Cancer

We also determined circulating CEA levels in the same population of patients with breast cancer (Table 6). Among normal control subjects, 90.6% are reported to have CEA values < 3.0 ng/ml, and 98.7% have CEA values < 5.0 ng/ml (62). Thus, CEA reference levels of 3.0 ng/ml and 5.0 ng/ml provide estimates of specificity comparable with CA15-3 reference levels of 22 U/ml and 30 U/ml in a normal population.

Significantly more patients with metastatic breast cancer had elevated CA15-3 antigen levels than had elevated CEA levels (see Table 6). Although only 87 of 158 patients (55%) had CEA levels

Table 5 Distribution of CA15-3 Levels in Patients with Breast Cancer

Stage	No. of patients	No. of patients (%) with CA15-3 levels					CA15-3 level[a]
		>22 U/ml	>25 U/ml	>30 U/ml	>35 U/ml	>40 U/ml	
Normal controls	1050	99 (9.4)	58 (5.5)	14 (1.3)	5 (0.5)	1 (0.09)	13.3 ± 6
Primary breast cancer	31	9 (29)	7 (23)	6 (20)	3 (10)	2 (7)	26.9 ± 30
stage I	3	0					12.1 ± 4
stage II	14	5 (36)	4 (29)	3 (21)	1 (7)	1 (7)	28.4 ± 14
stage III	7	0					17.6 ± 4
stage IV	7	4 (57)	3 (43)	3 (43)	2 (29)	1 (14)	37.5 ± 38
Metastatic breast cancer	158	115 (73)	109 (69)	99 (63)	88 (55)	82 (52)	175.4 ± 520
local only	26	13 (50)	12 (46)	10 (38)	7 (27)	6 (23)	34.4 ± 44
bone only	34	27 (79)	27 (79)	24 (71)	21 (62)	18 (53)	104.0 ± 137
liver	24	20 (83)	19 (79)	19 (79)	18 (75)	18 (75)	544.9 ± 1163

[a]Mean U/ml + SD.
Source: Ref. 61, reproduced with permission.

Table 6 Comparison of CA15-3 and CEA Levels in Patients with Breast Cancer

Stage	No. of patients	CEA level[a]	No. of patients (%) with CA15-3 levels >22 U/ml	No. of patients (%) with CEA levels >3.0 ng/ml	p value	No. of patients (%) with CA15-3 levels >30 U/ml	No. of patients (%) with CEA levels >5.0 ng/ml	p value
Normal controls			(9.4)	(9.4)		(1.3)	(1.3)	
Primary breast								
cancer	31	1.2 ± 1	9 (29)	2 (7)	$0.01 < p < 0.02$	6 (19)	0	$0.005 < p < 0.1$
stage I	2	0.6 ± 0.1	0	0	NS	0	0	NS
stage II	14	1.2 ± 1	5 (36)	2 (14)	NS	3 (21)	0	NS
stage III	7	1.3 ± 0.9	0	0	NS	0	0	NS
stage IV	7	1.3 ± 0.8	4 (57)	0	$0.005 < p < 0.01$	3 (43)	0	$0.02 < p < 0.05$
Metastatic breast								
cancer	158	24.0 ± 53	115 (73)	87 (55)	< 0.001	99 (63)	64 (41)	< 0.001
local only	26	2.9 ± 5	13 (50)	5 (19)	$0.01 < p < 0.02$	10 (38)	3 (12)	$0.02 < p < 0.05$
bone only	34	11.8 ± 17	27 (79)	20 (59)	NS (0.07)	24 (71)	15 (44)	0.02
liver	24	79 ± 104	20 (83)	21 (88)	NS	19 (79)	18 (75)	NS

[a]Mean ng/ml + SD.
Source: Ref. 61, reproduced with permission.

> 3.0 ng/ml and only 41% had CEA levels > 5.0 ng/ml, 115 (73%) and 99 (63%) had CA15-3 values > 22 U/ml and 30 U/ml, respectively. These differences were highly significant ($p < .001$) (see Table 6). Thirteen (50%) and 10 (38%) of 26 patients with only local recurrence had CA15-3 levels > 22 U/ml and 30 U/ml, respectively. Of these same 26 patients, only five (19%) and three (12%) had CEA levels > 3.0 ($0.01 < p < .02$) and 5.0 ng/ml ($0.02 < p < .05$), respectively. Of 34 patients with only bone metastases, 27 (79%) and 24 (71%) had CA15-3 levels > 22 U/ml and 30 U/ml, whereas 20 (59%) and 15 (44%) had CEA levels > 3.0 ng/ml and 5.0 ng/ml. The CA15-3 assay was significantly more sensitive than the CEA assay in patients with only bone metastases for the CA15-3 reference of 30 U/ml ($p = .02$). In contrast, over 80% of patients with hepatic metastases had elevations of both CA15-3 and CEA values (no significant difference). Finally, combining results of the two assays did not significantly increase the sensitivity when compared with CA15-3 alone for any patient group.

Thus, the CA15-3 IRMA is significantly more sensitive than the CEA-RIA in the evaluation of patients with both primary and metastatic breast cancer (see Table 6). Furthermore, the sensitivity of the CA15-3 assay is higher than the CEA assay in patients with only local metastases and in patients with only bone metastases. Levels of both antigens are elevated in most patients with hepatic metastases, and thus, the sensitivities of the assays are not statistically different in this subgroup. Importantly, combining results of the two assay does not enhance sensitivity compared with the CA15-3 assay alone. Thus, the use of both assays is not complementary.

Correlation of Circulating CA15-3 Antigen with the
Clinical Course of Patients with Breast Cancer

The CA15-3 assay was used to monitor serial samples during 57 clinical courses of patients with breast cancer (61). The CA15-3 levels increased by at least 25% of the original level in 19 of 21 patients (91%) with progressive disease. Furthermore, CA15-3 levels increased by at least 50% in 16 of these 21 patients (76%) and by at least 75% in 10 of these 21 patients (48%). In nine of these 21 patients (43%), the CA15-3 levels increased by a factor of 2, or more. Conversely, CA15-3 levels decreased, by at least

50%, in seven of nine patients (89%) with regressive disease. Finally, in 27 patients with stable disease, 16 (59%) had values that did not vary by more than ± 25% of the original CA15-3 value. Thus, serial CA15-3 levels correlated with changes in the clinical course in 42 of 57 patients (74%).

In summary, CA15-3 levels are more commonly elevated than CEA levels in patients with primary and metastatic breast cancers. Furthermore, sequential monitoring of CA15-3 levels in patients can be useful in evaluation of the clinical course of the disease.

RELATIONSHIP OF MONOCLONAL ANTIBODY DF3 TO OTHER MONOCLONAL ANTIBODIES PREPARED AGAINST BREAST CARCINOMA—ASSOCIATED ANTIGENS

Milk-fat globule membrane (MFGM) has been employed by other investigators as a source for the generation of MAbs. The MAbs prepared against human MFGM have detected tumor-associated antigenic determinants (3,4). One determinant was detectable in large glycoprotein molecules with complex carbohydrate side chains (63). Molecular weight determinations and lectin-blocking studies would suggest that this antigen (HMFG-1) is similar to the DF3 antigen, although the pattern of antibody binding to breast carcinoma lines is different (3,4,22). Another high-molecular-weight glycoprotein identified in MFGM and human mammary epithelial cell membranes has been partially characterized as having a high sugar content (8). This antigen (HMFG-Mc5) and the HMFG-1, however, have not been purified or characterized further.

A large glycoprotein, with a molecular weight similar to that of DF3, HMFG-1, and HMFG-Mc5, has been isolated from milk-fat globule (64). The results of that study suggested that this mucinlike glycoprotein contained approximately 50% carbohydrate. The antigen (PAS-0) was susceptible to Pronase and subtilisin BPN' digestion but was resistant to chymotrypsin. The PAS-0 bound both wheat germ agglutinin and peanut agglutinin. The PAS-0 glycoprotein, like DF3 antigen, was susceptible to alkaliborohydride treatment, indicating that the carbohydrate moiety was linked to the protein with O-glycosidic bonds. More recent studies (65) have demonstrated that PAS-0 carries antigenic determinants for epithelial membrane antigen, a glycoprotein detectable on epithelial cells (4,5,66).

Another MAb (F36/22), prepared against a human breast tumor cell line, identifies an antigen detectable in human breast carcinomas and in the circulation of breast cancer patients (12, 58). This antigen has been purified and was shown to be a high-molecular-weight glycoprotein (67). The F36/22 antigen bound strongly with wheat germ agglutinin but weakly with concanavalin A, lentil lectin, and peanut agglutinin. Furthermore, in contrast to DF3 antigen, F36/22 was not susceptible to pretease or neuraminidase treatments, whereas reactivity of both antigens was affected by alkaline conditions.

Other high-molecular-weight glycoproteins have been described as tumor-associted antigens. The cell membrane determinants defined by MAb Ca1, designated the CA antigen, are two major glycoproteins with estimated molecular weights of approximately 350,000 and 390,000 (68,69). In contrast to DF3 antigen and the other antigens defined by MAbs HMFG-1, HMFG-Mc5, and F36/22, the CA antigen has been detected on a wide range of human tumors (69). The CA antigen, however, is structurally similar to DF3 antigen in that most of the carbohydrate is O-glycosidically linked to a polypeptide and that antigenicity is partially destroyed by neuraminidase (68-70). Thus, together, these high-molecular-weight mucinlike glycoprotiens may represent a family of tumor-associated antigens. The purification and further identification of each of these components may provide certain insights into the extent of their biochemical and immunological similarities.

On the basis of the present studies, it would appear that the characteristics of the tumor-associated antigen defined by MAb DF3 are similar to those of the antigen in human milk. The determinant recognized by MAb DF3 in both antigens probably consists of several sialyl oligosaccharides on a peptide backbone. The purification of these antigens now provides an opportunity to prepare MAbs against other antigenic determinants on each of these molecules and to determine if there are specific sites on the tumor-associated antigen that could be exploited for the development of more specific immunologic assays.

SUMMARY

Major efforts are underway to develop MAbs with sufficient selectivity to impact on the diagnosis and therapy of breast cancer. A variety of MAbs have been produced that react with distinct antigens expressed by human mammary tissues. These antibodies are being employed in immunoperoxidase studies of breast carcinomas to determine if staining patterns relate to factors such as degree of tumor differentiation, ER status, and prognosis. These MAbs are also being used to detect breast cancer micrometastases in body fluids and bone marrow. Another in vitro diagnostic approach under study is the use of these MAbs to monitor circulating breast carcinoma-associated antigens. These areas of investigation are reviewed in this chapter with an emphasis on the MAb DF3 developed and characterized in our laboratories.

The murine MAb designated DF3, was prepared against a membrane-enriched fraction of a human breast carcinoma. Immunoperoxidase staining has demonstrated the presence of DF3 antigen on the apical borders of more-differentiated secretory mammary epithelial cells and in the cytosol of less-differentiated malignant cells. The expression of DF3 antigen also correlates with the degree of breast tumor differentiation and estrogen-receptor status. These findings have suggested that MAb DF3 reacts with a differentiation antigen detectable on the surface of human breast carcinoma cells. More importantly, the measurement of circulating DF3 antigen levels provides a useful marker to follow the clinical course of patients with metastatic breast cancer. We have purified the MAb DF3 cross-reacting antigens both from human milk and from malignant effusions. These antigens have been defined as high-molecular-weight mucinlike glycoproteins. The MAb DF3 is, thus, useful in in vitro diagnostic assays for human breast cancer. These findings with MAb DF3 are related to studies with other MAbs generated against human breast carcinoma-associated antigens.

REFERENCES

1. I. C. Henderson and G. Canellos, *N. Eng. J. Med. 302*:17,78 (1980).
2. G. Bonadonna and P. Valagussa, *J. Clin. Oncol. 3*:259 (1985).

3. J. J. A. Taylor-Papadimitriou, J. Peterson, J. Arklie, J. Burchell, R. L. Ceriani, and W. Bodmer, *Int. J. Cancer 28*:17 (1981).
4. J. J. A. Taylor-Papadimitriou, W. Bodmer, M. Egan, and R. Millis, *Int. J. Cancer 28*:23 (1982).
5. C. S. Foster, P. A. W. Edwards, E. A. Dinsdale, and A. M. Neville, *Virchows Arch. Pathol. Anat. 394*:279 (1982).
6. J. Hilkens, J. Hilgers, F. Buijs, P. Hageman, D. Schol, G. Van Doornewaard, and J. Van den Tweel, in *Protides of the Biol. Fluids Colloq.* (H. Peeters, ed.), Vol. 31, Pergamon Press, Oxford, p. 1013 (1983).
7. J. Hilkens, F. Buijs, J. Hilgers, P. Hageman, A. Sonneberg, and M. Van der Valk, *Int. J. Cancer 34*:197 (1984).
8. R. Ceriani, J. Peterson, J. Lee, R. Moncada, and E. W. Blank, *Somatic Cell Genet. 9*:415 (1983).
9. G. Greene, C. Nolan, J. Engler, and E. Jensen, *Proc. Natl. Acad. Sci. USA 77*:5115 (1980).
10. F. Hendler, D. Yuan, and E. Vitetta, *Trans. Assoc. Am. Phys. 94*:217 (1981).
11. D. Yuan, F. Hendler, and E. Vitetta, *J. Natl. Cancer Inst. 68*: 719 (1982).
12. L. D. Papsidero, G. A. Croghan, M. J. O'Connell, L. A. Valenzuela, T. Nemoto, and T. Ming Chu, *Cancer Res. 43*:1741 (1983).
13. G. Croghan, L. Papsidero, L. Valenzuela, T. Nemoto, R. Penegrante, and M. Chu, *Cancer Res. 43*:4980 (1983).
14. H. Soule, E. Linder, and T. Edgington, *Proc. Natl. Acad. Sci. USA 80*:1332 (1983).
15. S. Menard, E. Tagliabue, S. Canevari, G. Fossati, and M. Colnalghi, *Cancer Res. 43*:1295 (1983).
16. S. Canevari, G. Fossati, A. Balsari, S. Sonnino, and M. Colnaghi, *Cancer Res. 43*:1301 (1983).
17. D. Colcher, P. Horan-Hand, M. Nuti, and J. Schlom, *Proc. Natl. Acad. Sci. USA 78*:3199 (1981).
18. M. Nuti, Y. A. Tetramoto, R. Mariani-Costantini, P. Horan-Hand, D. Colcher, and J. Schlom, *Int. J. Cancer 29*:539 (1982).
19. P. Hand, M. Nuti, D. Colcher, and J. Schlom, *Cancer Res. 43*: 728 (1983).
20. D. Colcher, P. Horan-Hand, M. Nuti, and J. Schlom, *Cancer Invest. 1*:127 (1983).

21. J. Schlom, J. Greiner, P. Horan-Hand, D. Colcher, G. Inghirami, M. Weeks, S. Pestka, P. Fisher, P. Noguchi, and D. Kufe, *Cancer 54*:2777 (1984).
22. D. Kufe, G. Inghirami, M.Abe, D. Hayes, H. Justi-Wheeler, and J. Schlom, *Hybridoma 3*:223 (1984).
23. J. Lundy, A. Thor, R. Maenza, J. Schlom, F. Forouchar, M. Testa, and D. Kufe, *Breast Cancer Res. Treat. 5*:269 (1985).
24. E. R. Fisher, C. K. Redmond, H. Liu, H. Rockette, B. Fisher, *Cancer 45*:349 (1980).
25. W. A. Knight, B. Fisher, G. Bannayan, A. Walder, E. J. Gregory, A. Jacobson, D. M. Queen, D. E. Bennett, W. L. McGuire, C. K. Osborn, C. Redmond, and H. C. Ford, *Breast Cancer Res. Treat., 1*:37 (1981).
26. B. W. Davis, D. T. Zava, G. W. Locher, A. Goldhirsch, and W. H. Hartmann, *Eur. J. Cancer Clin. Oncol. 20*:375 (1984).
27. K. W. McCarty, T. K. Barton, B. F. Fetter, B. H. Woodard, J. A. Mossler, W. Reeves, J. Daly, W. E. Wilinson, and K. S. McCarty, *Cancer 46*:2851 (1980).
28. S. Thoresen, M. Tangen, K. F. Stoa, and F. Hartveit, *Histopathology 5*:257 (1981).
29. S. J. Schnitt, J. L. Connolly, J. R. Harris, S. Hellman, and R. B. Cohen, *Cancer 53*:1049 (1984).
30. B. B. Rasmussen, J. Hilkens, J. Hilgers, H. H. Nielsen, S. M. Thorpe, and C. Rose, *Breast Cancer Res. Treat. 2*:401 (1982).
31. B. Rasmussen, B. Pedersen, S. Thorpe, J. Hilkens, J. Hilgers, and R. Carsten, *Cancer Res. 45*:1424 (1985).
32. M. J. S. Wilkinson, A. Howell, M. Harris, J. T. Papadimitriou, R. Swindell, and R. A. Sellwood, *Int. J. Cancer 33*:299 (1984).
33. N. Berry, D. Jones, J. Smallwood, I. Taylor, N. Kirkham, and J. Taylor-Papadimitriou, *Br. J. Cancer 51*:179 (1985).
34. I. Ellis, C. Hinton, J. MacNay, C. Elson, A. Robins, A. Owainati, R. Blamey, R. Baldwin, and B. Ferry, *Br. Med. J. 20*:881 (1985).
35. J. C. Woods, A. I. Spriggs, H. Harris, and J. O. McGee, *Lancet 2*:512 (1982).
36. A. K. Ghosh, A. Spriggs, J. Taylor-Papidimitriou, and D. Mason, *J. Clin. Pathol. 36*:1154 (1983).
37. A. A. Epenetos, G. Canti, J. Taylor-Papidimitriou, M. Curling, and W. F. Bodmer, *Lancet 2*:1004 (1982).

38. S. Menard, F. Rilke, G. Torre, R. Mariani-Constantini, M. Regazzoni, E. Tagliabue, L. Alasio, and M. Colnaghi, *Am. J. Clin. Pathol. 83*:571 (1985).
39. A. Szpak, W. Johnson, S. Lottich, D. Kufe, A. Thor, and J. Schlom, *Acta Cytol. 28*:356 (1984).
40. H. B. Coakham, B. Brownell, E. I. Harper, J. A. Garson, P. M. Allan, E. B. Lane, and J. T. Kemshead, *Lancet 1*:1095 (1984).
41. M. P. Holley, G. F. Clough, H. L. D. Duguid, and A. Cuschieri, *Clin. Oncol. 9*:325 (1983).
42. W. Redding, P. Monaghan, S. Imrie, M. Ormerod, J-C. Gazet, R. Coombes, H. Clink, D. Dearnaley, J. Sloane, T. Powles, and A. M. Neville, *Lancet 2*:1271 (1983).
43. D. Dearnaley, J. Sloane, S. Imrie, R. C. Coombes, M. G. Ormerod, H. Lumley, M. Jones, and A. M. Neville, *J. R. Soc. Med. 76*:359 (1983).
44. A. K. Ghosh, W. N. Erber, S. R. Hatton, N. O'Connor, B. Falini, M. Osborn, and D. Y. Mason, *Br. J. Haematol. 61*:21 (1985).
45. W. Peters, J. Eder, W. Henner, S. Schryber, D. Wilmore, R. Finberg, D. Schoenfeld, R. Bast, B. Gargone, K. Antman, J. Anderson, K. Anderson, M. Kruskall, L. Schnipper, and E. Frei, III, *J. Clin. Oncol. 4*:646 (1986).
46. M. Abe and D. W. Kufe, *Cancer Res. 44*:4574 (1984).
47. M. Abe and D. W. Kufe, *J. Cell. Physiol. 126*:126 (1986).
48. H. Sekine, T. Ohno, and D. W. Kufe, *J. Immunol. 135*:3610 (1985).
49. P. Franchimont, P. R. Zangerle, J. C. Hendrick, A. Reuters, and C. Colin, *Cancer 39*:2806 (1977).
50. D. Kleinberg, *Science 190*:276 (1975).
51. I. Dao, C. Ip, and J. Patel, *J. Natl. Cancer Inst. 65*:529 (1980).
52. T. Kloppel, T. Keenan, M. Freeman, and J. Morre, *Proc. Natl. Acad. Sci. USA 74*:3011 (1977).
53. V. Skipsky, M. Barclay, F. M. Archibald, T. P. Lynch, and C. C. Stock, *Proc. Soc. Exp. Biol. Med. 136*:1261 (1971).
54. D. Haagensen, Jr., J. Kister, J. Panick, J. Giannola, H. H. Hansen, and S. Wells, Jr., *Cancer 42*(Suppl):1646 (1978).
55. D. Tormey and T. Waalkes, *Cancer 42*:1507 (1978).
56. R. Ceriani, M. Sasaki, H. Sussman, W. M. Wara, and E. Blank, *Proc. Natl. Acad. Sci. USA 79*:5420 (1982).

57. C. H. Thompson, S. L. Jones, R. H. Whitehead, and I. F. C. McKenzie, *J. Natl. Cncer Inst.* 70:409 (1983).
58. L. Papsidero, T. Nemoto, G. Croghan, and T. Chu, *Cancer Res.* 44:4653 (1984).
59. J. Hilkens, V. Kroezen, J. M. G. Bonfrer, M. De Jong-Bakker, and P. F. Bruning, *Cancer Res.* 46:2582 (1986).
60. D. F. Hayes, H. Sekine, T. Ohno, M. Abe, K. Keefe, and D. Kufe, *J. Clin. Invest.* 75:1671 (1985).
61. D. F. Hayes, D. Zarawski, and D. Kufe, *J. Clin. Oncol. 4*: 1542 (1986).
62. Abbott CEA-RIA Monoclonal: Package insert. Abbott Laboratories, Diagnostics Division, 1984.
63. J. Burchell, H. Durbin, and J. Taylor-Papadimitriou, *J. Immunol 131*:508 (1983).
64. M. Shimizu and K. Yamauchi, *J. Biochem 91*:515 (1982).
65. M. G. Ormerod, J. McIlhinney, K. Steele, and M. Shimizu, *Mol. Immunol. 22*:265 (1985).
66. J. P. Sloane, F. Hughes, and M. G. Ormerod, *Histochem J. 15*:645 (1983).
67. L. D. Papsidero, G. A. Croghan, E. A. Johnson, and T. M. Chu, *Mol. Immunol. 21*:955 (1984).
68. F. Ashall, M. E. Bramwell, and H. Harris, *Lancet 2*:1 (1982).
69. J. O. D. McGee, J. C. Woods, F. Ashall, M. E. Bramwell, and H. A. Harris, *Lancet 2*:7 (1982).
70. M. E. Bramwell, V. P. Bhavanandan, G. Wiseman, and H. Harris, *Br. J. Cancer 48*:177 (1983).

4
Monoclonal Antibody Assays for Lung Cancer

James A. Radosevich and Steven T. Rosen / Northwestern University / VA Lakeside Medical Center, Chicago, Illinois

Inchul Lee and Victor E. Gould / Rush-Presbyterian-St. Luke's Medical Center, Chicago, Illinois

INTRODUCTION

Lung carcinomas are a leading cause of death for both men and women in the United States. These malignancies will account for approximately 150,000 newly diagnosed cases per year, resulting in over 100,000 deaths annually (1). Despite warnings that emphasize the risk associated with tobacco abuse, air pollution, and some occupational practices, the incidence of this malignancy continues to rise. It has been estimated that even if all of these environmental exposure sources were removed today, the rise in lung cancer would continue well past the turn of this century. The latent period and exact causes of this disease have not been conclusively identified, and the incidence has gone from a rare malignancy in the early decades of this century, to epidemic porportions today.

Prevention programs including antismoking campaigns and clean air legislation have not affected the incidence of lung cancer. Mass screening of target populations have failed in altering the low overall (10%) cure rate for this heterogeneous group of neoplasms. Cytological screening of sputum and periodic chest x-rays of high risk patients have failed to alter substantially the statistics of this disease. New approaches for early detection and for therapy obviously are needed.

The major problem in the design of new treatment strategies is rooted in the initial pathological diagnosis of this disease. Because present treatment is based solely on this diagnosis, it is critical that a consistent classification system be established and used. Light and electron microscopic evaluation of lung tumors fail to allow consistent classification of these tumors, especially those of mixed cell types and those that lack salient features of any given tumor subtype. With the advent of monoclonal antibody (MAb) technology, the hope of overcoming this critical problem was raised. These tools have only begun to be produced and systematically used to analyze a large tumor panel. Our experience and that of others will be discussed and will reveal the tremendous amount of work that needs to be done to solve the requirements for early and accurate diagnosis and treatment of lung cancer.

HISTOLOGICAL AND IMMUNOHISTOCHEMICAL EVALUATION

Human lung cancer specimens, when hematoxylin-eosin stained, have characteristic features that allow most cases to be classified as a particular histological subtype. This has led to several classification schemes, all of which fail in cases with overlapping histologies or that lack differentiating features (2-4). Lung cancer has been traditionally divided into two major groups: small-cell lung cancer and non-small-cell lung cancer. Small-cell lung cancer is distinguished from other histological subtypes by a markedly different natural history and response to therapy. Because of the controversial nature of the definitions of the pathological entities of human lung cancer, a brief review of a classification system will be presented, after which the manner that specific MAbs are beginning to clarify the ambiguity of traditional definitions will be discussed.

Traditional Light and Electron Microscopy Definitions

The methods used for immunostaining have been greatly improved over the last few years. In particular, the use of the avidin-biotin complex method has greatly improved the sensitivity of this assay (5). Unfortunately, most MAbs do not work in paraffin sections, so frozen tissue must be used. Those MAbs that do work in fixed-embedded tissue, are beginning to show their utility as lung cancer markers. These will be of particular value because no special handling of the tissues will be required, and this will allow these reagents to become useful in routine tests. Retrospective studies can be done with ease on previously prepared tissues, making these reagents even more valuable in the clinical correlation of the lung cancer patients, histories and histologies.

Squamous Cell Carcinoma

Squamous cell carcinomas often progress from various degrees of dysplasia of basal cells of the bronchial epithelium. By light microscopy they show at least one of the three characteristic features of squamous cell carcinoma, i.e, extensive intercellular bridges, pearl formation, and keratinization of individual cells. The nuclei are often pleomorphic and hyperchromatic, with jagged borders. Necrotic keratinized cells also may be seen.

Adenocarcinoma

Adenocarcinomas generally arise in the peripheral areas of the lung and, characteristically, will form glandlike structures with or without mucin production. The degree of gland formation is an indication of the degree of differentiation. The cells are usually large, with abundant cytoplasms that frequently demonstrate mucus-containing vacuoles by electron microscopy. Tight junctions are common. The nuclei are large and clear, with prominent nucleoli. The nuclei appear similar to those seen in squamous cell carcinoma, but they lack the distinctive hyperchromasia and jagged characteristic of squamous cell carcinoma.

Bronchioloalveolar Carcinoma

Bronchioloalveolar carcinoma is classified as a subgroup of adenocarcinoma of the lung by the World Health Organization. It is defined as a tumor in which cylindrical tumor cells grow upon the walls of preexisting alveoli. These carcinomas may be indistinguishable by routine histological analysis from metastatic adenocarcinoma of the lung. Electron microscopy sometimes may be a useful tool, but it does not always accurately identify all types of this tumor. Cells resembling nonciliated, bronchiolar cells (Clara cells) are considered diagnostic for this tumor, but often these cells are not typical enough for positive identification. Some of these tumors have cells that secrete mucin and show differentiation toward cilia expression.

Large-Cell Carcinoma

The category of large-cell carcinoma is most likely not a true category, but in reality it is now a miscellaneous category for a group of tumors that express features found in several other subtypes of lung tumors. The cells are large like those of adenocarcinoma, but they do not form glandlike structures or acini, and they do not produce mucin. There is no pearl formation as in squamous cell carcinoma, nor are there extensive intercellular bridges of keratinization. However, ultrastructural studies have shown similarities of large-cell carcinomas to both squamous and adenocarcinoma cells. This type of tumor is best categorized by the lack of pure features seen in other subtypes.

Small-Cell Neuroendocrine Carcinoma

The small-cell neuroendocrine subclass was formerly called a typical "oat" cell carcinoma comprised of round or fusiform cells with scanty cytoplasm. Often, hyperchromatic nuclei devoid of a cytoplasmic component are seen. Nucleoli are rare, whereas

mitoses are abundant. Crushing artifact is so common a characteristic of this subclass that it is a useful diagnostic criterion. Electron
microscopic evaluation reveals tightly packed cells with many
poorly developed cell junctions and extensive interlacing of cytoplasmic processes.

Intermediate-Cell Neuroendocrine Carcinoma

The intermediate-cell neuroendocrine subclass of bronchopulmonary carcinomas is a variant of the aforementioned small-cell
neuroendocrine type. These cells appear about twice the size of
their small-cell neuroendocrine counterparts and have moderately
more cytoplasm. Their cell shape is polygonal or fusiform, and the
nuclei are frequently vesicular with irregular chromatin distribution and abundant mitoses. This subtype is further set apart
from the small-cell neuroendocrine subtype in that crushing artifact is not a prominent feature. The cells have an irregular clus-
tered pattern with central necrosis and peripheral palisading. By
electron microscopic evaluation, this subclass shares features with
both small-cell neuroendocrine and well-differentiated neuroendocrine lung carcinomas. Closely packed cells, with many cell
junctions and interlaced cytoplasms, are the rule for this subtype.

Well-Differentiated Neuroendocrine Carcinoma

As a subset of lung carcinomas, this class is similiar to the carcinoids, but express an unmistakable cellular and nuclear pleomor-
phism. Their overall growth pattern is similiar to carcinoids; however, mitoses may be readily found. The cytoplasm of these cells
are polygonal and show abundant pale to slightly eosinophilic
staining. Nucleoli and mitoses are not prominent landmarks, but
they can be found. Ultrastructurally, these tumors resemble true
carcinoids. The cells are large, closely packed, with moderately defined cell junctions and abundant cytoplasm. They share the
property of interlaced cytoplasms with intermediate-cell and
small-cell neuroendocrine carcinomas. Neurosecretory granules are
usually found in cytoplasmic extensions and are not as abundant,
overall, as in carcinoid tumors.

Carcinoid Tumors

Carcinoid tumors are marked by their rather indolent growth, but
they share many of the amine precursor uptake and decarboxy-

lation system properties of small-cell carcinomas. The cells are somewhat uniform, with abundant clear or lightly eosinophilic cytoplasm. The nuclei are central, are regular in shape, and have uniformly dispersed chromatin. The cells grow as a mosaic pattern with rare or no mitoses. Cords of cells, nests, trabeculae, and ribbons of cells may be seen alone or in combinations. Ultrastructually, carcinoids show abundant neurosecretory granules.

Mesotheliomas

Malignant mesotheliomas are classified into three histological subtypes: epithelial, spindle cell, and biphasic (mixed). Although these are not true lung tumors, their presentation and distinction from other lung tumors merits discussion. They may form glandular or tubular structures that resemble pulmonary adenocarcinomas which are metastatic to the pleura. Mesothelioma of the epithelial type may have cells arranged in solid, tubular, papillary, or reticular patterns. The nuclei are ovoid, centrally located, variable in size, and usually vesicular. A solitary nucleoli is often observed. Mitotic indexes and the amount of cytoplasm are variable. Necrosis may be present, but it is rarely extensive. Frequent and prominent desmosomes, ovoid nuclei with coarse chromatin, and prominent nucleoli are seen using ultrastructural analysis. The cytoplasm is abundant and may contain undulating intermediate filaments (tonofilaments). Microfilaments and microtubules, lysosomes, rough endoplasmic reticulum, and mitochrondria are rarely observed. Microvilli are prominent.

Spindle cell mesotheliomas form irregular intertwined bundles of cells. Mitoses are frequent with pleomorphic and hyperchromatic nuclei. Necrosis is often present and is extensive. In contrast to the epithelial type, spindle cell mesotheliomas generally lack cell junctions, have nuclei that are elongated and folded, frequently show free ribosomes, and rarely show tonofilament bundles by ultrastructural analysis.

The biphasic mesothelioma cell types are seen as an irregular intermixed population of both epithelial and spindle cell components. Ultrastructurally, biphasic mesotheliomas have tightly opposed, round, and spindle-shaped cells that appear to have features similar to those cells seen in epithelial and spindle cell mesotheliomas.

Monoclonal Antibodies

Over 200 MAbs have been reported to react with human lung tumors. Many of the reagents work only on frozen tissues and have not been extensively tested for their binding specificity to various subclasses of pulmonary carcinomas. Although a greater spectrum of antigens are preserved in frozen sections, these tissues are more difficult to process on a routine basis. Some of the reported MAbs have the particularly advantageous property of being able to recognize their respective antigen in formalin-fixed, paraffin-embedded tissues. In an attempt to standardize and test the utility of these MAbs, over 200 well-studied, human pulmonary tumors were designated as a core bank of tissues to be tested. These tumors were defined by traditional light and electron microscopic evaluation. Some of the following MAbs have been tested against this panel, thus allowing a direct comparison of their binding patterns. The results are summarized in Table 1. It is clear that these reagents will not replace light and electron microscopic evaluation, but they may serve as useful adjuncts in defining the subclasses of lung cancer.

624A12

The initial report of MAb technology used the hybridization of mouse spleen cells to a mouse myeloma cell line (6). Immunologists have long known that different species give different antibody responses to the same antigen. Accordingly, rats, rather than mice, were immunized with lung cancer cell lines in an attempt to elicit unique antibody responses not seen in mice. One such antibody is the rat IgM MAb, 624A12, which was raised against an intermediate small-cell line, NCI-H69 (7). This MAb recognizes the ceramide pentasaccharide that contains the lacto-*N*-fucopentose III (LNFP III) sequence of sugars, an isomere of the Lewis A blood group antigen. A mouse MAb, 534F8, also has been described that reacts with LNFP III (8).

The LNFP III sequence is well preserved in routine formalin-fixed, paraffin-embedded tissues. In a large study of over 200 patients, LNFP III was found to be expressed on adenocarcinomas, bronchioloalveolar carcinomas, and some squamous cell, large-cell, and intermediate neuroendocrine carcinomas (9). Small-cell neuroendocrine, well-differentiated neuroendocrine carci-

Table 1   Monoclonal Antibody-Binding Patterns

Tumor Type	MAb[a]				
	624A12	44-3A6	B72.3	RAP-5	DWP
Squamous cell carcinoma	11/38	0/39	2/36	23/33	3/29
Adenocarcinoma	49/50[b]	41/41	27/66	8/49	2/46
Large-cell carcinoma	11/30	21/27	8/22	11/18	3/25
Bronchioloalveolar	10/11	0/12	10/21	21/24	0/26
Small-cell neuroendocrine carcinoma	0/33	0/28	0/24	0/20	0/19
Intermediate neuroendocrine carcinoma	7/26	10/17	7/21	18/21	4/18
Well-differentiated neuroendocrine carcinoma	0/10	8/10	0/6	5/6	0/6
Carcinoid	0/21	10/10	0/16	11/13	0/13
Mesothelioma					
epithelial type	0/22	5/22[c]	0/12	2/16	1/16
biophasic type	0/15	4/15[c]	0/6	1/9	0/8
spindle type	0/6	1/6[c]	0/4	0/3	0/5

[a]Ratios represent the number of positive cases over total number of cases tested.
[b]The one negative case was irradiated before surgery.
[c]The staining pattern was confined to scattered single cells that were discernible from adenocarcinomas.

noma, carcinoid, and mesotheliomas all tested negative. Together, 624A12 in conjunction with another MAb, 44-3A6, have been shown to serve as useful diagnostic adjuncts in distinguishing adenocarcinoma from mesothelioma and adenocarcinomas from bronchioloalveolar carcinoma (10). A summary of this and other MAbs stained on this same panel of tumors is shown in Table 1.

The expression of the epitope recognized by 624A12 has been mapped through human fetal development, and the adult normal organ biodistribution has been determined (11). The tissues that stained were primarily of epithelial and neuroectodermal origin. The aberrant expression of blood group-related antigens has become of interest in studying tumor biology. A MAb related to 624A12, B72.3 recognizes TAG-72, which has been shown to contain a number of blood group epitopes and will be discussed later (12,13). These two MAbs have similar, but not identical, binding patterns when tested against a large panel of human lung cancer tumors.

44-3A6

Monoclonal antibody 44-3A6 is an IgG1 and was raised against the human lung adenocarcinoma cell line, A549 (14). It has been shown by Western blot analysis to react with a 40,000 dalton protein. By use of live cell radioimmunoassays and fluorescent activated cell sorter (FACS) analysis, the antibody has been found to react with the cell surface of human adenocarcinoma cell lines. The epitope recognized by 44-3A6 is well preserved in routine formalin-fixed, paraffin-embedded tissues. When the avidin-biotin complex method is used to stain paraffin sections, the antigen has been reported to appear at the cell surface and also weakly in the cytoplasm.

In a survey study of over 200 well-characterized human lung carcinomas, 44-3A6 was found to react with all adenocarcinomas, some large-cell carcinomas, as well as subsets of intermediate-neuroendocrine carcinomas, well-differentiated neuroendocrine carcinomas, and carcinoids, but not with mesotheliomas. It does not react with squamous cell carcinomas, bronchioloalveolar carcinomas or small-cell neuroendocrine carcinomas (15). In an immunocytochemical study of 35 bronchial brushings and their tissue correlates, 44-3A6 was found to react reproducibly in all positive cases (16). These two studies show that 44-3A6 will be a useful diagnostic adjuvant. When used in conjunction with 624A12 on daughter paraffin-embedded sections, it has been shown that mesothelioma can be distinguished from metastatic adenocarcinoma of the lung to the pleural wall. That is to say, all adenocarcinomas are positive for 44-3A6 and mesotheliomas are negative for 624A12 and 44-3A6 (10).

Immunohistochemical staining has also been seen on a wide range of tumor types arising in various human tissues. In a survey of over 300 such cases, 44-3A6 reacted with some, but not all, adenocarcinomas arising outside of the lung. The normal adult and fetal distribution has also been investigated and found to be expressed in a limited number of tissues and cell types.

The limited biodistribution of this antigen, as well as its inability to be detected in lung cancer patient serum, suggests that it may be useful in immunotherapy and immunodiagnosis. Radiolabeled $131I$ 44-3A6 has been shown to be localized in the tumor in male nude mice bearing A549 xenografts. The full potential of this antibody as a lung cancer tumor marker has yet to be realized and will require additional studies. Two other MAbs, KS 1/4 and KS 1/17, which react similarly to 44-346, have been reported and will now be discussed.

KS 1/4 and K 1/17

The MAbs KS 1/4 and KS 1/17 appear to recognize a similar cell surface glycoprotein of about 40,000 daltons found on adenocarcinomas (17). These two MAbs have properties similar to those of 44-3A6. The antigen(s) recognized by these three MAbs share many common properties that include: (1) the antigens appear not to be shed; (2) they are not related to the HLA-A,B antigens; and (3) they react with various other nonlung adenocarcinomas. Clearly, the antigen(s) that KS 1/4 and KS 1/17 recognize are of interest. Second-generation antibodies that work in paraffin or large survey studies of frozen sections will be useful in clarifying their usefulness as diagnostic reagents. It is now difficult to determine whether these three MAbs recognize different epitopes on the same antigen, or recognize a family of related molecules, or if they are a random set of proteins that share similar properties.

LuCa2, LuCa3, and LuCa4

The MAbs LuCa2, LuCa3, and LuCa4 have been shown to react with squamous cell tumor tissues, and with cell lines (18). Unfortunately, they do not work in formalin-fixed, paraffin-embedded tissues and have been tested only on a limited number of clinical specimens. LuCa2 was found to react with a 125,000 dalton protein, LuCa3 with a 230,000- and 240,000 dalton protein, and LuCa4 with 150,000- and a 300,000 dalton protein. Positive staining of squamous, adenocarcinoma, and adenosquamous carcinomas, as well as small-cell carcinoma was found for LUCa2. Both LuCa3 and LuCa4 had much more limited binding patterns to squamous cell carcinomas of lung, with LuCa4 staining only a select set of squamous cell carcinomas. Both LuCa3 and LuCa4 immunostained the squamous cell portion of the one adenosquamous tumor that was tested.

B72.3

The mouse MAb B72.3 is an IgG1 which was raised against a membrane-enriched fraction from a human mammary carcinoma metastasis (13,19). It recognizes a high-molecular-weight mucinlike molecule, TAG-72, which is resistant to chondroitinase digestion and contains blood group-related oligosaccharides. This marker is detected both extracellularly and intracytoplasmically in positively staining tumors using the avidin-biotin complex method. Monoclonal antibody B72.3 has been used to detect TAG-72 in the serum of patients with colon carcinomas (20). The expression of this antigen has been shown in a wide range of tumors arising from various tissues including breast, colon, pancreas, and prostate. The fetal and limited normal adult expression has been reported. Because of the limited distribution of the antigen and of its localization in tumor-bearing xenograft mice, this MAb has been used in clinical trials.

In a large study of over 200 bronchopulmonary neoplasms that were formalin-fixed and paraffin-embedded, B72.3 was found to stain only a subset of adenocarcinomas, large-cell carcinomas, bronchioloalveolar carcinomas, and intermediate-neuroendocrine carcinomas (21). Two squamous cell carcinomas also stained. Small-cell carcinomas, well-differentiated carcinomas, carcinoid, and mesotheliomas all tested negative. The staining pattern was reminiscent of 624A12 except that many fewer squamous cell carcinomas stained with B72.3. This MAb may also be useful to study the cell biology of lung cancer, especially to define the border between the adenocarcinoma-squamous cell subtypes.

SM1

A cell surface epitope that is present on both glycolipids and glycoproteins is detected by the MAb SM1 (22). This MAb was found to bind strongly to three small-cell lung carcinoma cell lines, but to a lesser degree to other non-small-cell lung cancer lines. In tissues, SM1 binding was demonstrated in more than 95% of the small-cell (WHO classification) tissues tested. No immunoreactivity was seen in a bronchial carcinoid. Both the reactivity and specificity of this MAb were affected by any type of fixation and by routine paraffin embedding. This has hampered its use in a large survey of tumor tissues. Interestingly, 80% of the SM1 antigen is associated with the glycolipid fraction, and it is poorly preserved in fixed tissue. The glycolipids detected by 624A12, and other by MAbs, are well preserved, suggesting that the epitope recognized by SM1 must have either unique properties or an extremely fragile conformation.

LAM-8

Western blot analysis, using small-cell lung cancer membrane extracts, shows that LAM-8 binds to a band of 135,000 daltons (23). This MAb binds to the cell surface of small-cell lung cancer cell lines and is sensitive to treatments that destroy carbohydrate. The epitope is well preserved in routine formalin-fixed, paraffin-embedded tissues and has been found to stain about 80% of the small-cell lung carcinoma tumors tested. Within this group of tumors, there is marked cellular heterogeneity in positive LAM-8 immunostaining. LAM-8 stained neither nonsmall-cell lung tumors nor a wide variety of other tumors from other organs.

RAP-5 and DWP

Since the discovery of human transformation-inducing genes (oncogenes), a great deal of effort has been put forth to understand their role in the transformation of normal cells into malignant cells. One family of oncogenes and their products, the *ras* family, has been extensively studied. This family of genes produces a protein product of 21,000 daltons, which has been found to have both GTP-binding activity, as well as GTPase activity (24, 25). The *ras p21* has been implicated as being associated with the inner surface of the plasma membrane and may play a role in signal transduction from extracellular stimuli . The increased expression of the normal *ras p21* gene product has been reported, as has the expression of mutated *ras p21* gene products containing altered amino acids at positions 12, 13, and 61.

The mouse MAb RAP-5 was produced against the amino acid sequence representing positions 10-17 of *ras p21* from T24 bladder carcinoma cells (26). It is known to react with mutated *ras p21* gene products and therefore is a "pan" *ras* MAb. A similar rat monoclonal, Y13-259, has also been reported (27). The fetal and normal organ distribution has been evaluated for this MAb. The expression of enhanced *ras p21*, as detected by RAP-5, has also been reported in breast, colon, and prostate cancer, with the general suggestion that enhanced expression correlates with more aggressive tumors.

The MAb DWP was produced against an amino acid sequence similar to that of RAP-5, except that a substitution of valine at position 12 was made for the usually occurring glycine. The MAb DWP has been shown to react specifically with this substitution and not with others, except for a slight reactivity to the cysteine substitution. (28).

Both of these MAbs react immunohistologially with formalin-fixed, paraffin-embedded tissue. In a comparative survey, over 200 primary lung tumors were studied for the expression of the normal and mutated *ras p21* gene products. RAP-5 bound to a subset of squamous cell carcinomas, adenocarcinomas, large-cell carcinomas, bronchioloalveolar carcinomas, intermediate and well-differentiated neuoendocrine carcinomas, as well as to carcinoids and mesotheliomas. No staining was found in small-cell neuroendocrine carcinomas. This pattern is quite contrary to other reports of a graded expression approximating the degree of malignancy found in other tumor systems.

DWP stained only a relatively few specimens of squamous cell carcinoma, adenocarcinoma, large-cell carcinoma, intermediate-cell carcinoma, and a mesothelioma. This restricted staining pattern was as expected because this specific mutation is only rarely found. Of interest are two cases, an adenocarcinoma and a squamous cell carcinoma of the lung, which were RAP-5-negative and DWP-positive. The biochemical confirmation of this finding remains to be done. The usefulness of these two MAbs in the immunodiagnosis of lung cancer is now unclear. As further clinical studies correlating patient history and staining pattern are carried out, these MAbs may distinguish select patient populations. DWP may be extremely valuable because of its selectivity.

Other Monoclonal Antibodies

Since the first report of MAbs, many have been produced that react against human lung cancer. These have been raised against a variety of human lung cancer cell lines, primary lung tumors, and isolated lung cancer tissue fractions. Many of these MAbs have been reported once in an initial publication, but they have since been lost in follow-up. Antigens recognized by these MAbs have been described as ranging from high-molecular-weight mucinlike molecules to small proteins. Many MAbs have never been successfully characterized in terms of the molecular nature of the antigen that they recognize. This is particularly important if we are to understand the biology of lung cancer.

Monoclonal antibodies E6 and H317 are directed against human placental alkaline phosphatase, and both have been reported to work in paraffin-embedded tissues (29). These two MAbs were tested, along with an MAb directed against CEA and the cancer antigen, CA 125, detected by OC125. Ten cases consisting of 3 epidermoid, 1 epidermoid/adenocarcinoma, 3 adenocarcinomas, and 1 bronchioloalveolar, 1 large-cell, and 1 small-cell carcinoma were tested. Human placental alkaline phosphatase was found in all of these, as was CEA, by use of these MAbs. The CA 125 antigen was found in only two epidermoid tumors. Again, it is unfortunate that a larger number of cases have not been investigated to determine if the epidermoid carcinomas could be further classified using this CA 125 antibody. Some antihuman placental alkaline phosphatase and CEA MAbs appear to be pan malignancy antibodies, and may be useful in distinguishing dysplasia from malignancy. Because various antigens and MAbs react with different CEA epitopes, it is important to recognize the particular staining pattern for each reagent. Polyclonal anti-CEA antiserum has been shown to correlate with longer survival in small-cell lung cancer but not with morphological subtypes as classified by 1977 WHO system. This antiserum reacts with CEA-s (a physiochemical subset of CEA) and NCA (nonspecific cross-reacting antigen). When MAbs against CEA are tested against a large panel of lung tumors, it seems reasonable that this marker will yield important data. Monoclonal antibodies to CEA are described more fully in Chapter 10.

The MAb HNK-1 detects an antigen on a subpopulation of large granular lymphocytes known to have natural killer cell function (30). All of the small-cell tumor cell lines tested were positive for the expression of this antigen. Several large-cell tumor lines were also positive, whereas adenocarcinomas and squamous cell carcinomas were negative. Like blood group markers and their related molecules, hemopoietic marker antigens have been reported to be expressed on nonhemopoietic tumors, but these have not been extensively studied in pulmonary carcinomas.

Cytoskeleton Markers

The cytoskeleton is a collection of tubular and filamentous components that include microtubules, microfilaments, and intermediate filaments. The intermediate filament family can be broken down into desmin, vimentin, glial, keratin, and neurofilaments, which are characteristic of muscle cells, mesenchymal cells, glial cells, epithelial cells, and neural cells, respectively. These filaments can all be immunologically distinguished. Polyclonal antisera to these components have been studied to various degrees in human lung cancer. Monoclonal antibodies have been produced against all of these but have not yet been tested on a large tumor panel (31). These markers will become increasingly more important as MAbs that work in paraffin sections become available. A clear example of this is that the criteria for the diagnosis of squamous cell carcinoma has long included "the presence of keratinization."

Neuroendocrine Markers

Dense-core granules have been reported in the normal bronchus, as well as in small-cell carcinoma and carcinoid tumors. All of these tumors contain neuron-specific enolase, which is one of the several isoenzymes of the glycolytic enzyme enolase, and they may also contain serotonin. These are not found in nondense-core granule tumors. Other histochemical markers, such as glycogen, mucosubstances, corticotropin, β-human chorionic gonadotropin, somatostatin, and calcitonin, have been found in both types of tumors. These are, however, more common on nondense-core granule-containing tumors. Monoclonal antibodies to neuron-specific enolase have been made but have not been fully tested on lung tumors (32). Other MAbs against these markers may be useful in defining those cases that are the exceptions to these generalities. Chromogranin A is a protein that is costored and coreleased with catecholomines, and synaptophysin is an integral membrane glyco-protein that occurs in presynoptic vesicles of neurons. These two markers have been reported to be produced by lung neoplasms (33,34). Monoclonal antibodies defining these have been pro-duced, but not extensively tested, against lung tumors. At present, these look promising as markers.

SEROLOGICAL ASSAYS

Lung cancer-associated serum tumor markers have not yet shown the degree of specificity or sensitivity needed in a diagnostic scre-ening assay. The use of tobacco and benign respiratory conditions are often associated with elevated marker levels. However, in select instances these tumor markers may aid in assessing the extent of disease and provide a tool for monitoring patient therapy. Mono-clonal antibodies are currently being used to measure several of these markers and can potentially be produced against the re-mainder.

Carcinoembryonic Antigen

Carcinoembryonic antigen is a β-migrating glycoprotein of about 180,000 daltons (35). A recent report evaluating 243 patients with untreated advanced lung cancer demonstrated elevated plasma levels ($\geqslant$ 5 mg/ml) in adenocarcinomas (54%), small-cell lung car-cinomas (35%), large-cell lung carcinomas (38%), and squamous cell carcinomas (53%). The authors noted both a relationship be-tween pretreatment CEA levels and the extent of disease and that serial measurements of plasma CEA correlated with response to therapy. This study confirms the observation that CEA levels may be useful in monitoring treatment in lung cancer patients (36).

Human Chorionic Gonadotropin and α-Fetoprotein

Human chorionic gonadotropin (HCG) is a glycoprotein of 45,000 daltons containing two dissimilar polypeptide subunits designated α and β (37). It is the β-chain that confers specificity. α-Fetoprotein (AFP) is an oncofetal antigen with physiocohemical properties similar to those of serum albumin (38). Elevated HCG and AFP levels may assist in identifying a subgroup of patients with chemotherapy-sensitive, poorly differentiated, or undifferentiated lung carcinomas. Eleven of 12 patients listed in one report had lung mediastinal involvement. Six of these patients obtained a complete remission with chemotherapy. The authors theorized that these therapy-responsive patients may have extragonadal germ cell tumors. Modest elevation of HCG and AFP can also be seen with small-cell and nonsmall-cell cancer histologies (38).

Calcitonin

Calcitonin is a 32-amino acid polypeptide that inhibits both calcium and phosphate release from bone (39). Ectopic production has been noted in patients with small-cell lung cancer. Elevated levels have been noted in about 45% of patients with extensive disease. It appears that calcitonin levels correlate with the extent of disease and may be of use in monitoring therapy (40).

Neuron-Specific Enolase

Neuron-specific enolase (NSE) is one of several isoenzymes of the glycolytic enzyme enolase (2-phospho-D-glycerate hydrolase, EC 4.2.1.1). The enolase isoenzymes are dimers of 100,000 daltons formed from various combinations of three subunits; a, β, and γ. Synthesis of the subunit is enhanced 10- to 100-fold in neural and neuroendocrine tissue (41). Neuron-specific enolase refers to both the γ-γ and a-γ dimers. Tumors originating within the amine precursor uptake and decarboxylation (APUD) network contain substantial amounts of NSE. In three large study series, 70% of patients with small-cell lung cancer had elevated levels of NSE (42). Mean NSE levels correlated with the extent of disease, and serial NSE measurements reflected the clinical response. No patient had a rising NSE level without eventual evidence of recurrent or progressive disease.

Creatine Kinase BB

Creatine kinase (CK; ATP-creatine N-phosphotranserase; EC 2.7. 3.2) also occurs in serum as different isoenzymes (43). It has been demonstrated that CK-BB determinations are of value in estimating tumor burden, assigning prognosis, and monitoring response to therapy in patients with small-cell lung cancer. Elevated levels ($\geqslant 10$ ug/ml) were listed in 41% of patients with extensive disease but in only 2% of patients with limited disease. In vitro production of CK-BB by established small-cell lung cancer cell lines has been demonstrated (44).

Sialosylated Lewis^x and Sialosylated Lewis^a

By use of MAbs CSLEX-1 (antisialosylated Le^x) and CSLEA-1 (antisialosylated Le^a), elevated levels of each were noted in 65% of 46 patients with untreated lung cancer (45). A similar percentage with marker elevation was seen with each histological subtype. Eighty-seven percent of the 46 patients showed positive results with at least one of the two antibodies. These antigens, as well as other oligosaccarides found on carbohydrate-rich, mucin-type glycoproteins in serum, may prove to be valuable markers for monitoring lung cancer patients.

SUMMARY

Human lung carcinomas are a heterogeneous group of tumors that have been, at best, difficult to consistently classify, diagnose, and treat. With the advent of MAb technology, there was great hope that reagents would be produced that would be useful in finding a cure for these malignancies. Great effort has been put forth to produce MAbs that will consistently recognize select populations of these tumors. There are, however, few reagents that appear to be potentially valuable for routine diagnosis. There are many reports of MAbs that demonstrate the selectivity needed for this task but that are not suitable for routine use. These reports give hope to the possibility of second-generation MAbs that will have both the selective properties and other qualities needed for them to be used in routine diagnosis of human lung cancer. As more of these reagents become available, our understanding of the basic biology of these malignancies will also improve. This will allow patient populations to be more consistently selected for specific treatment protocols and, therefore, to be more accurately tested for the efficacy of that treatment. Potentially, some of these MAbs will be important in the in vivo diagnosis and treatment of lung cancer, and their role in the treatment of human lung cancer is only now beginning to be appreciated. These reagents will become more valuable in the future and will be important weapons in the arsenal used to cure this disease.

ACKNOWLEDGMENT

This work was supported in part by a Veterans Administration Merit Review Grant to J.A.R. and S.T.R.

REFERENCES

1. E. Silverberg, CA-Cancer J. Clin. 32:15 (1982).
2. V. E. Gould, R. L. Linnoila, V. A. Memoli, and W. H. Warren, Lab. Invest. 49:519 (1983).
3. V. E. Gould, R. L. Linnolla, V. A. Memoli, and W. H. Warren, Pathol. Annu. 18:287 (1983).
4. World Health Organization, Am. J. Clin. Pathol. 77:123 (1982).
5. S. M. Hsu, L. Raine, and H. Fanger, J. Histochem. Cytochem. 29:577 (1981).
6. M. L. Gefter, D. H. Margulies, and J. D. Scharff, Somatic Cell Genet. 3: 231 (1977).
7. S. T. Rosen, J. L. Mulshine, F. Cuttitta, J. Fedorko, D. M. Carney, A. F. Gazdar, and J. D. Minna, Cancer Res. 44:2052 (1984).
8. F. Cuttitta, S. Rosen, A. Gazdar, and J. Minna, Proc. Natl. Acad. Sci. USA 78:4591 (1981).
9. I. Lee, J. A. Radosevich, Y. Ma, W. H. Warren, S. T. Rosen, and V. E. Gould, Pathol. Res. Pract. (in press).
10. I. Lee, J. A. Radosevich, G. Cheifec, Y. Ma, W. H. Warren, S. T. Rosen, and V. E. Gould, Am. J. Pathol. 123:497 (1986).
11. S. T. Rosen, S. Combs, R. Marder, J. Minna, J. Mulshine, M. Polovina, and J. A. Radosevich, Protides Biol. Fluids Proc. Colloq. 32:561 (H. Peeters, ed.) (1984).
12. V. G. Johnson, J. Schlom, A. J. Paterson, J. Bennett, J. L. Magnani, and D. Colcher, Cancer Res. 46:850 (1986).
13. D. Cohlcher, P. Horan Hand, M. Nuti, and J. Schlom, Proc. Natl. Acad. Sci. USA 78:3199 (1981).
14. J. A. Radosevich, Y. Ma, I. Lee, H. R. Salwen, V. E. Gould, and S. T. Rosen, Cancer Res. 45:5898 (1985).
15. I. Lee, J. A. Radosevich, S. T. Rosen, Y. Ma, S. G. Combs, and V. E. Gould, Cancer Res. 45:5813 (1985).
16. B. F. Banner, V. E. Gould, J. A. Radosevich, Y. Ma, I. Lee, and S. T. Rosen, Diagn. Cytopathol. 1:300 (1985).

17. N. M. Varki, R. A. Reisfeld, and L. E. Walker, *Cancer Res. 44*:681 (1984).
18. S. Kyoizumi, M. A. Kiyama, N. Kouno, K. Kobuke, M. Hakoda, S. L. Jones, and M. Yamakido, *Cancer Res. 45*:3274 (1985).
19. M. Nuti, Y. Teramoto, R. Mariani-Constantine, P. Horan Hand, D. Colcher, and J. Schlom, *Int. J. Cancer 29*:539 (1982).
20. D. Stragmignoni, R. Bowen, B. Atkinson, and J. Schlom. *Int. J. Cancer 31*:543 (1983).
21. C. A. Szpak, W. W. Johnston, V. Roggli, J. Kolbeck, S. C. Lottich, R. Vollmer, A. Thor, and J. Schlom, *Am. J. Pathol. 122*:252 (1986).
22. S. D. Bernal and J. A. Speak, *Cancer Res. 44*:265 (1984).
23. R. A. Stahel, C. J. O'Hara, M. Mabry, R. Waibel, K. Sabbath, J. A. Speak, and S. D. Bernal, *Cancer Res. 46*:2077 (1986).
24. R. Sweet, S. Yokoyama, T. Kamata, J. R. Feramisco, M. Rosenberg, and M. Gross, *Nature 311*:273 (1984).
25. A. Papageorge, D. Lwry, and E. Scholnick, *J. Virol. 44*:509 (1984).
26. P. Horan Hand, A. Thor, D. Wunderlich, R. Muraro, A. Caruso, and J. Schlom, *Proc. Natl. Acad. Sci. USA 81*:5227 (1984).
27. R. W. Ellis, D. Defeo, T. Y. Shih, M. A. Gonda, H. A. Young, N. Tsuchida, D. R. Lowry, and E. M. Scholnick, *Nature 292*:506 (1981).
28. W. P. Carney, H. J. Wolfe, D. Petit, L. Bator, R. DeLellis, A. S. Tischler, Y. Dayal, P. Hamer, G. Cooper, and H. Rabin, *Monoclonal Antibodies and Cancer Therapy*. Alan R. Liss, New York 1985.
29. E. J. Norwen, D. E. Pollet, M. W. Eedekens, P. G. Hendrix, T. W. Briers, and M. E. DeBroe, *Cancer Res. 46*:866 (1986).
30. S. P. C. Cole, S. Mirski, R. C. McGarry, R. Cheng, B. G. Campling, and J. C. Roder, *Cancer Res. 45*:4285 (1985).
31. G. N. P. van Muijen, D. J. Ruiter, C. van Leeuwen, F. A. Prins, D. Rietsema, S. O. Warnaar, *Am. J. Pathol. 116*:363 (1984).
32. P. J. Maranjos, A. J. Gazdar, and D. N. Carney, *Cancer Lett. 15*:67 (1982).
33. D. T. O'Connor and L. J. Deftos, *N. Engl. J. Med. 314*:1145 (1986).
34. B. Wiedenmann, W. W., Franke, C. Kurn, R. Moll, and V. E. Gould, *Proc. Natl. Acad. Sci. USA 83*:3500 (1986).
35. H. S. Slayter and J. E. Coligan, *Biochemistry 14*:2323 (1975).
36. T. Shinkai, N. Saijo, K. Tominago, K. Eguchi, E. Shimizer, Y. Sasaki, J. Fujita, H. Futami, H. Ohkura, and K. Suemasu, *Cancer 7*:1318 (1986).
37. G. B. Pierce, F. J. Dixon, and E. Verney, *Arch. Pathol. 67*:204 (1959).
38. D. Gitlin and M. Boesman, *J. Clin. Invest. 46*:1010 (1967).
39. K. E. W. Melvin, A. H. Tashjian, and H. H. Miller, *Recent Prog. Horm. Res. 28*:399 (1972).
40. C. C. Cate, E. B. Douple, K. M. Andrews, O. S. Pettengill, T. J. Curphey, G. D. Sorenson, and L. H. Mauer, *Cancer Res. 44*:949 (1984).

41. D. A. Hullin, K. Brown, P. A. M. Kynoch, C. Smith, and R. J. Thompson, *Biochim. Biophys. Acta 628*:98 (1980).
42. D. N. Carney, P. J. Maragos, D. C. Ihde, M. H. Cohen, P. J. Marangos, P. A. Bunn, J. D. Minna, and Adi F. Gazdar, *Lancet 1*:583 (1982).
43. D. Thompson and J. Haddow, *Cancer 43*:1820 (1979).
44. A. F. Gazdar, M. H. Zweig, D. M. Carney, A. C. Von Steirteghen, S. B. Baylin, and J. D. Minna, *Cancer Res. 41*:5399 (1984).
45. M. Hirota, K. Fukushima, P. I. Terasaki, G. Y. Terashita, J. Galton, and M. Kawahara, *Cancer Res. 45*:6453 (1985).

5
Diagnostic Uses
of Antimelanoma Antibodies

Ingegerd Hellström and Karl Erik Hellström / ONCOGEN, and University of
Washington, Seattle, Washington

INTRODUCTION

Melanomas are among the human tumors studied most intensely
with monoclonal antibody (MAb) technology, and a variety of
melanoma-associated cell surface antigens have been demonstrated, as well as several cytoplasmic antigens that have strong association with melanomas (1-4).

Most of the specificity studies have been done on the cell surface antigens, because these can be more easily measured by
quantitative-binding assays. Although none of the surface antigens
yet identified has absolute selectivity for melanoma cells, several

of them are expressed much more strongly in melanomas than in normal tissues. For example, most melanomas express 50,000-500,000 molecules per cell of p97, a transferrinlike glycoprotein (5-8), whereas there are fewer than 8000 molecules of p97 per cell in normal tissues. Other relatively melanoma-specific surface antigens include a GD3 ganglioside (9-12), sometimes present in an O-acetylated form (13), a proteoglycan (14,15), an antigen that is the receptor for nerve growth factor (16), as well as GD2 and GM3 ganglioside antigens (17-19). The quantitatively increased amounts of these antigens in melanoma appear to be sufficient for tumor "targeting" of therapeutic agents (20-24).

Within the first couple of years of MAb-related work on melanoma, the p97, proteoglycan, and GD3 antigens were identified independently in several laboratories, whereas few equally specific antigens have since been detected, in spite of intense efforts by a large number of investigators over a 6-year period. Whether or not antigens of greater specificity can be detected by using human MAb is difficult to predict, but given the experience from comparing anti-HLA MAb of mouse or human origin, a higher specificity of the human MAb is not to be expected. Furthermore, no tumor-associated cell surface antigen of remarkably better specificity than those defined by mouse MAb has yet been identified by human MAb (25). It is also noteworthy that melanoma-associated GD2 and GM3 antigens, as defined by mouse MAb, had been previously demonstrated by antibodies in the sera of patients with melanoma (18). This suggests that there is only a limited number of cell surface antigens that can be demonstrated on human melanoma. Therefore, it makes more sense to develop the best possible approach for applying the already known antigens to various clinical purposes than to hunt for an entirely melanoma-specific antigen (if such an antigen would be ultimately discovered, so much the better).

Diagnostic approaches of the antimelanoma MAb available today include the detection of melanoma cells in histological specimens, development of serum assays for melanoma, and the in vivo "imaging" of melanoma with radiolabeled MAb or antibody fragments. We shall discuss these approaches, emphasizing the experience of our own group.

DETECTION OF MELANOMA CELLS IN HISTOLOGICAL SPECIMENS

The diagnostic goal of the immunohistological assays are, first, to demonstrate melanoma cells metastatic to various organs, including lymph nodes; second, to differentiate between melanomas and other types of neoplasms, to provide the correct diagnosis of a metastatic tumor whose primary origin is unknown; and, third, to distinguish between (malignant) melanomas and (benign) nevi. Because pathologists routinely work with formalin-fixed, paraffin-embedded sections, techniques applicable to such material are preferred. A priori, both cell surface antigens and cytoplasmic antigens may be considered as suitable markers.

Because immunohistology lends itself to demonstrating antibody binding to tumor cells in vivo, it is often part of the screening by which new MAbs are identified. For this purpose, our laboratory is using a variant of the Sternberger peroxidase-antiperoxidase (PAP) technique (26), which has been described in detail (15,27), and similar techniques (often based on avidin-biotin reactions) are widely employed. Many tumor antigens identified by MAb are sensitive to paraffin embedding, hence, the procedure for immunostaining uses acetone-fixed sections prepared from frozen tissue, which is later followed by tests on sections from paraffin-embedded tissues. In view of our interests in tumor targeting, we have focused on cell surface antigens, as will be described first. However, as we shall then discuss, the cytoplasmic antigens appear to be better diagnostic markers for immunohistology, as applied to clinical problems.

Cell Surface Antigens

Several melanoma-associated cell surface antigens, including p97, a proteoglycan, and the GD3 antigens, have been studied extensively in sections from primary and metastatic melanoma. In one study (15), for example, all of four primary melanomas and 21 of 30 metastatic melanomas were stained by the antiproteoglycan antibody 48.7, as were six of six compound nevi. The degree of staining of the melanomas varied from weak to very strong, and there was also an intercellular variability among cells from the same melanoma. Tissues from 10 different nonmelanoma tumors were also tested, as were 24 different samples of normal tissues. All were negative with the exception of a weak staining of some normal (probably endothelial) cells in the walls of blood vessels. Skin biopsies from 17 patients were cut to preserve the dermoepidermal junction and stained by MAb 48.7. Melanocytes, which could be identified by the DOPA-oxidase reaction, were unstained.

The MAb 96.5, which is specific for p97, was also tested in the study referred to (15). This MAb stained melanoma and nevi but did not react appreciably with other neoplastic or normal cells, including skin melanocytes. When 25 melanoma samples were studied in parallel with both MAb 48.7 and 96.5, nine were stained with both, seven were stained only with MAb 48.7, and six only with MAB 96.5. The staining was sometimes strong with one MAb and weak with the other. Only three of the 25 melanomas were not stained by either MAb. A subsequent study (28,29) showed that MAb 2B2, which is specific for the melanoma-associated GD3 antigen, bound to 26 of 27 metastatic melanomas tested. Fifty-five percent of melanomas, compared with 0% of other tumors (mostly carcinomas), were stained by three MAbs, 96.5, 48.7, and 2B2, whereas 96% of melanomas and 20% of other tumors were stained by at least two of these MAbs (29).

Other investigators have identified similar cell membrane-associated tumor antigens in both melanomas and benign nevi (30, 31), and they have emphasized the variability in antigen expression between different melanomas as well as between different cells from the same melanoma (29,31-34). Furthermore, HLA-DR antigens have been commonly identified on the malignant lesions, hence, their presence may have diagnostic significance (30,31,35). The proteoglycan antigen appears to be a particularly good marker because of its frequent expression (31).

These data indicate that MAbs to melanoma-associated cell surface antigens react with frozen sections of melanoma in a pattern that is relatively, but not absolutely, specific for melanomas and nevi. It follows that as most melanomas express high amounts of these antigens in vivo and as the antigens are localized at the cell surface, they may be suitable markers for nuclear imaging (discussed later) and also be good targets for MAb-based therapy. However, because there is a variation between the expression of the antigens in different melanomas, and also between different cells from the same melanoma, the use of MAb "cocktails" is probably needed for most clinical purposes (29,31,33). It is encouraging that at least one melanoma antigen was detected in all of the metastatic melanomas studied, when the same samples were tested with MAbs to three different such antigens (29).

The value, for immunohistological diagnosis, of MAbs to the three antigens on which our group has concentrated (and other melanoma-associated cell surface antigens, as well) is hampered by the variability in antigen expression between different melanomas, the presence of the antigens in nevi, and the failure of most of the MAbs to stain routinely prepared, i.e., formalin-fixed, paraffin-embedded, sections. Furthermore, distinction between melanomas and other neoplasms is limited because essentially all the MAbs also react with some carcinomas. The role of immunohistological assays with these MAbs is, therefore, primarily for screening of which tumors express the corresponding antigens as a basis for selecting an MAb for tumor imaging or therapy.

Cytoplasmic Antigens

A better approach for immunohistological diagnosis is to use MAbs to certain melanoma-associated cytoplasmic antigens, which are preserved in paraffin-embedded tissue sections, are more melanoma-specific, and also show less variability than the surface antigens referred to (36-44). One such antigen (and the one studied the most) is S-100, which is expressed in virtually all melanomas and in some nonmelanocytic tumors, including gliomas, salivary gland tumors, and a subset of breast carcinomas (36,37,40). By combining anti-S-100 MAb and MAbs to cytoskeletal proteins present in epithelial cells and absent from melanomas, a high degree of diagnostic precision can be obtained (41). Still, there may be difficulties by this approach in distinguishing between gliomas and melanomas metastatic to the brain.

Several other MAbs to cytoplasmic antigens also deserve attention, and some may be better than MAbs to S-100. The MAb 8-1H has been used to detect cells from ocular melanoma that have metastasized to the liver, and it has, thereby, proved to be clinically useful (42). The MAb HMSA-1 (36), which was developed against purified melanosomal fractions of human melanoma, stains melanomas, including amelanotic lesions, as well as melanocytic nevi, but does not react with normal melanocytes, various normal tissues, or with most nonmelanocytic tumors. The

MAb HMB-45, recently developed by Vogel and Gown (43), shows exquisite selectivity for melanoma (60 of 62 stained) compared with other tumors (none of 168 stained). It does not stain intradermal nevi or melanocytes. In view of its selectivity, MAb HMB-45 might become a reagent of choice for distinguishing among poorly differentiated tumors of uncertain origin. An MAb developed by Ruiter et al. (44) is interesting because it can, like MAb HMB-45, discriminate between melanomas and nevocellular nevi. Two human MAbs, which were obtained by Kan-Mitchell et al. (45), react with cytoplasmic antigens of melanomas and some carcinomas. They do not stain compound nevi and appear to be diagnostically useful.

It is clear from these facts that there are several MAbs that react to cytoplasmic antigens in formalin-fixed, paraffin-embedded sections that can be employed both for distinguishing melanomas from other tumors and for detecting melanoma cells metastatic to various organs, e.g., to lymph nodes and liver. If the preliminary evidence can be confirmed that there are MAbs that stain melanoma and not benign nevi, these particular MAbs will extend the use of immunohistology for melanoma diagnosis to include those cases in whom it is difficult to morphologically differentiate between a nevus and a melanoma. Immunostaining of cytological specimens obtained by needle biopsy may further add to the use of MAbs for tumor diagnosis by making possible the testing of metastases that are not easily accessible to surgical removal; however, such studies have not yet been reported for melanoma.

SERUM ASSAYS FOR DIAGNOSTIC PURPOSES

Monoclonal antibody-based techniques may be used to detect antigens, antibodies, or immune complexes in the sera of patients with melanoma. The goal is to develop assays that aid in the "staging" of patients, i.e., in the assessment of the degree of tumor spread, as well as in their clinical "monitoring," for example, during therapy. Serum assays might also contribute to establishing a primary diagnosis, but this is a much more difficult task.

Antigens in Serum

Assays for measuring the levels of known antigens in the circulation come first to mind, because they are most straightforward

and allow a high level of precision. The key problem is to identify
an antigen that is secreted (or "shed") from tumor cells to such an
extent that the amount of antigen that is derived from a relatively
small tumor (which may consist of 10^9 or fewer cells) can be detected above a background derived from the approximately 5 x
10^{13} normal cells in the body. The antigen must, therefore, either
have exquisite specificity for neoplastic cells, or it must be released from such cells to a much larger extent than from any
normal cells. The problem is particularly great when attempting to
establish a diagnosis of melanoma at an early enough point to be
clinically useful, because melanomas often metastasize even when
they are minute. No melanoma antigen meeting these high de-
mands for specificity has yet been identified, with the possible exception of the O-acetylated form of the GD3 antigen. However,
this antigen is expressed in only a relatively small percentage of
melanomas (13), and there is no published evidence that it is released to the circulation in sufficiently high amounts to be a good
diagnostic marker. There are cytoplasmic antigens that have been
claimed to be highly specific for melanoma (see earlier discussion).
Nevertheless, their expression on various normal cells has not been
studied by very sensitive and quantitative techniques, and it is uncertain to what extent they are released from living melanoma
cells.

Serum assays have been performed to detect circulating p97,
proteoglycan, or GD3 antigens, because these are among the more
specific and common antigens of human melanoma and easily
adapt themselves to sensitive and quantitative assays. Unfortunately, the results have not been encouraging. By using a double-
determinant test (46) with MAbs to two different epitopes of the
p97 antigen, nanogram quantitites of p97 could easily be measured in patient serum. Some patients with disseminated (stage III
or IV) melanoma were found to have higher levels of circulating
p97 than did patients free of the disease. However, normal
controls had approximately 5 ng of p97 per milliliter of serum,
and the level of p97 in patients with a small tumor load (as in
primary melanoma and in most cases of stage II disease) was no
different. Hence, a serum assay based on measurement of p97
levels is not likely to be clinically useful. The situation is similar
for the melanoma-associated proteoglycan antigen, which has been
reported to be increased in patients with stage IV melanoma but

not in patients with less-advanced disease (47), and it was also the same for the GD3 antigen (I. Hellström et al., unpublished findings). Likewise, a 100-kD tumor-associated cytoplasmic protein, which is secreted into the circulation, was not present at significantly increased levels in the sera of patients with tumors (including melanoma) until these were widely disseminated (47, 48). Thus, measurement of antigens in serum has been less rewarding in melanoma than has, for example, the monitoring of certain tumor-associated mucins in the sera of patients with breast carcinoma (49).

It may be possible, however, that a series of consecutive tests on sera from the same melanoma patient will yield clinically important information much earlier in the disease than when the antigen level in one serum sample from a particular patient is compared with a "normal" standard. Indeed, as a tumor grows, there might be a small, but still measureable, increase in the amount of circulating antigen over the baseline for the given patient, hence, the detection of such a gradual increase would indicate tumor recurrence.

Assays Based on Immune Responses to Tumor

When considering an immunological approach to diagnosis, one should be aware of the possibility that the patient's immune system can recognize the presence of a tumor, as suggested by some of the early immunological work on human cancers (50). If, indeed, this is true, circulating immune cells, antitumor antibodies, anti-idiotypic antibodies, suppressor factors, or helper factors may be identified. This might already occur early in the disease because the immune system (as represented by lymphocytes in the area of a tumor) may be perturbed by the presence of tumor cells expressing large amounts of an antigen that is normally expressed at a very low level.

Only a small fraction of patients with growing melanoma or whose melanomas have been removed, appear to have circulating antibodies that can be detected by binding assays and are directed toward tumor antigens that are either individually unique or shared by many melanomas and some other tumors (51). However, cell-mediated immune reactions to melanoma-associated antigens have been described as occurring much more frequently

(52-55), as have lymphocyte-dependent antibodies (56) and "blocking" serum factors suppressing the cell-mediated reactions (52,54,56). There is, in fact, reported evidence that the presence of blocking factors some of which are immune complexes (57-59), correlates with a poor prognosis (53,54,58-61), and that lymphocyte-dependent antibodies are associated with a good prognosis (56). It has not been proved, however, that measuring either blocking factors or lymphocyte-dependent antibodies is useful clinically, because the differences that have been described have been based on comparisons between groups of patients with, or without, disease, rather than on prospective double-blind studies (55). Another approach may be to look for anti-idiotypic antibodies in patient sera (62) because these may reflect an ongoing immune response to tumor antigens. Such antibodies (63) may also be employed diagnostically to detect circulating lymphocytes, antibodies, or suppressor factors that express idiotypes involved in an immune response to tumor antigens. Currently, there are no diagnostic tests based on anti-idiotypic antibodies.

Recent work from Kirkwood and Vlock (64,65) provides perhaps the greatest promise, so far, toward the development of clinically useful serum assays for melanoma. Using ultrafiltration at low pH for breaking up immune complexes, as first suggested by Sjögren et al. (66), most patients with growing melanoma had circulating antibodies to melanoma antigens (64,65). The data indicated, therefore, that past failures to detect antitumor antibodies in melanoma patients were due to complex formation between the antibodies and shed tumor antigen.

In a subsequent study (67), Kirkwood's group investigated the reactivity of serum antibody against a cultured allogeneic melanoma by testing sera from 43 patients with either stage I or stage II melanoma. Of these patients, 15 relapsed and 28 remained disease-free over the course of evaluation. Serum samples were obtained within 2 months of surgery when all patients were free of disease by physical examination and routine radiologic and laboratory evaluation. Antibody reactivity was measured by protein A hemadsorption before and after acid dissociation and ultrafiltration. The titer of antimelanoma antibody in either native serum or serum disassociated from immune complexes was associated with eventual relapse (P = 0.0001), implying that antibody reactivity against melanoma was an important prognostic factor. Because the antibodies could already be detected in stage I and II patients, the findings are of obvious clinical interest.

Kirkwood and Vlock did not detect reactivity against normal cells, using absorption analysis (64), but they did not study the specificity of the antimelanoma antibodies to the same extent as, for example, was done in a careful study by Shiku et al. (51), who only infrequently found such antibodies. It would be useful to have MAbs to the antigen(s) that are recognizable in the patients, because that would make possible definitive studies on the specificity of the reactions measured. Such studies are particularly needed because the measurement of antibody responses to cultivated, allogeneic melanoma cells is certainly less precise than, for example, the measurement of circulating tumor antigen and is much less adaptable to the clinical monitoring of large numbers of patients.

RADIOIMMUNODIAGNOSIS OF TUMORS IN VIVO

The presence of cell surface antigens that are expressed at higher levels in melanomas than in normal tissues suggests that MAbs can be used for in vivo diagnosis of tumors. The clinical goal of this approach is to obtain information contributing to patient staging and also to follow the in vivo expression of tumor antigens that can be targeted by injected antibodies.

Experiments were first carried out to test the localization of injected antibodies in nude mice that had received human melanoma transplants. These studies showed that melanoma-specific MAbs selectively localized to tumors expressing the relevant antigens (68-70). The level of tumor antigen expression, as assessed in vitro by using a cell-binding assay, correlated with the extent to which a given MAb bound to the tumor in vivo (69).

Studies performed by Larson et al. (68) in patients with metastatic melanoma showed that intravenously injected radiolabeled MAbs, which were specific for p97, could be used to image tumors as detected by using a gamma camera. The level of in vivo binding of MAb to a tumor nodule correlated with the amount of p97 antigen that it expressed (24). The Fab fragments appeared to be preferable to whole MAb, because they imaged tumor more quickly and they were less prone to induce an antibody response to immunoglobulin antigens of mouse origin. Approximately 80%

of metastases were detected, as long as they were positive for p97 and were at least about 10 mm in diameter. This included some metastases that had not been previously observed with other techniques. Subcutaneous metastases, as well as metastases in lung, liver, mesenterium, and brain, were demonstrated (24,68).

The specificity of the MAb localization was established in two ways. First, experiments were performed on biopsies from patients who had received ^{131}I-labeled anti-p97 fragments in parallel with ^{125}I-fragments prepared from an MAb directed to an irrelevant antigen. In tumors, the specific fragments localized some three to 10 times better than the control fragments, whereas both localized to approximately the same extent in normal tissues. Second, the same patient was imaged on three subsequent occasions; (1) after having received p97-specific MAb fragments; (2) about 1 month later, after injection of nonspecific (control) fragments; and (3) an additional month later, after another injection of p97-specific fragments. Only the p97-specific fragments localized selectively to tumor (24).

Two subsequent studies have shown that MAbs, specific for the melanoma-associated proteoglycan antigen (and Fab fragments prepared from such MAbs), localize more to metastatic melanoma than to normal tissues (71,72). In the latter of these two studies (72), a large group of patients were investigated at several different centers. Imaging of tumor was observed to about the same extent as that reported from the p97 system. In addition, the important observation was made that some previously unknown metastases were first detected by imaging and subsequently confirmed by other techniques.

In most of the currently published work, the MAbs (fragments) were labeled with ^{131}I. In one study described by Larson et al. (73), they were labeled instead with ^{123}I after which the uptake was measured by single-photon tomography. It was possible to image smaller tumors and to get better resolution, a finding supported by subsequent studies of Delaloye et al. (74) on MAbs to human colon carcinoma. In work by Fawwaz et al. (72), MAbs were labeled with either technetium or indium. Both of these two isotopes seemed to have advantages over ^{131}I, for which one of the problems is deiodination in vivo and another is that the energy level is not ideal for use with existing γ-cameras (for which an isotope such as technetium is better).

Evidence that injected MAbs localize to melanoma cells, and not to normal stroma within the tumors, come from work in which unlabeled MAbs, specific for either p97 or the proteoglycan antigen, have been given to patients with metastatic disease. In patients receiving approximately 200 mg of MAb, or more, clear-cut binding of mouse immunoglobulin to the surface of melanoma cells was observed, whereas there was little binding to normal cells in the stroma (75,76).

Nuclear imaging after intravenous injection of radiolabeled MAbs (or fragments) is clinically promising (77). It can demonstrate not only that there is a "suspect" tissue but that this tissue expresses a known tumor marker, and it can also reveal the in vivo distribution of MAb preparations that are aimed for tumor targeting (24,78). There are some drawbacks, however. A tumor nodule must be at least some 10 mm in diameter to be detectable, and even then, some nodules are not; thus, the imaging approach suffers from the same weakness as serum assays that are based on antigen detection, namely, that this method detects the tumor only when it is relatively large. It is not yet clear if imaging with radiolabeled antimelanoma MAbs (or fragments) has any real clinical value by providing information on which some patients can be cured who, otherwise, would not be. To improve this situation, work is needed to improve the quality of the nuclear imaging by use of isotopes, such as technetium, that give better images with available equipment. Ultimately, it may become possible to detect the localization of antibodies to tumors by a technique, such as nuclear magnetic resonance, that has better resolution.

Another problem is that almost all patients injected with mouse MAbs develop antimouse antibodies, particularly if they are injected repeatedly. These antibodies can interefere with subsequent injections of mouse MAbs. Although the antimouse antibodies develop a longer time after the patients receive MAb fragments rather than whole MAb, they do appear fairly regularly after injection of fragments as well. By using chimeric (mouse-human) MAb (79), it should be possible to decrease the immunogenicity of a whole MAb preparation to approximately that of Fab fragments, and with human MAb (25), the problem should decrease further. The human MAbs, however, may still be immunogenic by inducing the formation of antibodies to their allotypic and idiotypic determinants. Such antibodies might also interfere with repeated injection. Thus, methods for decreasing the immuno-genicity of injected MAb (fragments) are needed.

CONCLUSIONS

Several antigens have been found that are expressed at high levels in human melanoma and in trace amounts in normal tissues. Some of these antigens are localized at the cell surface, and others are cytoplasmic. The cell surface antigens are of potential interest for a whole variety of diagnostic and therapeutic purposes, whereas the cytoplasmic antigens are primarily interesting as markers for im-munohistological diagnosis.

There are three potential diagnostic uses of melanoma-specific MAb: to facilitate the histopathological diagnosis of primary and metastatic melanoma, to develop serum assays for monitoring melanoma patients, and to aid in the staging and monitoring of patients by nuclear imaging. For immunohistology, MAbs to intracellular antigens, such as S-100, used alone or in combination, now provide the best approach. Diagnostic studies based on com-parisons of the level of melanoma antigens in serum with the levels in various control groups have not been rewarding because they have detected only late stages of the disease; it remains to be seen whether "longitudinal" studies on sera from individual patients, over the course of disease, will be more informative. Recent reports on antibodies circulating in the form of immune com-plexes are most promising because they indicate that progno-stically useful information can be obtained as early as stages I and II. Radioimmunodiagnosis has demonstrated some melanoma metastases that were not recognized by other approaches. This technique should also provide the needed background for targeting MAbs for therapy.

ACKNOWLEDGMENTS

The authors gratefully acknowledge collaboration with Dr. J. P. Brown, Dr. P. L. Beaumier, Dr. S. M. Larson, Dr. M.-Y. Yeh, and Dr. H. J. Garrigues. The authors also thank Dr. E. Lavie and Dr. P. S. Linsley for valuable discussions and Phyllis Harps for her as-sistance in the preparation of the manuscript. The work of the authors has been supported by ONCOGEN, and by National Cancer Institute grant CA 38011.

REFERENCES

1. H. Koprowski and Z. Steplewski, in *Monoclonal Antibodies and T-Cell Hybridomas* (G. J. Hammerling, U. Hammerling, and J. F. Kearney, eds.), Elsevier, Amsterdam (1981), p. 161.
2. R. A. Reisfeld and S. Ferone (eds.), in *Melanoma Antigens and Antibodies*, Plenum Press, New York/London (1982).
3. F. X. Real, A. N. Houghton, A. P. Albino, C. Cordon-Cardo, M. R. Melamed, H. F. Oettgen, and L. J. Old, *Cancer Res. 45*:4401 (1985).
4. K. E. Hellström and I. Hellström, in *Monoclonal Antibodies for Tumour Detection and Drug Targeting* R. W. Baldwin and V. S. Byers, eds.), Academic Press, New York, (1985), p. 17.
5. R. G. Woodbury, J. P. Brown, M. -Y. Yeh, I. Hellström, and K. E. Hellström, *Proc. Natl. Acad. Sci. USA 77*:2183 (1980).
6. J. P. Brown, K. Nishiyama, I. Hellström, and K. E. Hellström, *J. Immunol. 127*:539 (1981).
7. J. P. Brown, R. M. Hewick, I. Hellström, K. E. Hellström, R. F. Doolittle, and W. J. Dreyer, *Nature 296*:171 (1982).
8. T. M. Rose, G. D. Plowman, D. B. Teplow, W. J. Dreyer, K. E. Hellström, and J. P. Brown, *Proc. Natl. Acad. Sci. USA 83*:1261 (1986).
9. W. G. Dippold, W. G., K. O. Lloyd, L. T. C. Li, H. Ikeda, H. F. Oettgen, and L. J. Old, *Proc. Natl. Acad. Sci. USA 77*:6114 (1980).
10. M. -Y, I. Hellström, K. Abe, S. Hakomori, and K. E. Hellström, *Int. J. Cancer 29*:269 (1982).
11. C. S. Pukel, K. O. Lloyd, L. R. Trabassos, W. G. Dippold, H. F. Oettgen, and L. J. Old, *J. Exp. Med. 155*:1133 (1982).
12. E. Nudelman, S. Hakomori, R. Kannagi, S. Levery, M. -Y. Yeh, K. E. Hellström, and I. Hellström, *J. Biol. Chem. 257*:12752 (1982).
13. D. A. Cheresh and R. A. Reisfeld, *Science 24*:844 (1984).
14. A. C. Morgan, Jr., Dr. R. Galloway, K. Imai, and R. A. Reisfeld, *J. Immunol. 126*:365 (1981).
15. I. Hellström, H. J. Garrigues, L. Cabasco, G. H. Mosely, J. P. Brown, and K. E. Hellström, *J. Immunol. 130*:1467 (1983).
16. P. M. Grob, A. H. Ross, H. Koprowski, and M. Bothwell, *J. Biol. Chem. 260*:8044 (1985).
17. G. Schulz, D. A. Cheresh, N. M. Varki, A. Yu, L. K. Staffileno, and R. A. Reisfeld, *Cancer Res. 44*:5914 (1984).
18. T. Tai, L. D. Cahan, T. Tsuchida, R. E. Saxton, R. F. Irie, and D. L. Morton, *Int. J. Cancer 35*:607 (1985).
19. J. M. Carubia, R. K. Yu, L. J. Macala, J. M. Kirkwood, and J. M. Varga, *Biochem. Biophys. Res. Commun. 120*:500 (1984).
20. G. F. Rowland, C. A. Axton, R. W. Baldwin, J. P. Brown, J. R. F. Corvalan, M. J. Embleton, V. A. Gore, I. Hellström, K. E. Hellström, E. Jacobs, C. H. Marsden, M. V. Pimm, R. G. Simmonds, and W. Smith, *Cancer Immunol. Immunother. 19*:1 (1985).

21. P. Casellas, J. P. Brown, O. Gros, P. Gros, I. Hellström, R. K. Jansen, P. Poncelet, H. Vidal, and K. E. Hellström, *Int. J. Cancer 30*:437 (1982).
22. J. A. Carrasquillo, K. A. Krohn, P. Beaumier, R. W. McGuffin, J. P. Brown, K. E. Hellström, I. Hellström, and S. M. Larson, *Cancer Treat. Rep. 68*:317 (1984).
23. A. N. Houghton, D. Mintzer, C. Cordon-Cardo, S. Welt, B. Fliegel, S. Vadham, E. Carswell, M. R. Melamed, H. F. Oettgen, and L. J. Old, *Proc. Natl. Acad. Sci. USA 82*:1242 (1985).
24. S. M. Larson, J. A. Carrasquillo, K. A. Krohn, J. P. Brown, R. W. Mc-Guffin, J. M. Ferens, M. M. Graham, L. D. Hill, P. L. Beaumier, K. E. Hellström, and I. Hellström, *J. Clin. Invest. 72*:2101 (1983).
25. R. J. Cote, D. M. Morrissey, H. F. Oettgen, and L. J. Old, *Fed. Proc. 43*:2465 (1984).
26. L. A. Sternberger (ed.), in *Immunocytochemistry*, John Wiley & Sons, New York (1979), p. 104.
27. H. J. Garrigues, W. Tilgen, I. Hellström, W. Franke, and K. E. Hellström, *Int. J. Cancer 29*:511 (1982).
28. I. Hellström, K. E. Hellström, and J. P. Brown, in *Progress in Cancer Research and Therapy* (S. R. Wolman and A. J. Mastromarino, eds.) Raven Press, New York (1984), p. 185.
29. K. E. Hellström, I. Hellström, J. P. Brown, S. M. Larson, G. T. Nepom, and J. A. Carrasquillo, in *Genes and Antigens in Cancer Cells, Contributions to Oncology Series* (G. Riethmüller, H. Koprowski, S. von-Kleist, and K. Munk, eds.), Vol. 19, Karger, Basel (1984), p. 121.
30. M. S. Ernstoff, P. Duray, K. Stenn, and J. M. Kirkwood, *J. Invest. Dermatol. 84*:430 (1985).
31. P. Natali, A. Bigotti, R. Cavaliere, S. K. Liao, M. Taniguchi, M. Matsui, and S. Ferrone, *Cancer Res. 45*:2883 (1985).
32. A. P. Albino, K. O. Lloyd, A. N. Houghton, F. F. Oettgen, and L. J. Old, *J. Exp. Med. 154*:1764 (1981).
33. M. -Y. Yeh, I. Hellström, and K. E. Hellström, *J. Immunol. 126*:1312 (1981).
34. C. Cillo, J. P. Mach, M. Schreyer, and S. Carrel, *Int. J. Cancer 34*:11 (1984).
35. P. G. Natali, A. Bigotti, R. Cavaliere, M. R. Nicotra, and S. Ferrone, *J. Natl. Cancer Inst. 73*:13 (1984).
36. A. J. Cochran, D. R. Wen, and H. R. Herschman, *Int. J. Cancer 15*: 159 (1984).
37. A. J. Cochran and D. R. Wen, *Pathology 17*:340 (1985).
38. T. Kageshita, M. Johno, T. Ono, T. Arao, and K. Imai, *Arch. Dermatol. Res. 277*:334 (1985).
39. Y. Akutsu and K. Kimbow, *Cancer Res. 46*:2904 (1986).
40. A. J. Cochran, W. S. Foulds, B. E. Damato, G. E. Trope, L. Morrison, and W. R. Lee, Br. J. Ophthalmol. 69:171 (1985).

41. K. C. Gatter, E. Ralfkiaer, J. Skinner, D. Brown, A. Heryet, K. A. Pulford, K. Hou-Jensen, and D. Y. Mason, *J. Clin. Pathol. 38*:1353 (1985).
42. L. A. Donoso, R. Folberg, R. Naids, J. J. Augsburger, A. A. Shields, and B. Atkinson, *Arch. Optholmol. 103*:799 (1985).
43. A. M. Gown, A. M. Vogel, D. Hoak, F. Gough, and M. A. McNutt, *Am. J. Pathol. 123*:195 (1986).
44. D. J. Ruiter, G. M. Dingjan, P. M. Steijlen, M. van Beveren-Hooyer, C. B. deGraaff-Reistma, W. Bergman, G. N. P. van Muijen, and S. O. Warnaar, *J. Invest. Dermatol. 85*:4 (1985).
45. J. Kan-Mitchell, A. Imam, R. A. Kempf, C. R. Taylor, and M. S. Mitchell, *Cancer Res. 46*:2490 (1980).
46. J. P. Brown, R. G. Woodbury, C. E. Hart, I. Hellström, and K. E. Hellström, *Proc. Natl. Acad. Sci. USA 78*:539 (1981).
47. P. Giacomini, F. Veglia, P. Cordiali Fei, T. Rehle, P. G. Natali, and S. Ferrone, *Cancer Res. 44*:1281 (1984).
48. P. S. Linsley, D. Horn, H. Marquardt, J. P. Brown, I. Hellström, K. E. Hellström, V. Ochs, and E. Tolentino, *Biochemistry 25*:2978 (1986).
49. P. S. Linsley, V. Ochs, S. Laska, D. Horn, D. Ring, A. E. Frankel, and J. P. Brown, *Cancer Res. 46*:3917 (1986).
50. I. Hellström, K. E. Hellström, H. O. Sjögren, and G. A. Warner, *Int. J. Cancer 7*:1 (1971).
51. H. Shiku, T. Takahashi, H. F. Oettgen, and L. J. Old, *J. Exp. Med. 144*: 873 (1976).
52. J. L. McCoy, L. F. Jerome, J. H. Dean, E. Pferlin, R. K. Oldham, K. H. Char, M. H. Cohen, E. L. Felix, and R. B. Herberman, *J. Natl. Cancer Inst. 55*:19 (1975).
53. I. Hellström, H. O. Sjögren, G. A. Warner, and K. E. Hellström, *Int. J. Cancer 7*:226 (1971).
54. W. J. Halliday, A. E. Maluish, J. H. Little, and N. C. Davis, *Int. J. Cancer 16*:645 (1975).
55. I. Hellström and K. E. Hellström, *J. Biol. Resp. Mod. 2*:310 (1983).
56. P. A. Hersey, A. Edwards, E. Murray, W. H. McCarthy and G. W. Milstron, *J. Natl. Cancer Inst. 71*:45 (1983).
57. W. C. Cheng, R. K. Gupta, and D. L. Morton, *Immunol. Invest. 14*:367 (1995).
58. R. K. Gupta and D. L. Morton, *Contemp. Top. Immunobiol. 15*:1 (1985).
59. R. D. Rossen, M. M. Crane, A. C. Morgan, E. H. Giannini, B. C. Giovanella, J. S. Stehlin, J. J. Twomey, and E. M. Hersh, *Cancer Res. 43*:422 (1983).
60. I. Hellström, G. A. Warner, K. E. Hellström, and H. O. Sjögren, *Int. J. Cancer 11*:280 (1973).
61. E. W. Murray, H. McCarthy, and P. Hersey, *Br. J. Cancer 36*:7 (1977).

62. M. G. Lewis, T. M. Phillips, K. B. Cook, and J. Blake, *Nature 232*:52 (1971).
63. G. T. Nepom, K. A. Nelson, S. L. Holbeck, I. Hellström, and K. E. Hellström, *Proc. Natl. Acad. Sci. USA 81*:2864 (1984).
64. J. M. Kirkwood and D. R. Vlock, *Cancer Res. 44*:4177 (1984).
65. D. R. Vlock and J. M. Kirkwood, *J. Clin. Invest. 76*:849 (1985).
66. H. O. Sjögren, I. Hellström, S. C. Bansal, and K. E. Hellström, *Proc. Natl. Acad. Sci. USA 68*:1372 (1971).
67. D. R. Vlock, R. DerSimonian, and J. M. Kirkwood, *J. Clin. Invest 77*: 1116 (1986).
68. S. M. Larson, J. P. Brown, P. W. Wright, J. A. Carrasquillo, I. Hellström, and K. E. Hellström, *J. Nucl. Med. 24*:123 (1983).
69. P. Beaumier, K. Krohn, J. A. Carrasquillo, J. Eary, K. E. Hellström, I. Hellström, W. Nelp, and S. M. Larson, *J. Nucl. Med. 26*:1172 (1985).
70. S. Matzku, J. Mattern, P. George, and I. Hellström, Gastenier Internationales Symposium, Radioaktive Isotope in Klinik and Forschung (1982), p. 295.
71. S. M. Larson, J. A. Carrasquillo, R. W. McGuffin, L. A. Krohn, J. M. Ferens, L. D. Hill, P. L. Beaumier, J. C. Reynolds, K. E. Hellström and I, Hellström, *Radiology 155*:487 (1985).
72. R. A. Fawwaz, T. S. Wang, A. Estabrook, J. M. Rosen, M. A. Hardy, P. O. Alderson, S. C. Srivastava, P. Richards, and S. Ferrone, *J. Nucl. Med. 26*:488 (1985).
73. S. M. Larson, J. A. Carrasquillo, K. A. Krohn, R. W. McGiffin, I. Hellström, K. E. Hellström, and D. Lister, *J. Am. Med. Assoc. 249*:811 (1983).
74. B. Delaloye, A. Bischof-Delaloye, F. Buchegger, V. von Fliedner, J. P. Grob, J. C. Volant, J. Pettavel, and J. P. Mach, *J. Clin. Invest. 77*:301 (1986).
75. R. Oldham, C. Woodhouse, R. Schruff et al., *Proc. Am. Soc. Clin. Oncol 3*:65 (1984) (abstr.).
76. G. E. Goodman, P. L. Beaumier, I. Hellström, B. Fernyhough, and K. E. Hellström, *J. Clin. Oncol. 3*:340 (1985).
77. M. T. Lotze, J. A. Carrasquillo, J. N. Weinstein, G. J. Bryant, P. Perentesis, J. C. Reynolds, L. A. Matis, R. R. Eger, A. M. Keenan, I. Hellström, K. E. Hellström, and S. M. Larson, *Ann. Surg. 204*:223 (1986).
78. R. F. Schmelter, G. D. Friefeld, J. Thomas, and W. A. Robinson, *Drug Intell. Clin. Pharm. 20*:125 (1986).
79. S. L. Morrison, M. J. Johnson, L. A. Herzenberg, and V. T. Oi, *Proc. Natl. Acad. Sci. USA 81*:6851 (1984).

6

Monoclonal Antibodies in Ovarian Cancer

Neil J. Finkler and Robert C. Knapp / Brigham and Women's Hospital, Harvard Medical School, Boston, Massachusetts

Robert C. Bast, Jr./ Duke University Medical Center, Durham, North Carolina

INTRODUCTION

The most fatal gynecological malignancy, ovarian cancer, claims approximately 11,000 lives annually in the United States. Ovarian carcinomas arise from the surface epithelium, stroma, or germ cells. In adults, about 90% of ovarian cancers are derived from surface epithelium or epithelium that lines subcapsular cysts. Although the use of tumor markers and advances in chemotherapy have dramatically changed the prognosis for patients with germ cell tumors, the outlook for patients with epithelial ovarian carcinoma has changed little since the advent of cytotoxic chemotherapy.

Ovarian cancer is staged according to the FIGO system (Table 1). Epithelial ovarian cancers can metastasize hematogenously or through lymphatics but are most frequently spread by surface contiguity over the peritoneum, studding serosal surfaces, blocking diaphragmatic lymphatics, and producing ascites. The majority of epithelial ovarian cancers are diagnosed in late stages, after they have spread throughout the abdominal cavity.

Despite adequate surgical cytoreduction, including total abdominal hysterectomy, bilateral salpingo-oophorectomy, and omentectomy, many tumor nodules are often left on the serosal surface of the bowel and peritoneium. Although cytotoxic chemotherapy leads to regression of residual tumor in approximately 70% of the patients, response to treatment is difficult to monitor. Often, "second-look" surgical procedures are required to assess tumor status after many months of cytotoxic therapy. Thus, a serum marker that could be used to monitor tumor status during and upon completion of primary treatment would be valuable in this setting.

Although response to treatment may appear to be beneficial, as documented histologically by negative results after a second-look procedure, tumor may recur in 40% of these women. Overall, less than 20% of patients with stage III or IV disease are cured.

The major clinical problem in ovarian cancer is the late stage of diagnosis in two-thirds of the patients. Early detection by means of a serum marker may permit diagnosis at a time when the tumor is confined to the ovaries (stage I) and when the prognosis for cure is still good. In addition, monoclonal antibodies (MAbs)

Table 1   FIGO Staging of Ovarian Cancer

Stage	Description
Stage I	Growth limited to the ovaries
Stage Ia	Growth limited to one ovary; no ascites 1. No tumor on the external surface; capsule intact 2. Tumor present on the external surface and/or capsule ruptured
Stage Ib	Growth limited to both ovaries; no ascites 1. No tumor on the external surface, capsule intact 2. Tumor present on the external surface and/or capsule ruptured
Stage Ic	Tumor either Ia or stage Ib, but with ascites present or positive peritoneal washings
Stage II	Growth involving one or both ovaries with pelvic extension
Stage IIa	Extension and/or metastases to the uterus and/or tubes
Stages IIb	Extension to other pelvic tissues
Stage IIc	Tumor either stage IIa or stage IIb but with ascites present or positive peritoneal washings
Stage III	Growth involving one or both ovaries with intraperitoneal metastases outside the pelvis and/or positive retroperitoneal nodes; tumor limited to the true pelvis with histologically proved malignant extension to small bowel or omentum
Stage IV	Growth involving one or both ovaries with distant metastases; If pleural effusion present, positive cytology required to assign a case to stage IV, parenchymal liver metastases equals stage IV
Special category	Unexplored cases thought to be ovarian carcinoma

may permit primary or recurrent disease to be localized   through
imaging of radionuclide-antibody conjugates and may provide
a system for targeted delivery of cytoxic drugs, toxins, and radioisotopes for more effective treatment of residual disease.

CA 125 ANTIGEN

The murine MAb OC-125 was the first murine antibody reported to react with human ovarian carcinoma (1). Antibody OC-125 recognizes a determinant designated CA 125, originally associated with a serous cystadenocarcinoma cell line. Determinants of CA 125 are found on a high-molecular-weight glycoprotein that is expressed by more than 80% of nonmucinous carcinomas (2-4). By use of biotin-avidin immunoperoxidase, Kabawat et al. (5) have demonstrated CA 125 in pleura, pericardium, peritoneum, amnion, and mullerian duct, as well as in the epithelial lining of the fallopian tube, endometrium, and endocervix. The antigen is present in epithelium during embryonic development but has not been detected in fetal or adult ovaries. Recent studies suggest that CA 125 may also be found in tracheobronchial epithelium and glands (6).

The activity of CA 125 in serum and body fluids is associated with complexes of a relative molecular mass (M_r) greater than 300,000 and greater than 500,000 (3). The smallest subunit of CA 125 that retains antigenic activity is approximately 200,000 M_r. Whether the CA 125 determinant is a carbohydrate or a protein remains to be resolved. Although the evidence is conflicting with regard to antigenic activity after various treatments (7,8), the protein structure appears to be important for CA 125 activity. However, a role for carbohydrate in the antigen structure has not been ruled out.

A radioimmunometric assay has recently been developed to monitor CA 125 levels in serum and body fluid (9,10), and a kit is now available from Centocor, Inc. (Malvern, Pennsylvania), to simplify clinical investigation. Antigen in 1000 μl of serum is bound to the OC-125 antibody on a polystyrene bead. Bound antigen may be detected by simultaneous incubation with 130,000 dpm of iodine-125 (^{125}I) and 1000 μl of trace buffer. Antigen units are arbitrarily defined relative to a standard specimen of CA 125. The assay can detect 1.4 U CA 125/ml and is linear up to 500 U/ml. The day-to-day coefficient of variation is 12-15%, and a doubling or halving of antigen levels is considered significant.

This assay has shown that only 1% of normal individuals have serum CA 125 levels higher than 35 U/ml, whereas more than 80% of ovarian cancer patients have antigen levels that exceed this value (9). Elevated levels of CA 125 can be found in most patients with recurrent carcinoma of the endometrium, fallopian tube, and endocervix, as well as other malignancies, including primary pancreatic, lung, breast, and colorectal lesions (9,11). As a result, serum CA 125 has not yet proved useful for the differential diagnosis of metastatic tumors of unknown origin. The highest serum CA 125 values, however, have been reported in patients with ovarian cancer, with values ranging to more than 8000 U/ml (9).

The level of CA 125 is not affected by smoking (12) but may be elevated in a number of benign conditions such as pregnancy (13), menstruation (14), endometriosis (13,15), adenomyosis (14), pelvic inflammatory disease, renal failure (16), pancreatitis (16), peritonitis (16), and chronic alcoholic hepatitis (16). However, physicians who are monitoring patients with previously diagnosed ovarian cancer or who present with an adnexal mass are not likely to be confused by other conditions.

CA 125 As a Screen for Ovarian Cancer

Because of the late stage of diagnosis in two-thirds of the patients with ovarian carcinoma, tumor usually has come to involve the upper abdomen by the time of initial exploration. Standard therapy would be more efficacious and cure rates higher if ovarian cancer were detected while it was still localized to the pelvis. Early studies by Knauf and Urbach (17) found that markers defined by heteroantisera were elevated in 70% of patients with stage I or stage II disease. Antigen from exophytic lesions or within cysts may enter the circulation before metastases have occurred. In exophytic lesions, antigens shed from surface excrescences are cleared by the diaphragmatic lymphatics and enter the circulation through the alternative thoracic duct. Within cysts, a steep concentration gradient favors diffusion of antigen across the cyst wall into the ovarian stroma. A rich microvasculature and lymphatic supply within the stroma could clear antigen from the ovary, accounting in part for the elevated antigen levels in serum from patients with stage I disease.

In one fortuitous cases, monitored retrospectively, an elevated level of CA 125 was noted 10-12 months before clinically apparent stage III epithelial ovarian carcinoma (18). A diagnosis of stage I and II disease has been associated with CA 125 levels higher than 35 U/ml in 72% and higher than 65 U/ml in 56% of the patients (range: 9-3774 U/ml) (19).

To screen large populations to detect patients with ovarian cancer, the level of false-positive values must be acceptable. The cost and morbidity of exposing patients with elevated CA 125 values who do not have cancer to either laparoscopy or some other surgical intervention are high. In an early study, CA 125 levels were measured in 1020 patients with benign disease attending a gynecology clinic in Boston (13). Among these women, CA 125 values were higher than 65 U/ml in 1.8% of the patients. When pregnant patients were excluded, the CA 125 level exceeded 65 U/ml in 1%. When a second antigen determination was obtained, CA 125 exceeded 65 U/ml in 0.5% of patients. In a recent clinical screening trial, CA 125 was evaluated in 917 nuns from the Philadelphia Archdiocese (20). Median age was 55 years, and CA 125 levels tended to decline with advancing age. In the entire group, a single determination revealed levels above 65 U/ml in 0.8%. If only patients over 40 years of age were considered, the positive rate would have dropped to 0.6%.

Even with this relatively low false-positive rate (0.6%), effective screening would require the development of confirmatory assays to eliminate false-positive values, given the low prevalence of ovarian carcinoma. Two strategies have been developed toward this goal, both of which depend upon additional serum markers using MAb technology. The first has identified epitopes aberrantly coexpressed on molecules that bear CA 125; the second uses simultaneous evaluation of antigens not affected by benign conditions that elevate CA 125.

The epitope CA 19-9 is a sialylated Lewis blood group determinant that can be found in tissue sections from most of gastrointestinal cancers and as many as 40% of ovarian carcinomas (21). Elevated serum antigen levels were found in up to 29% of patients with ovarian cancer (22,23). The CA 125 and CA 19-9 epitopes are antigenically distinct (24). On Western blot analysis, CA 125 was associated with complexes exceeding 300,000 and 500,000 M_r. CA 19-9 migrates with the larger moiety, suggesting a similar origin in some supramolecular complex. Novel MAbs have been sought that would bind epitopes of CA-125-positive mucin and would be associated with different lineages when expressed by normal tissues. Such antibodies have been found and are now being investigated.

Antigens not affected by those benign conditions that elevate CA 125 have also been employed, with major attention focused on CA 72.3 and CA 15-3. The determinant CA 72.3 is expressed on a high-molecular-weight glycoprotein and is associated with breast, lung, colon, and ovarian carcinomas but not with mesothelial cells (25,26). Levels above 10 U/ml are found in patients with colorectal, lung, and ovarian carcinoma. Tumor-associated CA 15-3 is detected in a heterodeterminant sandwich radioimmunometric assay utilizing an immunoabsorbent (27) and a radiolabeled probe (25). Elevated serum values of CA 15-3 above 30 U/ml are found in patients with breast, lung, ovarian, and prostate carcinoma. In recent studies monitoring patients with breast cancer, CA 15-3 proved to be more sensitive than carcinoembryonic antigen (CEA) as a monitoring tool. When sera from 57 patients with ovarian carcinoma were recently assayed, elevated levels were found for CA 125 (higher than 65 U/ml in 82%), CA 15-3 (higher than 30 U/ml in 60%), CA 72.3 (higher than 10 U/ml in 47%), and NB/70K (higher than 45 U/ml in 59%) (28). All patients with elevated CA 15-3 or CA 72.3 levels also had elevated CA 125.

In the same collaborative study, 50 serum samples showing elevated CA 125 levels were identified among several thousand specimens from patients with benign disease seen at the Mayo Clinic (28). These false-positive sera were assayed using the same panel of four antibodies. The CA 125 level exceeded 35 U/ml in all the selected samples and 65 U/ml in 42%. Although B-72.3 and CA 15-3 were elevated in only 6% and 2%, respectively, the value of NB/70K was elevated in 62% of patients with benign disease. In patients with elevated CA 125 and ovarian cancer, one of the two tests for B-72.3 or CA 15-3 was positive in 83% of the patients but in only 5% of the patients with benign disease. It should be noted that CA 125 levels were substantially higher in patients with cancer than in patients with benign disease.

With CA 125 levels above 65 U/ml, the risk that the patient, in retrospect, actually has ovarian cancer should be increased 100-fold. If elevations in CA-72.3 and CA 15-3 are also noted, the relative risk would increase to approximately 1000-fold. By using these data and extrapolating an incidence of ovarian cancer of 20:100,000 in patients over 40 years of age, five to ten false-positive results should be identified for every true-positive. In this high-risk population, ultrasound examination and careful physical examination should be considered. In addition, the use of MAbs may help identify the source of elevated CA 125 through radio-nuclide imaging.

   With ovarian carcinoma, then, it is possible to imagine a strategy to identify patients at risk for occult ovarian cancer by means of a single marker such as CA 125. Patients at even higher risk could then be identified by means of confirmatory assays and, if necessary, the site of elevated CA 125 could be determined either on noninvasive examination such as ultrasound or by the injection of radiolabeled MAbs for radionuclide imaging.

CA 125 in the Differential Diagnosis of Pelvic Masses

Patients presenting with pelvic masses for exploratory laparotomy would benefit from the preoperative diagnosis of cancer. In such instances, patients may be referred for primary exploration to an institution capable of performing definitive cytoreductive surgery. Repeat laparotomy for adequate cytoreduction could thus be avoided and primary cytotoxic therapy could be instituted promptly.

   Two major prospective studies have been conducted in such patients. At the Karolinska Institute in Stockholm, CA 125 values were determined in 100 patients before exploratory laparotomy (29). In 76 of 77 patients with benign disease, CA 125 levels were less than 65 U/ml. Consistent with previous observations, CA 125 was not elevated in patients with mucinous or borderline tumors, but was elevated in nine of 11 patients with ovarian cancer and in four of five patients with nonovarian gynecological malignancies. Overall, 13 of 14 patients with an elevated CA 125 levels and pelvic mass had some form of gynecological cancer. Similar results were obtained in a multicenter prospective trial in the United States (30). In patients with a pelvic mass, CA 125 higher than 50-65 U/ml predicted malignancy 80-90% of the women. Investigations are now under way to determine whether or not noninvasive preoperative evaluation of a pelvic mass (i.e., with ultrasound) in combination with CA 125 levels can better predict patients with ovarian cancer than does either modality alone.

   Thus, an elevated CA 125 level in a patient with a pelvic mass should heighten clinical suspicion of ovarian or nonovarian gyne-cological malignancies. Widespread use of the CA 125 assay may identify patients who should be referred to major institutions capable of carrying out first-line treatment.

Monitoring Tumor Status with CA 125 During Primary Therapy

The ability to monitor tumor status during primary therapy would provide the clinician with evidence of therapeutic efficacy. If elevated levels of CA 125 during primary therapy could predict a subset of patients whose tumor has not responded to standard cytotoxic chemotherapy, a more aggressive form of treatment may be considered. A multitude of studies from Europe, Japan, and the United States have confirmed that in approximately 80% of the patients with ovarian cancer serum CA 125 is elevated. (Table 2) (9,31-42). In a retrospective analysis, a remarkably good correlation was noted between stable, progressive, and regressive disease and stable, rising, and falling antigen levels, respectively (Figure 1). In the initial report in which OC-125 was used to monitor epithelial ovarian cancer, changes in antigen levels correlated with the disease course in 93% of the instances studied (9). Transient elevations in CA 125 have been observed after tumor lysis (18,33), but levels then decline, with a half-life of 4.8 days (33). Tumor regression has been associated with a decrease in antigen levels as much as 1000-fold.

In a double-blind collaborative study of 31 patients with epithelial ovarian cancer, serum CA 125 levels were monitored prospectively to assess the role of this antigenic marker in predicting persistent tumor (43). At 3 months, CA 125 values were found to be a highly significant prognostic factor. Failure of CA 125 to fall below 35 U/ml by 3 months correlated strongly with persistent disease at second-look operation after 9-12 months of cytotoxic therapy. All 13 patients whose CA 125 levels exceeded 35 U/ml at 3 months had persistent disease. It is important that persistent tumor was noted in some cases, even when CA 125 subsequently fell to less than 35 U/ml. The extent of decrease in CA 125 levels during the first 3 months of therapy was also predictive of clinical outcome. Levels were found to be reduced by at least 80% in 13 of 15 patients clinically free of disease at second-look operation; in the two patients who did not show this reduction, preoperative CA 125 levels had been less than 35 U/ml. Only five of 13 patients with clinically positive outcomes showed an 80% reduction in CA 125 levels.

Table 2 CA 125 Levels in Ovarian Cancer Patients

Investigators	Antigen levels (U/ml)	No. positive/ no. studied	Positive %
Bast et al. (9)	35	84/101	83
Chatal et al. (31)	30	35/38	92
Sarmini et al. (32)	35	14/27	52
Canney et al. (33)	35	45/58	83
Crombach et al. (34)	35	71/91	78
Auvray et al. (35)	35	43/49	83
Kreienberg and Melchart (36)	65	36/57	63
Lien (37)	65	29/30	97
Kimura et al. (38)	35	19/23	83
Eerdekens et al. (39)	35	10/20	50
Van Dalen et al. (40)	35	13/14	92
Heinonen et al. (41)	35	9/12	75%
Total		408/520	78.5%

Source: Ref. 42.

In summary, it appears that CA 125 levels are an effective indicator of tumor status in patients undergoing primary therapy.
Furthermore, stable, falling, and rising titers correlate with tumor
status. Failure of CA 125 to fall below 35 U/ml after 3 months of
treatment has been highly predictive of positive results on second-
look operation. If CA 125 fails to normalize after 3 months of
cytotoxic therapy, the patient may be considered for more aggressive treatment, such as intraperitoneal therapy or autologous
bone marrow transplantation.

Correlating Tumor Status with CA 125 at Second-Look Procedures

It has been customary practice to proceed with the second-look
surveillance procedure upon completion of primary treatment to

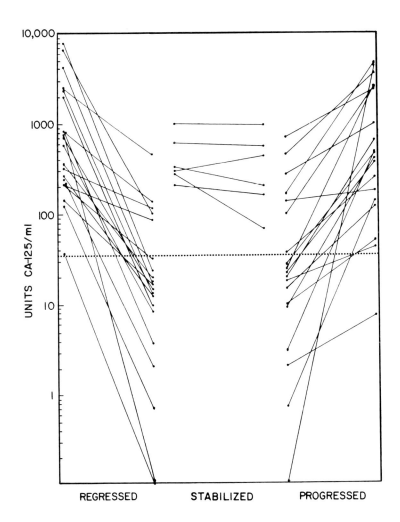

Figure 1   CA 125 levels in patients in whom disease has regressed, stabilized, or progressed (*Source*: Ref. 9.)

assess tumor status, and the role of CA 125 monitoring at this stage has been well studied. In several recent reports (44,45), serum CA 125 levels have been correlated with tumor status at second-look operations in patients with ovarian cancer. In one multicenter study, tumor status was correlated with CA 125 levels determined within 1 week of the second-look procedure in 81 patients (46). Seventeen patients with CA 125 levels higher than 35 U/ml all had tumor at second-look procedure, whereas 22 of 64 patients with levels below 35 U/ml were found to have tumor. The predictive values for positive and negative results on CA 125 assay were 100% and 65.6%, respectively.

Berek et al. (45) reported similar results in 55 patients in clinical remission who underwent second-look operation to assess disease status after chemotherapy (Table 3). Disease was discovered in all 12 patients with an elevated CA 125 level. The predictive value of a positive test result was 100%. Serum CA 125 levels less than 35 U/ml were found in 44% of patients with positive results on second-look, thus rendering a predictive value of 56% for a negative test result.

More recently, at the Brigham and Women's Hospital two patients were identified in whom CA 125 values were elevated months after cytotoxic chemotherapy (47). Evaluation by clinical examination, laparoscopy, and radiographic studies using CT scans failed to identify the source of these elevated antigen levels. On laparotomy and retroperitoneal dissection, metastatic tumors were found in retrocaval and paracaval lymph nodes.

These studies indicate that CA 125 levels above 35 U/ml correlate strongly with the presence of tumor upon completion of primary therapy. Although the specificity of this assay approaches 100%, its sensitivity remains low. When serum CA 125 levels return to less than 35 U/ml, small amounts of residual disease may be found in as many as 60% of patients. Greater sensitivity might be achieved if antigen levels in peritoneal fluid are measured. In one recent report from the National Cancer Institute, CA 125 levels were evaluated in 1500 ml of periotenal lavage fluid at the time of second-look laparoscopy (48). Antigen levels higher than 35 U/ml predicted disease status in 80% of the patients. The predictive value of a positive test result was 86% and that of a negative test result 72%.

Table 3 Correlation Between CA 125 Level and Residual Disease at Second-Look Examination

CA 125 assay	Residual disease at second look ($n = 54$)	
	No	Yes
Negative	24	18
Positive	0	12
Total	24	30

Sensitivity 12/30 = 40%; specificity 24/24 = 100%; predictive value of a positive result 12/12 = 100%; predictive value of a negative result 24/52 = 57.1%
Source: Ref. 45.

Preliminary data from the Brigham and Women's Hospital and Duke University Medical Center suggest that the level of CA 125 in a small amount of undiluted peritoneal fluid in healthy individuals with benign disease exceeds 200 U/ml in 2% of the patients (49); in malignant ascites, the value exceeds 200 U/ml in 80% of the patients. If these data are confirmed, residual disease may be documented by assaying CA 125 in fluid obtained by culdocentesis before second-look procedures.

An elevated serum CA 125 at the time of second-look procedure may, therefore, be considered presumptive evidence of persistent tumor. If false-positive results can be excluded, a second-look procedure may not be necessary to prove the presence of tumor. In this setting, the challenge is to identify the location of the tumor noninvasively and to treat the recurrent or persistent disease effectively.

CA 125 as a Predictor of Clinical Recurrence

Although elevated CA-125 levels at time of second-look surgery appear to indicate persistent tumor, the absence or presence of tumor at second-look may not be the most important factor for survival (50,51). Because survival is the most important variable, and is closely associated with the interval to clinical recurrence, it would be useful to have a tumor marker that could predict recurrence and, therefore, provide sufficient lead time to allow the oncologist to institute second-line therapy at an optimal time in selected patients.

In one multicenter study, serum CA 125 levels were followed in 55 patients with epithelial ovarian cancer who were clinically and radiographically free of tumor at time of second-look surgery (52). An elevated CA 125 level at second-look surgery was associated with a 60% chance of clinical recurrence within 4 months, compared with a 5% chance of recurrence for levels less than 35 U/ml. In patients with CA 125 levels above 35 U/ml, the risk for recurrence was greatest between 2 and 4 months after such surgery. Thirty-five patients had clinical recurrence after second-look surgery, with a mean lead time before recurrence of 3 months; in over 90% of patients, the mean lead time was at least 2 months (Figure 2). These results have been confirmed in separate reports (53).

Serum CA 125 and Survival

The ultimate goal in patients with ovarian cancer is to predict prognosis and to initiate effective therapy to achieve cure. Through the use of MAbs, clinicians can monitor patients with epithelial ovarian cancer during and at the completion of primary therapy. Monoclonal antibody testing can effectively predict tumor persistence and recurrence and may provide lead time during which second-line therapy can be initiated.

Studies are under way to determine whether CA 125 can be used to predict survival (54). In a preliminary investigation, survival correlated with CA 125 levels in patients undergoing second-look procedures (Figure 3). Survival was worse in patients with proven tumor and elevated CA 125 levels than in those whose CA 125 levels were below 35 U/ml with or without recurrence. It should be noted that the difference in survival rates between patients who had negative results on CA 125 assay with and without tumor recurrence was not statistically significant. This preliminary report suggests that CA 125 levels above 35 U/ml upon completion of therapy is a better predictor of survival than is the presence or absence of tumor alone.

Studies are now under way to assess the ability of "up-front" CA 125 levels to predict survival. The impact of surgical cytoreduction and cytotoxic chemotherapy on CA 125 levels and survival statistics needs to be examined.

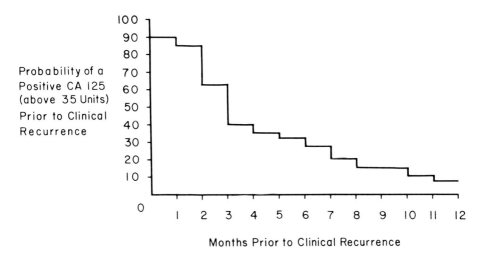

Figure 2   CA 125 lead time for patients with clinical recurrence (*Source*: J. M. Niloff, et al. The CA 125 assay as a predictor of clinical recurrence in epithelial ovarian cancer. *Am. J. Obstet. Gynecol. 155*: 56-60 (1986), with permission from the C. V. Mosby Co).

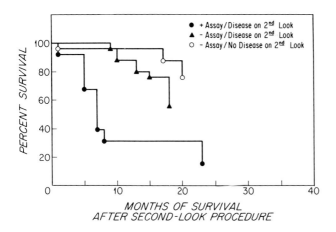

Figure 3   CA 125 and the presence or absence of disease at second-look procedure as correlated with survival (*Source*: courtesy of Centocor, Inc., Malvern, Pennsylvania).

MONOCLONAL ANTIBODIES TO OTHER OVARIAN CANCER-ASSOCIATED ANTIGENS

Since the first report of CA 125, a number of other MAbs that bind to both mucinous and nonmucinous tumors have been developed against ovarian cancer (Table 4) (55-85). In addition, a number of antibodies raised against other carcinomas and sarcomas have been found to react with ovarian cancers. Monoclonal antibodies associated with ovarian cancer have been used to detect major histocompatibility complex determinants (86), placental alkaline phosphatase (81,82), and estrogen receptors (87,88). Reagents have all been murine immunoglobulins except for one report of a human MAb (89).

The antigenic heterogeneity of ovarian tumors was examined in a recent report in which primary tumor and metastatic lesions from 21 patients were tested against a panel of eight different determinants defined by MAbs (90). The antigen profiles of the metastatic tumors differed from those of primary tumors in 10 patients, and not all the cells within a tumor bound antibody. When ascitic fluid from one patient was examined on five different occasions, variations were observed in antigen expression over time. Antigenic heterogeneity and the selection of antigenic variants over time must be considered when one is developing new approaches to immunodiagnosis or immunotherapy utilizing MAbs.

Ovarian carcinoma-associated antigens defined by MAbs have been described. Some of these antigens have proved to be carbohydrate epitopes expressed on high-molecular-weight glycoproteins and glycolipids. These may represent aberrant glycosal transferase or glycosidase activity of tumor cells (91,92). Among these carbohydrate determinants are CA 19-9 (66,67), MOV-2 (56,57), DUPAN-2 (68,69), F 36/27 (70,71), and DF-3 (72,74). Antigens, such as CA 125, CA 19-9, MOV-2, and B-72.3, may be coexpressed on the same high-molecular-weight glycoprotein.

Complementary Sera Markers

By measuring different antigens concurrently, researchers have hoped to monitor a great variety of histological tumors and attain greater sensitivity in detecting residual tumor. In an early study, the combined use of CEA, CA 125, and CA 19-19 was no more effective in monitoring ovarian tumor burdens than was CA 125

Table 4 Monoclonal Antibodies Reactive with Epithelial Ovarian Carcinomas

Source of immunogen	Antibody	Investigators
Ovarian carcinoma	OC-125	Bast et al. (1)
	ID3	Bhattacharya et al. (55,56)
	MOV-2	Tagliabue et al. (57,58)
	OC-133	Berkowitz et al. (59)
	MD144	Mattes et al. (60)
	MF61	Mattes et al. (60)
	MF116	Mattes et al. (60)
	632	Fleuren et al. (61)
	$4F_4, 7A_{10}$	Bhattacharya et al (62)
	$2C_8, 2F_7$	Bhattacharya et al. (63)
	3C2, 4C7	Tsuji et al. (64)
	WB12123	Knauf et al. (65)
	OVTL-3	Poels et al. (66)
	UMNMWR-2	Wahl and Piko (67)
	8C, 10B	Baumal et al. (68)
Endometrial carcinoma	MC55	Mattes et al. (60)
	MH94	Mattes et al. (60)
Colorectal carcinoma	19-9	Koprowski et al. (69, 70)
Pancreatic carcinoma	DU-PAN-2	Metzgar et al. (21,71)
Breast carcinoma	F36/22	Croghan et al. (72-74)
	DF3	Sekine et al. (25,26,75)
	B72.3	Colcher et al. (76,77)
	260F9	Frankel et al. (78,79)
	454C11	Frankel et al. (78,79)
	280D11	Frankel et al. (78,79)
	245E7	Frankel et al. (78,79)
Milk-fat globule protein	HMFG2	Epenetos et al.(80)
	AUA1	
Placental alkaline phosphase	NDOG2	Sunderland et al. (81)
	E6	Degroote et al. (82)
Laryngeal carcinoma	Ca-1	Woods et al. (83,84)
Osteogenic sarcoma	791-T/36	Embelton et al. (85)

Source: Ref. 42

alone (22). The antigens (CA 125) and NB/70K are distinct antigenic markers (93). Although each of these antigens alone is elevated in 80% of ovarian cancer patients, up to 98% of patients show elevated levels of at least one marker when these antigens are used in combination (94). A new assay using MAbs antibodies reactive with NB/70K is now under investigation. Several markers appear to complement CA 125, including MOV-2 (95), DF-3 (25), placental alkaline phosphatase (39,40), galactosyl transferse (96), and lipid-associated sialic acid (97). Assay of CA 125 has been shown to be more effective in monitoring epithelial ovarian cancer than are measurements of circulating immune complexes (98).

Immunocytochemical Detection of Malignancy

Monoclonal antibodies to several different tumor types have been examined in an effort to discriminate malignant from benign cells in cytological preparations. By use of HMFG-2 and AUAI antibodies, malignant cells were identified in 28 of 34 effusions and proved to be malignant histologically. Malignant cells were absent in 27 of 28 specimens examined (99). One specimen considered positive, based on antibody testing, was reexamined histologically and malignant cells were found. In a recent study of MOV-2, false-negative results were reported in 8% of the specimens (96). The antibodies F36-22 and B-72.3 react with ovarian tumor cells but not with benign mesothelial cells, suggesting a potential role in immunocytochemical studies (75,78).

It would be useful if individual MAbs could aid in the diagnosis of unknown primary tumors. At present, the available MAbs react with cells of primary tumors from different sites. Phenotypes defined with multiple MAbs might allow more effective discrimination of tumor cells at different primary sites.

RADIONUCLIDE IMAGING OF OVARIAN CANCER WITH MONO-CLONAL ANTIBODIES

The ability to conjugate isotopes to antibodies of different specificity has allowed radiounclide imaging of human ovarian carcinoma. Conjugates have been prepared utilizing iodine-131, iodine-123, and indium-111 to label polyclonal antibodies or MAbs reactive with human milk-fat globulin (HMFG) (80,100,101), placental alkaline phosphatase (102-104), carcinoembryonic antigen (CEA; 105), CA 125 (106,107), and osteogenic sarcoma-related antigen (104). In reports to date, tumors of the pelvis have been more readily identified than have para-aortic or diaphragmatic metastases. Because of the antigenic heterogeneity of these tumors, it has been suggested that a cocktail of labeled MAbs might provide better visualization than would use of a single MAb.

Several limitations need to be overcome before radionuclide imaging can be considered clinically useful. In the case of ^{131}I-labeled OC-125, the serum half-life of the MAb is prolonged by the formation of complexes with circulating antigen and may limit detection of small metastases (108). With other MAb conjugates, uptake of the label by the gut mucosa and urine has created artifacts. Conjugate uptake by the liver and ascitic fluid has also made localization of small tumor nodules difficult. Finally, although the sensitivity of immunoscintigraphy is promising, its specificity has not been satisfactory. By use of ^{123}I-labeled HMFG-2, scanning successfully localized ovarian cancer in 19 of 20 patients (101). Scans were also positive in 50% of patients studied who did not have ovarian cancer. If these limitations of radiolabeled MAb conjugates can be overcome, radionuclide imaging of ovarian cancer may greatly aid in the diagnosis of malignancy and the detection of recurrent or persistent disease.

SEROTHERAPY OF OVARIAN CARCINOMA WITH MONOCLONAL ANTIBODIES

The use of MAbs to ovarian cancer may also provide an avenue for effective therapy in augmenting antibody-dependent cell-mediated cytotoxicity (ADCC) or in delivering direct toxins, even in the presence of inadequate host-effector mechanisms.

Evidence for antitumor activity following contact between antibody and tumor cells has been obtained in animal models. Bast et al. (109) have shown that the addition of *Cornebacterium parvum* to a heteroantigen against a murine ovarian carcinoma eliminates more tumor cells than does injection of heteroantigen alone. *Corynebacterium parvum* increased the number and activity of effector cells capable of ADCC. Targeting effectors may require different strategies. Recent cell culture studies using the chemo-attractant formyl-methionyl-leucyl-phenylalanine linked to MAbs

OC-125 and OC-133 suggest that lymphocytes and macrophages can be attracted to these targets (110). It remains to be seen if these effectors of ADCC can lyse human epithelial ovarian tumor cells in situ. One of the main drawbacks may be a reduction in effectors for ADCC noted in patients with ovarian cancer. The effector formation may also be inhibited by the levels of circulating immune complexes, which are often elevated in ovarian cancer patients.

Because of the problem with effector function, an alternative serotherapeutic approach might be the delivery of cytotoxic drug, plant toxins, or radionuclides. Hamilton et al. (111) have described a xenograft model of human ovarian cancer that produces ascites and intraabdominal carcinomatosis in mice . Monoclonal antibody-plant toxin conjugates have been evaluated in tumor heterografts grown intraperitoneally in nude mice. Using this model, ricin-A conjugated to an antibody against human transferrin receptor has inhibited the growth of up to 10^7 human ovarian cancer cells and has significantly prolonged the survival of mice (112). Conjugates containing pseudomonal exotoxin were even more effective than conjugates containing the ricin-A chain.

A clinical study of ^{131}I conjugated to HMFG has been reported from Hammersmith Hospital in London (113,114). Twelve patients received intraperitoneal injections of a radionuclide conjugate with tolerable hematological and gastrointestinal toxicities. Doses as high as 150 mCi were administered to patients with ascites. In patients with stage IV disease, three of four patients reported symptomatic improvement but died within 6 months. In two patients with large-volume stage III disease, tumor stabilized for 6-8 months. Six patients with tumor volumes less than 2 cm were treated, with a complete response in four patients; two of these patients have remained in remission for more than 2 years after therapy.

Because ovarian cancer frequently spreads by surface continiguity over the peritoneum, intraperitoneal administration of immunoconjugate is likely to be more effective than intravenous administration. A higher concentration of drug can be targeted in the abdominal cavity and less toxicity will be encountered owing to intraperitoneal pharmacokinetics.

In recent phase I studies at the Brigham and Women's Hospital, ^{131}I-labeled OC-125 has been given intraperitoneally and intravenously to patients undergoing second-look procedures (115). In these early studies, intraperitoneal therapy has yielded a lower percentage of injected dose/per kilogram in blood and marrow when compared with intravenous administration. In addition, up to 10% of the dose per kilogram can be recovered in the tumor after intraperitoneal administration compared with 1-5% after intravenous administration. From these studies, it would appear that intraperitoneal therapy with radioisotope-labeled OC-125 may result in lower systemic toxicities and higher absorption of immunoconjugate by the tumor.

In the laboratory at the Brigham and Women's Hospital, OC-125 has recently been conjugated to chromophores. It is hoped that light activation of chromophore-antibody conjugate will lead to tumor cell lysis. Although this novel approach to tumoricidal activity may be futuristic, the use of MAb conjugates holds great promise for targeted delivery of various agents to tumor cells. It is also within reason to think that tumor cell uptake by a chromophore-MAb conjugate can effectively lead to tumor lysis.

Clinical trials should now be undertaken in patients who have residual disease after conventional cytoreduction and chemotherapy. These clinical trials should include immunotherapy utilizing MAbs and various MAb conjugates to determine the effective agents. Again, antigenic heterogeneity of tumors in different patients and of metastases within the same patient pose potential problems. If therapy is to be effective, it will certainly require a mixture of MAb/conjugates containing MAbs to a variety of different specificities.

CONCLUSION

Monoclonal antibody technology has begun to have some impact on the course and treatment of ovarian cancer. Cytotoxic chemotherapy has given the gynecological oncologist a means of producing tumor regression in most patients. Still, the overall survival of patients with stage III or IV ovarian cancer remains poor. The major frontiers in ovarian cancer are the ability to diagnose cancer when the tumor is asymptomatic and confined to the ovary and the ability to treat persistent residual or recurrent disease effectively. Monoclonal antibody and the development of MAbs reactive with ovarian cancer offer great promise toward realizing the goals.

REFERENCES

1. R. C. Bast, Jr., M. Feeney, H. Lazarus, L. Nadler, R. B. Colvin, and R. C. Knapp, *J. Clin. Invest. 68*:1331 (1981).
2. Y. Musuho, M. Zalutsky, R. C. Knapp, and R. C. Bast, Jr., *Cancer Res. 44*:2813 (1984).
3. H. M. Davis, V. R. Zurawski, Jr., R. C. Bast, Jr., and T. C. Klug. Isolation and partial characterization of an antigen associated with human epithelial ovarian carcinomas *Cancer Res. 46*:6143 (1986).
4. S. E. Kabawat, R. C. Bast, Jr., W. R. Welch, R. C. Knapp, and R. B. Colvin, *Am. J. Clin. Pathol. 79*:98 (1983).
5. S. E. Kabawat, R. C. Bast, Jr., A. K. Bhan, W. R. Welch, R. C. Knapp, and R. B. Colvin, *Int. J. Gynecol. Pathol. 2*:275 (1983).
6. E. J. Nouwen, D. E. Pollet, M. W. Eerdekens, P. G. Hendrix, T. W. Briers, and M. E. DeBroe, *Cancer Res. 46*:866 (1986).
7. J. Shishi, M. Ghazizadeh, T. Oguro, K. Aihara, and T. Araki, *Am. J. Clin. Pathol. 85*:595 (1986).
8. F. G. Hanisch, G. Uhlenbruck, C. Dienst, M. Strottrop, and E. Hippauf, *Eur. J. Biochem. 149*:323 (1985).
9. R. C. Bast, Jr., T. L. Klug, E. St. John, E. Jenison, J. Niloff, H. Lazarus, R. S. Berkowitz, T. Leavitt, C. T. Griffiths, L. Parker, V. R. Zurawski, and R. C. Knapp, *N. Engl. J. Med. 309*:883 (1983).
10. T. L. Klug, R. C. Bast, Jr., J. M. Niloff, R. C. Knapp, and V. R. Zurawski, *Cancer Res. 44*:1048 (1984).
11. J. M. Niloff, T. L. Klug, E. Schaetzl, V. R. Zurawski, R. C. Knapp, and R. C. Bast, Jr., *Am. J. Obstet. Gynecol. 148*:1057 (1985).
12. P. J. Green, S. K. Ballas, P. Westkaemper, H. G. Schwart, T. L. Klug, and V. R. Zurawski, *J. Natl. Cancer Inst. 77*:(2):337 (1986).
13. J. M. Niloff, R. C. Knapp, E. Schaetzl, C. Reynolds, and R. C. Bast, Jr., *Obstet. Gynecol. 64*:703 (1985).
14. M. Suzuki, I. Sekiguchi, M. Ohwada, T. Tamada, I. Sakurabayashi, and T. Kawai, *Rinsho Biyori 33*:285 (1985).
15. R. L. Barbieri, J. M. Niloff, R. C. Bast, Jr., E. Schaetzl, R. W. Kistner, and R. C. Knapp, *Fertil. Steril. 45*:630 (1986).
16. A. Ruibal, G. Encabo, J. A. Capdevila, S. Aguade, R. Gefaell, E. Ribera, and J. M. Martinez-Vasquez, *Med. Clin. 82*:560 (1984).
17. S. Knauf and G. I. Urbach, *Am. J. Obstet. Gynecol. 138*:1222 (1980).
18. R. C. Bast, Jr., F. P. Siegal, C. Runowicz, T. L. Klug, V. R. Zurawski, D. Schonholz, C. J. Cohen, and R. C. Knapp, *Gyecol. Oncol. 22*:115 (1985).
19. V. R. Zurawski, Jr., (Personal communication—data from Centocor).
20. V. R. Zurawski, S. F. Broderick, P. T. Lavin, P. Pickens, R. C. Knapp, and R. C. Bast, Jr., Serum CA 125 in a large group of non-hospitalized women: Relevance for the early detection of ovarian cancer *Obstet. Gynecol.* (in press).

21. R. S. Metzgar, M. T. Gaillard, S. J. Levine, F. L. Tuck, E. H. Bossen, and M. J. Borowitz, *Cancer Res.* 42:601 (1982).
22. R. C. Bast, Jr., T. L. Klug, E. Schaetzl, P. Lavin, J. M. Niloff, T. F. Greber, V. R. Zurawski, Jr., and R. C. Knapp, *Am. J. Obstet. Gynecol.* 149:553 (1984).
23. P. A. Canney, P. M. Wilkinson, R. D. James, and M. Moore, *Br. J. Cancer* 52:131 (1985).
24. R. C. Bast, Jr., T. Klug, A. Rheinhardt-Clark, C. Harrison, R. C. Knapp, and V. R. Zurawski, Jr., Coexpression of carbohydrate determinants on CA-125 positive moieties (in preparation).
25. H. Sekine, D. F. Hayes, K. A. Keefe, E. Schaetzl, R. C. Bast, Jr., R. C. Knapp, and D. W. Kufe, *J. Clin. Oncol.* 3:1355 (1985).
26. H. Sekine, T. Ohno, and D. W. Kufe, *J. Immunol.* 135:3610 (1985).
27. J. Hilkens, F. Bulis, J. Hilgers, P. H. Hageman, J. Calafat, A. Sonneburg, and B. Van der Valk, *Int. J. Cancer* 34:197 (1984).
28. R. C. Bast, Jr., A. Rheinhardt-Clark, D. Kufe, J. Schlom, V. R. Zurawski, Jr., R. C. Knapp, and R. E. Ritts, Development of confirmatory assays for the presence of ovarian cancer in patients with elevated CA 125 (in preparation).
29. N. Einhorn, R. C. Bast, Jr., R. C. Knapp, B. Tjernberg, and V. R. Zurawski, *Obstet. Gynecol.* 67:414 (1986).
30. G. D. Malkasian, R. C. Knapp, V. R. Zurawski, Jr., C. K. Podratz, C. R. Stanhope, R. Mortel, J. S. Berek, and R. C. Bast, Jr., Preoperative elevation of serum CA 125 levels in patients with pelvic masses — a discriminatory evaluation (submitted for publication).
31. J. F. Chatal, G. Ricolleau, P. Fumoleau, M. Kramer, C. Curtet, and J. Y. Douillard, *Cancer Detect. Pre.* 6:624 (1983).
32. H. Sarmini, M. Scalet, P. Pouillart, D. Robinet, A. Mazabraud, J. Bon, and A. Funes, *Monoclonal Antibodies in Oncology: Clinical Applications* (J. F. Chatal, M. Davis, and R. C. Angers, eds.) Nantes, (France) (1985).
33. P. A. Canney, M. Moore, P. M. Wilkinson, and R. D. James, *Br. J. Cancer* 50:765 (1984).
34. G. Crombach, H. H. Zippel, and H. Wurz, *Cancer Detect. Prev.* 6:623 (1983).
35. E. Auvray, P. Kerbrat, J. de Certaines, and C. Benoist, *Clin. Appl.* (Nantes) (1984).
36. R. Kreienberg and F. Melchart, *Cancer Detect. Prev.* 6:619 (1983).
37. L. C. Lien, F. X. Hu, and W. S. Liu, *Chin. J. Obstet. Gynecol.* 20:257 (1985).
38. E. Kinura, M. Murae, R. Koga, Y. Odawara, Y. Kakakayashi, K. Yokiyama, H. Nakata, T. Totake, K. Ochiai, M. Yasuda, Y. Tereshima, and S. Hachiya, *Acta Obstet. Gynecol. Jpn.* 26:2121 (1984).
39. M. W. Eerdekens, E. J. Nouwen, D. E. Pollet, T. W. Briers, and M. E. DeBroe, *Clin. Chem.* 3:687 (91985).

40. M. E. L. van den Burg, W. L. J. van Putten, P. H. Cox, and W. C. Haije, *ECCO 3*, Stockholm, Sweden, p. 135 (1985).

41. P. K. Heinonen, K. Tontti, T. Koivula, and P. Pystynen, *Br. J. Obstet. Gynecol. 92*:528 (1985).

42. R. C. Bast, Jr. and R. C. Knapp, in *Important Advances in Oncology* (W. Devita, S. Hellman, S. Rosenberg, eds.), J. P. Lippincott, Philadelphia (1987), pp. 39-53.

43. P. T. Lavin, R. C. Knapp, G. Malkasian, R. F. Mortel, E. Schaetzl, J. C. Berek, V. R. Zurawski, and R. C. Bast, Jr., CA-125 for monitoring of ovarian carcinoma during primary therapy (*Obstet. Gynecol. 69*:223 (1987).

44. J. M. Niloff, R. C. Bast, Jr., E. M. Schaetzl, and R. C. Knapp, *Am. J. Obstet. Gynecol. 151*:981 (1985).

45. J. S. Berek, R. C. Knapp, G. D. Malkasian, P. T. Lavin, N. F. Hacker, C. Whitney, J. M. Niloff, and R. C. Bast, Jr., *Obstet. Gynecol. 67*:685 (1986).

46. V. R. Zurawski, personal communication.

47. N. J. Finkler, S. J. Kapnick, C. T. Griffiths, and R. C. Knapp, Elevated serum CA-125 and epithelial ovarian cancer metastatic to retroperitoneal lymph nodes *Gyn. Onc.* (in press).

48. C. J. Allegra, R. L. Fine, B. C. Behrens, M. H. Zweic, Y. Ostcheg, R. F. Ozols, and R. C. Young, *Proc. Am. Soc. Clin. Oncol. 5*:118 (1986).

49. R. C. Bast, Jr., J. B. Weinberg, C. Haney, J. Soper, W. Creasman, V. R. Zurawski, Jr., and R. C. Knapp, CA-125 levels in peritoneal fluid in benign and malignant disease (in preparation).

50. J. S. Berek, N. F. Hacker, and L. D. Lagasse, *Obstet. Gynecol. 64*:207 (1984).

51. J. T. Wharton, C. L. Edwards, and F. N. Rutledge, *Am. J. Obstet. Gynecol. 148*:997 (1984).

52. J. M. Niloff, R. C. Knapp, P. T. Lavin. G. D. Malkasian, J. S. Berek, R. Mortel, V. R. Zurawski, Jr., and R. C. Bast, Jr., *Am. J. Obstet. Gynecol. 155*:56 (1986).

53. R. C. Knapp, P. T. Lavin, E. Schaetzl, J. M. Niloff, and R. C. Bast, Jr., *Proc. Soc. Gynecol. Oncol. 16*:30 (1985).

54. J. M. Niloff and R. C. Knapp, personal communication.

55. M. Bhattacharya, S. K. Chatterjee, J. J. Barlow, and H. Fuki, *Cancer Res. 42*:1650 (1982).

56. A. Gangopadhyay, M. Bhattacharya, S. K. Chatterjee, J. J. Barlow, and Y. Tsukada, *Cancer Res. 45*:1744 (1985).

57. E. Tagliabue, S. Menard, G. Della Torre, P. Barbanti, R. Miriani-Costantini, G. Porro, and M. I. Colanghi, *Cancer Res. 45*:379 (1985).

58. S. Miotti, S. Aguanno, S. Canevari, A. Diotti, R. Orlandi, S. Sonnino, and M. I. Colnaghi, *Cancer Res. 45*:826 (1985).

59. R. S. Berkowitz, S. Kabawat, H. Lazarus, R. C. Colvin, R. C. Knapp, and R. C. Bast, Jr., *Am. J. Obstet. Gynecol. 146*:607 (1983).
60. M. J. Mattes, C. Cordon-Cardo, J. L. Lewis, Jr., L. J. Old, and K. O. Lloyd, *Proc. Natl. Acad. Sci. USA 81*:568 (1984).
61. G. Fleuren, E. Coerkamp, M. Nap, and S. Warnaar, *Clin. Appl.* (Nantes) (1984).
62. M. Bhattacharya, S. K. Chatterjee, and J. J. Barlow, *Cancer Res. 44*:4528 (1984).
63. M. Battacharya, S. K. Chatterjee, A. Gangopadhyay, and J. J. Barlow, *Hybridoma 4*:49 (1985).
64. Y. Tsuji, T. Suzuki, H. Nishiura, T. Takemura, and S. Isojima, *Cancer Res. 45*:2358 (1985).
65. S. Knauf, J. Kalwas, B. F. Helkamp, L. W. Harwell, J. Beecham, and E. M. Lord, *Cancer Immunol. Immunother. 21*:217 (1986).
66. L. Poels, D. Peters, Y. van Megen, G. P. Vooijs, R. N. M. Berheyan, A. Willemen, C. C. van Nierkerk, P. H. K. Jap, G. Mungyer, and P. Kenemans, *J. Natl. Cancer Inst. 76*:781 (1986).
67. R. Wahl, and C. Piko, *Proc. Am. Assoc. Cancer Res. 26*:298 (1985).
68. R. Baumal, J. Law, R. N. Buick, H. Kahn, H. Yeger, K. Sheldon, T. Colgan, and A. Marks, Monoclonal antibodies to an epithelial ovarian adenocarcinoma: Distinctive reactivity with xenografts of the original tumor and a cultured cell line (submitted for publication).
69. H. Koprowski, Z. Stelewski, K. Mitchell, M. Herlyn, D. Herlyn, and J. P. Fuhrer, *Somatic Cell Genet. 5*:957 (1979).
70. C. Charpin, A. K. Bhan, and V. Zurawski, *Int. J. Gynecol. Pathol. 1*:231 (1982).
71. M. S. Lan, O. J. Finn, P. D. Fernsten, and R. S. Metzgar, *Cancer Res. 45*: 305 (1985).
72. L. D. Papsidero, G. A. Croghan, J. J. O'Connell, L. A. Valenzuela, T. Nemoto, and T. M. Chu, *Cancer Res. 43*:1741 (1983).
73. G. A. Croghan, L. D. Papsidero, L. A. Valenzuela, T. Nemoto, R. Penetrante, and T. M. Chu, *Cancer Res. 43*:4980 (1983).
74. G. A. Crohan, M. B. Wingate, M. Gamarra, E. Johnson, M. Chut, H. Allen, L. Valenzuela, Y. Tsukada, and L. D. Papsidero, *Cancer Res. 44*: 1954 (1984).
75. D. Kufe, G. Inghirami, M. Abe, D. Hayes, H. Justin-Wheeler, and J. Schlom, *Hybridoma 3*:223 (1984).
76. D. Colcher, P. Horan Hand, J. Nutim, and J. Schlom, *Cancer Invest. 1*: 127 (1983).
77. W. W. Johnston, C. A. Szapk, S. C. Lottich, A. Thor, and J. Schlom, *Cancer Res. 45*:1894 (1985).
78. A. E. Frankel, D. B. Ring, E. Tringale, and S. T. Hsieh-Ma, *J. Biol. Resp. Mod. 4*:273 (1985).

79. R. Pirker, D. J. P. Fitzgerald, T. C. Hamilton, R. F. Ozols, W. Laird, A.
     E. Frankel, M. C. Willingham, and I. Paston, *J. Clin. Invest. 76*:1261
     (1985).
80. A. E. Epenetos, S. Mather, M. Granowska, C. C. Nimmon, L. R. Haw-
     kins, K. E. Britton, J. Shepherd, J. Taylor-Papadimitriou, H. Durbin, J.
     S. Malpas, and W. F. Bodmer, *Lancet 2*:999 (1982).
81. C. A. Sunderland, J. O. Davies, and G. M. Stirrat, *Cancer Res. 44*:96
     (1984).
82. G. DeGroote, P. DeWade, A. van de Voorde, M. L. DeBroe, and W.
     Fiers, *Clin. Chem. 29*:115 (1983).
83. F. Ahsall, M. E. Bramwell, and H. Harris, *Lancet 2*:1 (1982).
84. J. C. Woods, A. I. Spriggs, H. Harris, and J. O. D. McGee, *Lancet 2*:
     512 (1982).
85. M. J. Embleton, B. Gunn, V. S. Byers, and R. W. Baldwin, *Br. J. Cancer
     43*:582 (1981).
86. S. E. Kabawat, R. C. Bast, Jr., W. R. Welch, R. C. Knapp, and A. K.
     Bhan, *Int. J. Cancer 32*:547 (1983).
87. M. F. Press, J. A. Holt, A. L. Herbst, and G. L. Greene, *Lab.Invest. 53*:
     349 (1985).
88. M. A. Lorincz, J. A. Holt, and G. L. Greene, *J. Clin. Endocrinol. Metab.
     61*:412 (1985).
89. W. H. Stomson and F. Al-Azzawi, *Ovarian Cancer Symposium*, Glasgow
     2.8 (1985).
90. J. M. Niloff, W. Welch, S. Taylor, A. Battaile, D. Anderson, R. C.
     Knapp, and R. C. Bast, Jr., *Gynecol. Oncol. 23*:246 (1986).
91. H. G. Rittenhouse, G. L. Manderino, G. M. Hass, *Lab. Med. 16*:556
     (1985).
92. T. Feizi, *Nature 314*:53 (1985).
93. S. Knauf, D. Andeson, R. C. Knapp, R. C. Bast, Jr., *Am. J. Obstet.
     Gynecol. 152*:911 (1985).
94. A. J. Dembo, D. L. Chany, A. Malkin, and G. I. Urbach, *Proc. Soc.
     Gynecol. Oncol. 16*:30 (1985).
95. M. J. Colnaghi, S. Canavari, S. Menard, S. Miotti, and F. L. Rilke,
     Monoclonal Antibodies (1984); Florence.
96. P. Gauduchon, J. Goussard, J. F. Heron, C. Bouvet, C. Tillier, E. Bar,
     and J. Y. LeTalaer, *Ovarian Cancer Symposium*, Glasgow 2.24 (1985).
97. P. E. Schwartz, S. K. Chambers, J. T. Chambers, J. Gutmann, R. S.
     Foemmel, and A. R. Beherman, *Proc. Am. Soc. Clinc. Oncol. 4*:118
     (1985).
98. J. Dodd, J. P. P. Tyler, A. J. Crandon, N. J. Blumenthal, R. A. Fay, P.
     J. Baird, L. J. Hicks, and C. N. Hudson, *Br. J. Obstet. Gynecol. 92*:
     1054 (1985).
99. R. C. Bast and R. C. Knapp, in *Monoclonal Antibodies for the Diagno-
     sis and Therapy of Cancer* (J. A. Roth, ed.), Future Publishing Co. (in
     press).

100. A. A. Epenetos, J. Shepherd, K. E. Britton, S. Mather, J. Taylor-Papadi-mitriou, M. Granowska, H. Durbin, C. C. Nimmon, L. R. Hawkins, J. S. Malpas, and W. F. Bodmer, *Cancer 55*:984 (1985).
101. M. Granowska, K. E. Britton, J. H. Shepherd, C. C. Nimmon, S. Mather, B. Ward, R. J. Osborne, and M. L. Slevin, *J. Clin. Oncol. 4*:730 (1986).
102. A. A. Epenetos, D. Snook, G. Hooker, R. Begent, H. Durbin, R. T. D. Oliver, W. F. Bodmer, and J. P. Lavender, *Lancet 2*:350 (1985).
103. J. O. Davies, E. R. Davies, K. Howe, P. C. Jackson, E. M. Pitcher, C. S. Sadowski, G. M. Stirrat, and C. A. Sunderland, *Br. J. Obstet. Gynecol. 92*:277 (1985).
104. E. M. Symonds, A. C. Perkins, M. V. Pimm, R. W. Baldwin, J. G. Hardy, and D. A. Williams, *Br. J. Obstet. Gynecol. 92*:270 (1985).
105. J. R. van Nagell, Jr., E. Kim, S. Casper, F. S. Primus, S. Bennett, F. H. Deland, and D. M. Goldenberg, *Cancer Res. 40*:502 (1980).
106. J. F. Chatal, P. Fumoleau, J. C. Saccavini, A. Bianco-Arco, A. Chet-taneau, P. Peltier, M. Kremer, Y. Guillard, A. Becam, and B. L. Mevel, Diagnostic value of emission-computed tomography using ^{131}I-labeled F (ab|) $_2$ fragments from monoclonal antibodies including OC-125 in the prospective detection of recurrences of gynecological carcinomas, *J. Clin. Inves.* (in press).
107. D. J. Hantowich, T. W. Griffin, J. McGann, M. Rusckowski, M. Gionet, R. Hunter, and P. W. Doherty, *International Conference on Monoclonal Antibody Immunoconjugates for Cancer*. San Diego, (1986), p. 40.
108. H. J. Haisma, A. Battaile, R. C. Knapp, and V. R. Zurawski, Jr., *International Conference on Monoclonal Antibody Immunoconjugates for Cancer*. Sand Diego, (1986), p. 44.
109. R. C. Bast, Jr., R. C. Knapp, A. Mitchell, J. Thurston, R. Tucker, and S. F. Schlossman, *J. Immunol. 123*:19145 (1979).
110. R. Obrist, R. Reilly, T. Leavitt, R. C. Knapp, and R. C. Bast, Jr., *Int. J. Immunopharmacol. 5*:307 (1983).
111. T. C. Hamilton, R. C. Young, K. G. Louie, B. C. Behrens, W. M. Mc-Koy, K. R. Grotzinger, and R. F. Ozols, *Cancer Res. 44*:5286 (1985).
112. D. J. Fitzgerald, M. J. Bjorn, R. J. Ferris, J. L. Winkelhake, A. E. Frankel, T. C. Hamilton, R. F. Ozols, M. C. Willingham, and I. Pastan, anti-tumor activity of an immunotoxin directed against the transferrin receptor of human ovarian cancer cells in nude mice (submitted for publication).
113. Hammersmith Oncology Group, *Lancet 1*:441 (1984).
114. A. A. Epenetos, *International Conference on Monoclonal Antibody Immunoconjugates for Cancer*. San Diego, (1986), p. 17.
115. H. Haisma, personal communication.

7
Monoclonal Antibody Assays for Pancreatic Cancer

Richard S. Metzgar, Michael J. Borowitz, Michael A. Hollingsworth, Young Woo Kim, and Michael S. Lan / Duke University Medical Center, Durham, North Carolina

INTRODUCTION

Human pancreatic adenocarcinoma has been a difficult malignancy to diagnose and study for a number of reasons. Among these difficulties, the inaccessible anatomical location of the pancreas is preeminent. Because the pancreas is sequestered among other organs of the gut, most previous attempts at early diagnosis have not been successful. Nevertheless, because the 2% of pancreatic adenocarcinoma patients who survive are those whose tumors are discovered fortuitously and surgically excised at a premetastatic stage, there is still considerable motivation for early diagnostic procedures. Most recently, modern immunological techniques using polyclonal and monoclonal antibodies (MAbs) have been applied to this problem.

The use of polyclonal antibodies in serological assays for pancreatic cancer started with the carcinoembryotic antigen (CEA) and was followed by the pancreatic oncofetal antigen (POA) and the 'PCAA assays (1,2). More recently, considerable attention has been given to the 19-9 and DU-PAN-2 antigens defined by murine MAbs (3,4) (for a review, see Ref. 5). In some instances, such as DU-PAN-2 and POA, the antibodies were elicited to pancreatic tumor material, whereas the CEA and 19-9 antibodies were elicited to colon tumors. One implication of these studies was that few, or none, of the antigens studied demonstrated organ specificity for the pancreas. This has been confirmed by the recent description of other MAbs elicited to breast and colorectal tumors, which also showed reactivity with adenocarcinomas from other organ sites (3,6). Moreover, the antigens of pancreatic tumors defined by most MAbs can usually be found on a variety of normal secretory tissues. Most pancreatic tumor markers defined by MAbs are, like CEA, also classified as oncofetal or developmental antigens. The rationale for classifying the antigens as oncofetal or developmental was: (1) there were often distinct differences in the distribution of the antigens between fetal and normal adult tissues; (2) a high percentage of tumors expressed the antigens to a greater degree than seen in normal adult tissues; (3) there was significant intertumor and intratumor heterogeneity of antigen expression, although, this heterogeneity has never been directly related to a stage of differentiation; and (4) serum assays for DU-PAN-2 and 19-9 antigens showed that fetal and newborn sera exhibited significantly higher levels than did sera of adults (7,8).

In contrast to the lack of specificity of pancreatic tumor antigens, early studies of normal exocrine pancreatic antigens demonstrated that a number of these antigens showed organ specificity (9,10). Many of these antigens, defined by polyclonal antisera, were associated with acinar cell secretory activity (11,12). Although most human exocrine pancreatic tumors are assumed to be of ductal cell origin, it is still disappointing that none of the antigens associated with this malignancy demonstrate specificity for the pancreas. However, because pure or enriched ductal cell populations were not tested with the polyclonal antibodies to pancreatic organ-specific antigens, the presence of these antigens on this cell type was never well documented.

Although a common embryonic origin of normal ductal and acinar cells is well documented, well-differentiated ductal and acinar cells usually express rather distinct biochemical or antigenic properties (13). The principal function of the differentiated acinar cell is to secrete digestive enzymes, whereas the major function of the ductal cells is transport of these enzymes. Many of the diagnostically useful pancreatic tumor-associated antigens now defined by MAbs have been highly glycosylated molecules with mucinlike biochemical characteristics (14,15). These antigens have not been functionally characterized, but some of the mucin-type antigens are secreted by normal and malignant cells and are assumed to have the usual protective and lubricative functions of these types of molecules. The functional properties are probably common to ductal or secretory epithelial cells from other organs, thus accounting for the observed tissue distribution of this class of pancreatic tumor antigens.

Some of the antigenic epitopes defined by murine MAbs reactive with pancreatic adenocarcinomas have been defined biochemically. These epitopes are often blood group antigens and have been relatively easy to define because they are expressed on glycolipids as well as on glycoproteins. In contrast, the DU-PAN-2 epitope has, thus far, been found only in its mucinous form (14). The structure of the DU-PAN-2 epitope has been difficult to establish because all efforts to degrade the molecule into subunits have resulted in a loss of antibody-binding activity. However, these large mucinlike glycoproteins have been useful for immunodiagnosis because they are readily detectable in body fluids. Many of the epitopes are stable to formalin fixation, making them amenable to extensive immunohistological studies.

The possible functional role of structural alterations in glycoproteins during differentiation or oncogenesis has been the topic of several recent reviews (16,17). Differences in the expression of blood group antigens between normal and malignant gastrointestinal tract tissues has been recently reported (18,19). Monoclonal antibodies to 19-9 and to ABO and Lewis blood group antigens have also been used in immunohistological studies to demonstrate heterogeneity of human pancreatic acinar cell populations.

The results of this latter study indicate that there may be several regulatory systems that can influence or regulate blood group antigen expression in a tissue-specific or cell-specific pattern (20).

Monoclonal antibodies have also been characterized that react with polypeptide and other glycoprotein molecules of pancreatic tumors (21-23). These MAbs and their antigens will be discussed in this chapter only if they have been tested in a diagnostic clinical setting.

The two major diagnostic applications of MAbs to exocrine pancreatic cancer include the use of immunohistological techniques at the tissue level and the detection by immunoassay of soluble antigens shed or released by tumor cells into body fluids. Because the 19-9 and CEA antigens are covered by separate chapters in this volume, the examples and technology in this chapter will be related to our experience and that of others with the DU-PAN series of MAbs to pancreatic tumor antigens (4,24). Some data and discussion of the use of multiple serum assays for the immunodiagnosis of pancreatic and hepatic tumors will be considered below. The limitations of the immunohistology and the serum marker assays will be considered and discussed in the appropriate sections.

IMMUNOHISTOCHEMICAL ANALYSIS OF PANCREATIC CARCINOMA BY MONOCLONAL ANTIBODIES

Immunohistochemistry in tumor diagnosis has, in general, been more concerned with classification of malignancies than with the diagnosis of malignancy per se. In large part, this has been due to the lack of availability of absolutely tumor-specific reagents. Immunohistochemistry has clearly been useful in distinguishing among carcinomas, melanomas, or lymphomas, or in subclassifying tumors, particularly lymphomas. However, its utility in subclassifying epithelial malignancies is less well established.

Pancreatic carcinomas are often difficult to diagnose by routine morphological means, particularly as inflammatory conditions of the pancreas, which may mimic carcinoma clinically, may also produce an atypical morphological appearance. Although some pancreatic carcinoma-associated MAbs show a degree of selectivity for carcinoma over chronic pancreatitis (see following discussion), these have not been tested in appropriate clinical situations mainly because diagnostic material is usually scant in these conditions. Another potential use of immunohistochemistry derives from the fact that pancreatic cancer is often occult at the time of diagnosis and may appear as a metastatic adenocarcinoma with no apparent primary tumor. Under these circumstances, a reagent with tissue specificity for the pancreas might help verify the existence of a pancreatic primary tumor.

Several groups have produced MAbs against pancreatic carcinoma, and other antibodies, such as 19-9, have been shown to react with pancreatic carcinoma as well as other tumors (Table 1 and 2). Most of these antibodies detect antigens that are denatured by routine formalin fixation and paraffin embedding, so that immunohistochemical surveys of their tumor and tissue reactivity have been performed on frozen sections. Other antibodies such as DU-PAN-2, C1-N3, and ARI-28 react with formalin-fixed tissues, hence, larger numbers of tissues and tumors have been screened. The immunohistochemical reactivity of pancreatic carcinoma-associated MAbs with fresh or fixed tumors and normal tissues is summarized in Table 1 and 2.

Some MAbs show no reactivity with any normal tissues under conditions in which they will react with pancreatic carcinoma. These include AR1-28, from Chin and coworkers (22), and C1-PB3 from Schmiegel et al. (23). Other antibodies, including DU-PAN-1 and DU-PAN-5, and Schmiegel's C1-N3 react with some normal tissues, but not with normal pancreatic epithelia. Antibody YPan2, from Yuan and coworkers (25), reacted only rarely and weakly with normal pancreatic tissue but not with other normal tissues (see Table 1).

To be considered a tumor-specific marker, it is necessary, but not sufficient, that an antibody fail to react with the normal pancreas. It is also necessary that such a marker not be present on benign lesions mimicking pancreatic carcinoma. Unfortunately, there are few reports addressing reactivity of pancreatic carcinoma MAbs with such lesions. DU-PAN-1 and DU-PAN-5 both react with most cases of chronic pancreatitis, as does antibody C1-N3. However, C1-PB3 was reported to react with 10 of 10 cases of pancreatic carcinoma and 0 of 4 cases of chronic pancreatitis. This antibody, perhaps in conjunction with antibody AR1-28, may become useful in helping to diagnose pancreatic carcinoma in difficult cases, but given the limited data currently available and

Table 1 Immunohistochemical Reactivity of Pancreatic Carcinoma MAbs with Normal Tissues

Type of tissue	Antibody										
	DU-PAN-1	DU-PAN-2	DU-PAN-3	DU-PAN-5	19/9	AR1-28	C54-0	C1-N3	C1-P8	YPan1	YPan2
Pancreas	-	+	+	-	+	-	+	-	-	+	-[a]
Chronic pancreatitis	+	+	+	+	NR[c]	+	+	-	NR	NR	NR
Colon	+	+	+	+	+	-	NR	NR	NR	-	-
Stomach	+	+	+	+	+	-	+	-	-	-	-
Small intestine	+	+	-	+	NR	-	NR	NR	NR	+[b]	-
Breast	-	-	-	-	NR	-	NR	NR	NR	-	-
Prostate	+	-	+	+	NR	-	+	-	-	+	-
Kidney	-	-	-	+	NR	-	+	-	-	-	-
Liver	-	-	-	-	NR	-	+	+	-	+	-
Salivary gland	+	+	+	+	+	NR	NR	NR	NR	-	-
Bladder	+	-	-	-	NR	-	NR	NR	NR	NR	NR
Bronchus	+	+	+	+	NR	-	NR	NR	NR	+	-
Lymph node	-	-	-	-	NR	-	-	-	-	-	-

[a]One-sixteenth of specimens positive.
[b]Duodenum only.
[c]NR, not reported.

174

Table 2 Immunohistochemical Reactivity of Pancreatic Carcinoma MAbs with Human Tumors[a]

Type of tissue	Antibody										
	DU-PAN-1	DU-PAN-2	DU-PAN-3	DU-PAN-5	19/9	AR1-28	C54-0	C1-N3	C1-P83	YPan1	YPan2
Pancreas	6/8[b]	29/30	8/8	7/8	2/3	23/27	10/10	10/10	10/10	17/19	14/19
Colorectal	4/9	6/15	6/9	6/9	38/54	NR[c]	4/4	4/4	3/3	6/13	4/13
Stomach	0/2	18/21	0/2	NR	7/13	NR	1/1	1/1	1/1	9/10	2/10
Breast	2/11	5/22	2/11	2/7	1/10	NR	1/1	1/1	1/1	6/10	3/10
Prostate	16/32	3/26	6/26	7/7	0/2	NR	0/1	0/1	0/1	2/6	1/6
Kidney	0/9	0/15	0/9	2/9	0/2	NR	NR	NR	NR	1/4	3/4
Bladder	6/10	3/10	4/10	1/9	NR	NR	2/2	0/2	1/2	4/5	0/5
Lung	0/5	4/16	0/5	0/5	NR	NR	1/2	0/2	1/2	2/11	0/11
Biliary	NR	5/5	NR	NR	1/2	NR	1/1	1/1	0/1	NR	NR

[a]Results obtained using a frozen section immunoperoxidase method, except for DU-PAN-2 and AR1-28 which used fixed, paraffin-embedded tissues.
[b]No. positive/no. tested.
[c]NR, not reported.

the poor track record of other immunologically defined "tumor-specific" markers, it seems unlikely that immunohistochemistry will replace conventional morphological studies in this area.

The other major application of immunohistochemistry is in distinguishing pancreatic carcinoma from other adenocarcinomas. Many pancreatic carcinoma-associated antigens resemble oncofetal or developmental markers in that their expression is stronger on tumor or fetal tissues compared with adult tissues. However, there has been considerable conservation of antigen expression throughout tissues derived from embryological endoderm, hence, tissue-specific markers have not been found.

One of the most extensively studied MAbs to pancreatic tumor antigens is DU-PAN-2, in part because of the stability of the antigen to routine formalin fixation. It is present in essentially 100% of the patients with pancreatic carcinoma and in almost 90% of gastric or biliary carcinomas, but detected much less frequently on other adenocarcinomas (see Table 2). Similar results were seen with this antibody in a series of Japanese patients (Sawabu et al., personal communication), except that only about half of the gastric carcinomas tested were positive. Although only a limited number of patients have been studied, the reactivity of metastatic lesions is largely similar to that of primary tumors. This relative selectivity is in contrast to colorectal carcinoma-associated antigens, such as 19-9, which react with similar percentages of colonic and pancreatic cancer (26). DU-PAN-2 showed more selective reactivity for carcinomas arising in tissues derived from the embryonic foregut in patients in the United States and Japan.

Most of the other pancreatic carcinoma-associated antibodies react with 75-100% of pancreatic carcinoma tissues, although the number of tumors studied was often limited by the lack of available frozen material (see Table 2). There is also considerable cross-reactivity of these antibodies with nonpancreatic tumors, although different antibodies show different patterns of cross-reactivity. These different patterns have not yet been explored for their diagnostic potential. For example, DU-PAN-4 and C54-0 react with almost all epithelial tumors and thus are of no help in differential diagnosis. However, DU-PAN-1, 3, and 5 react with a significant percentage of colorectal or genitourinary cancer, but not with lung, kidney, or breast cancer. Similarly, YPan1 is co-expressed by gastric, bladder, and, to a lesser extent, colorectal and breast cancer, whereas YPan2 reacts mainly with kidney tumors. From these patterns of cross-reactivity, it is possible to infer that a tumor reacting with several antibodies is much more likely to be pancreatic cancer than to be lung, breast, kidney, or prostate cancer. However, gastric carcinoma, biliary cancer, and even colorectal carcinoma are much more difficult to exclude because all markers show some cross-reactivity with these tumors.

This lack of specificity of MAb reactivity at the tissue level does not necessarily imply that these reagents cannot be used diagnostically. The factors governing secretion of many of these antigens are clearly different from those that govern their expression in a tumor, thus, an assay may be more specific when serum and not tissue is used as a substrate. This, in fact, is true of DU-PAN-2 (as described later).

From a practical standpoint, another possible application of immunohistochemistry is in helping to exclude pancreatic carcinoma. In our hands, a tumor that fails to react with DU-PAN-2 is unlikely to be pancreatic cancer; if it also fails to react with DU-PAN-1 it almost certainly is not. One caution that must be stressed before using antibodies in this manner is that one must have a good-sized sample of tumor. Many pancreatic carcinoma antigens show significant intratumor heterogeneity, with the percentage of positive tumor cells ranging from less than 10% up to 100% in different circumstances. DU-PAN-2 expression has shown heterogeneity, and there has been no correlation between the morphological appearance and antigen expression. Other antibodies, such as YPan1 and C1-N3 have shown a greater correlation between staining and the degree of differentiation of the tumor. Areas of poorly differentiated pancreatic adenocarcinoma showed the least amount of staining.

In summary, immunohistochemistry has contributed greatly to our understanding of the tissue distribution and the specificity of antigens defined by pancreatic carcinoma MAbs. In some instances, patterns of reactivity detected in tissue sections have given us clues to the physiology of some of the antigens, particularly those with mucinlike properties. The reagents currently available, however, do not provide the pathologist with a tool of sufficient specificity to use to solve routine clinical problems. Panels of MAbs with different patterns of cross-reactivity may help in recognizing pancreatic cancer and in excluding at least some other types of tumors from the differential diagnosis. Moreover, different MAbs in the degree to which they stain membrane, cytoplasm, or lumenal contents in different types of tumors, and these staining patterns have not been fully exploited in trying to increase specificity. However, better reagents are needed before immunohistochemistry becomes routine in diagnosing pancreatic carcinoma in difficult cases.

ASSAYS FOR PANCREATIC TUMOR-ASSOCIATED ANTIGENS IN BODY FLUIDS

Radioimmunoassays

The introduction of the radioimmunoassay (RIA) by Berson and Yalow (27) has made a major contribution to both basic science research and the diagnosis of disease. However, the use of RIA for the diagnosis of cancer is still in the early stages of development, largely because of lack of a tumor-specific antibody or of an antigen source for the assay. Our laboratory has been investigating the DU-PAN-2 glycoprotein antigen because its biochemical characteristics make it suitable for use in an RIA for the detection and monitoring of antigen levels in serum samples (28).

We know very little about the physiology of the DU-PAN-2 molecule or about the cause of elevated levels of this antigen in body fluids of certain patients with benign or malignant disease. Most of the initial studies on the tissue distribution of the DU-PAN-2 antigen were retrospective and were done on tissue sections of patients whose body fluids had not been tested for antigen levels. Although we initially reported that all pancreatic cancer tissue sections tested in a small study were positive for DU-PAN-2 (29), we later reported that only 60-70% of patients with this disease had elevated serum levels of this antigen (28). Again, the tissue and serum studies were not done on the same patients at the same time. However, recent unpublished studies from Japanese workers (Sawabu, personal communication) demonstrated that in a small study of 28 gastric, 12 colorectal, and 3 pancreatic cancer patients, 46% of patients with serum DU-PAN-2 values in the normal range expressed antigen that could be readily detected in tumor sections. Moreover, in approximately 50% of the ovarian carcinoma patients studied in our own laboratory, antigen could be detected in the tissue sample without being elevated in serum samples. Thus, the mere presence of the DU-PAN-2 antigen in diseased cells or tissue does not necessarily mean that serum levels of this antigen will be increased.

Although the antigen recognized by DU-PAN-2 is not tumor-specific, it is usually elevated in patients with pancreatic cancer. The DU-PAN-2 antigen levels in the sera and ascites of patients with malignant and nonmalignant disease were analyzed in our laboratory using a competition RIA. The detailed methods for the DU-PAN-2 competition RIA have been published previously (28). Briefly, a test sample is mixed with a predetermined amount of DU-PAN-2 MAb, incubated overnight, and then added to plates coated with a standardized amount of partially purified DU-PAN-2 antigens. Free antibody binds to the immobilized antigen on the plate, whereas the DU-PAN-2 antibody-antigen complex remains in solution and can be washed off. The amount of antibody remaining on the plate is then determined using radiolabeled goat antimouse antibody. The percentage of inhibition caused by the presence of DU-PAN-2 antigen in the test sample is converted to arbitrary units per milliliter based on a standard antigen reference sample. The amount of DU-PAN-2 antigen in 20 μl of 1:500 dilution of standard preparation was designated as 100 U/ml. The percentage inhibition in the RIA showed a reproducible and linear relationship with the amount of antigen up to 200 U/ml (28).

Results of the assay on serum samples from patients with malignant and benign disease, as well as those of normal volunteers, are summarized in Table 3. The mean DU-PAN-2 level from 274 healthy donors was 124 U/ml, whereas the mean value from 203 pancreatic cancer patients was 10,134 U/ml. Approximately 66% of the pancreatic cancer patient samples exceeded the arbitrary cutoff value of 400 U/ml, in contrast to only 1% of normal healthy subjects. Gastric cancer patients also showed high serum levels of DU-PAN-2 antigen, but the percentage of patients having DU-PAN-2 antigen levels higher than 400 U/ml was less than half that for patients with pancreatic cancer. Although the number of samples tested was small, gallbladder cancer and hepatoma patients expressed high mean values of DU-PAN-2, with the percentage of patients showing antigens levels exceeding 400 U/ml being 46% for gallbladder cancer patients and 48% for hepatoma patients. In contrast, serum samples from patients with bladder cancer, breast cancer, ovarian cancer, malignant melanoma, and naso-

Table 3   DU-PAN-2 Serum Values[a] of Healthy Donors, Cancer, and Non-tumor Patients

Group studied	No. of patients tested	Mean DU-PAN-2 (U/ml)	% of sera with DU-PAN-2 values >400
Healthy subjects	274	124	1
Benign genitourinary disease	40	265	2
Pancreatitis	31	212	3
Pancreatic cancer	203	10,134	66
Benign gastric disease	58	203	4
Gastric cancer	78	15,942[b]	31
Benign small-intestine disease	47	236	9
Small-intestine cancer	34	6,505	21
Gallbladder cancer	13	8,280	46
Benign liver disease	85	1,446	46
Hepatoma	21	7,747	48
Colorectal cancer	188	567	13
Bladder cancer	41	195	5
Breast cancer	40	173	5
Ovarian cancer	55	119	0
Melanoma (stage III)	19	92	0
Nasopharyngeal cancer	21	89	0

[a]Determined by competition RIA.
[b]One serum sample had a value $>10^6$ U/ml.

pharyngeal carcinoma showed antigen levels similar to those found in the healthy donors. Similar findings of DU-PAN-2 levels by RIA in sera of 139 patients, mainly with digestive cancer, were recently reported by Sawabu et al. (30). Less than 10% of patients with pancreatitis, benign gastric disease, and benign small-intestine disease had DU-PAN-2 levels above the 400 U/ml cutoff (see Table 3). However, 46% of patients with benign liver disease demonstrated elevated antigen levels. Most categories of benign liver disease showed some increase in mean unit per milliliter serum

DU-PAN-2 levels. The highest levels were in primary biliary cirrhosis and sclerosing cholangitis. Most patients with stable cirrhosis had serum values in the upper-normal range, 200-400 U/ml (31). One explanation for the elevated DU-PAN-2 antigen values in benign and, perhaps, in malignant diseases is that the antigen is a normal constituent of ductal cells of the pancreas, gallbladder, and especially, the liver. The normal tissue distribution studies also show heterogeneity in the expression of the DU-PAN-2 antigen on these ductal cells. This heterogeneity of antigen expression has not, as yet, been correlated with differentiation, although this is a distinct possibility. Thus, any perturbation of ductal cells, either by benign or malignant disease or perhaps by enhanced production or secretion during regeneration, could cause elevated levels of DU-PAN-2 in the lymphatic and vascular systems. Immunoperoxidase staining of regional nodes in patients with pancreatitis and of noninvolved nodes of pancreatic adenocarcinoma patients has demonstrated the presence of DU-PAN-2 antigen (unpublished data). In malignancy, a large tumor burden secreting or shedding DU-PAN-2 could also contribute to elevated levels in body fluids. Because the DU-PAN-2 mucin is probably metabolized in the liver, poor liver function could additionally enhance the levels that were already elevated by the mechanisms just cited.

The DU-PAN-2 levels in cord blood samples and sera from infants (under 6 months of age) were also significantly elevated (Figure 1). However, the mean values of DU-PAN-2 in infants' sera gradually decreased below the arbitrary cutoff level (400 U/ml) by 11 months of age. This confirms the oncofetal nature of the DU-PAN-2 antigen that was suggested by its immunohistology (7).

By use of competition RIA, Mahvi et al. (32) analyzed DU-PAN-2 antigen levels from patients with adenocarcinoma of the pancreas who underwent a variety of therapeutic treatments. Although the patients sample size was small, all six of the patients who underwent surgical resection demonstrated declining DU-PAN-2 serum levels postoperatively, with normal values being achieved within 6 weeks after resection (Figure 2). The DU-PAN-2 serum levels from patients who responded to adjuvant chemotherapy and radiation declined in all patients after initiation of therapy (Figure 3). However, the serum DU-PAN-2 antigen level rose again when advanced disease was noted clinically.

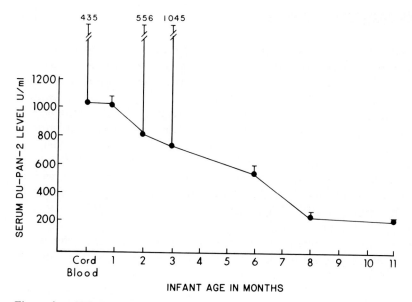

Figure 1   DU-PAN-2 levels in cord blood and infants' serum. The DU-PAN-2 levels are expresseed in arbitrary units per milliliter by competition RIA, as defined in Ref. 28.

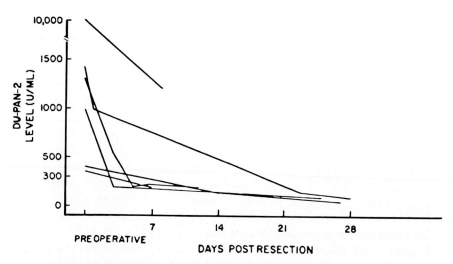

Figure 2   DU-PAN-2 serum levels following pancreatic cancer resection in six patients. The DU-PAN-2 levels are expressed in arbitrary units per milliliter by competition RIA, as defined in Ref. 28. (*Source*: Ref. 32.)

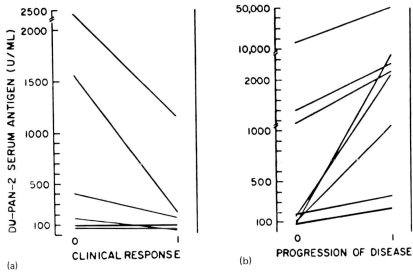

Figure 3   (a) Changes in DU-PAN-2 serum levels in patients who responded to nonsurgical therapy. Point 0 is the initiation of chemotherapy/radiation therapy. Point 1 is the DU-PAN-2 levels when the patients was noted to have a clinical response. (b) Changes in DU-PAN-2 with clinical progression of disease. Point 0 is the DU-PAN-2 level during each patients' remission or stabilization. Point 1 is the DU-PAN-2 level when progressive disease was first noted. The DU-PAN-2 levels are expressed in arbitrary units per milliliter by competition RIA, as defined in Ref. 28. (*Source*: Ref. 32.)

Moreover, in three of six patients with clinically documented tumor regression or stabilization, an elevated DU-PAN-2 serum level was noted 1 to 7 months before clinical evidence of progressive disease. These results suggest that monitoring the DU-PAN-2 antigen levels in serum could be a useful measurement to determine the response of pancreatic cancer patients to the therapy.

Enzyme-Linked Immunoassay

The enzyme-linked immunosorbent assay (ELISA) developed by Engvall et al. (33) has also been useful for diagnostic and research purposes. Recently, the sensitivity of ELISA has approached that of the RIA by using secondary and tertiary antibodies to enhance the sensitivity. An obvious advantage of ELISA over RIA is that it eliminates the handling of radioisotopes. Additionally, the ELISA reagents are less expensive, easier to prepare, and more stable than the radiolabeled reagents. The colored products of ELISA can be read either visually or quantitatively by spectrophotometry.

The DU-PAN-2 antigen in body fluids was analyzed by ELISA using monomeric DU-PAN-2 antibody coupled to horseradish peroxidase. The expression of multiple epitopes on the DU-PAN-2 antigen molecule allowed Bayashi and Kawai (34) to develop a double-determinant ELISA for the detection of DU-PAN-2 antigen in the samples. Briefly, 96-well microtiter plates were coated with DU-PAN-2 antibody. Diluted test samples were added to each well monomeric DU-PAN-2 antibody conjugated to horseradish peroxidase was added and allowed to react with the bound antigen. After washing off the unbound conjugates, enzyme substrate was added to wells and the amount of enzyme present, which was proported to antigen, was determined colorimetrically on an ELISA plate reader. The ELISA absorbance showed a linear relationship with the amount of added DU-PAN-2 antigen standard. Also, a linear regression analysis of 96 independently tested samples using ELISA and RIA showed a good correlation between these two assay methods with a correlation coefficient of 0.925 (Figure 4). As yet, there have been no published data on DU-PAN-2 ELISA testing. However, our laboratory and others in Japan are currently using this assay for routine clinical DU-PAN-2 antigen testing.

We cannot rule out the possibility that some serum or body fluid components other than the DU-PAN-2 antigen could inhibit the DU-PAN-2 MAb from binding to its natural antigen. In this regard, the chances of obtaining false-positive determinations of DU-PAN-2 antigen by the double-determinant ELISA is less than by a competition RIA.

COMPARISON OF ANTIGENS AND ASSAYS FOR PANCREATIC CANCER

The available studies using polyclonal antibodies and MAbs that detect serum antigens and show promise in aiding the diagnosis, classification, and clinical management of patients with pancreatic and other gastrointestinal tract malignancies have indicated that

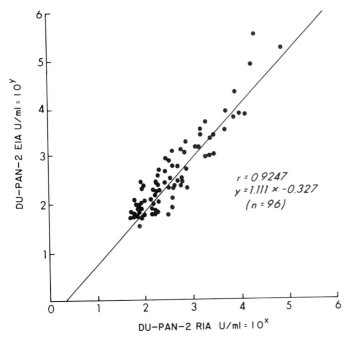

Figure 4   Correlation of DU-PAN-2 serum levels determined by RIA and
ELISA (EIA) (*Source*: unpublished data proved by Kyowa Medex Co.
Ltd., Tokyo, Japan and by Dr. N. Hattori and Dr. N. Sawabu of Kanazawa
University, Kanazawa, Japan).

different cancer markers are usually complementary. Thus, multiple antigen assays improve the chance of finding a useful marker
for classifying or monitoring a patient's disease. Recently Sawabu
et al. (30) evaluated the usefulness of DU-PAN-2 together with
other serum markers for digestive tract malignancies with emphasis on pancreatic cancer. These investigators compared serum
levels of 19-9 and CEA with DU-PAN-2. Figure 5 shows the relationship of DU-PAN-2 and CEA in patients with pancreatic and
other types of malignancies. No significant correlation between
these two markers was observed. In this study, five of eight pancreatic cancer patients with CEA values below 5 µg/ml had elevated DU-PAN-2 values. When DU-PAN-2 serum levels were compared with 19-9 values in a simialr group of patients, a value of

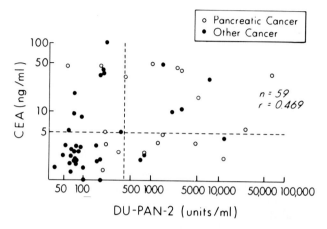

Figure 5   The relationship between individual serum levels of DU-PAN-2 and CEA in pancreatic and other cancer patients. The DU-PAN-2 levels were determined by competition RIA, as defined in Ref. 28. CEA levels were determined by the RIA kit of Dainabot, Tokyo, Japan (*Source*: Ref. 30).

0.349 was observed (Figure 6). Using these two markers, only seven of 39 pancreatic cancer patients were negative for both DU-PAN-2 and 19-9 antigens at the cutoff values used for these studies. The overall incidence of pancreatic cancer patients who fail to develop elevated 19-9 levels has been reported to be 20-30% (35,36). Thus, the combination of CEA, 19-9, and DU-PAN-2 assay may substantially enhance the sensitivity of testing for a pancreatic cancer as well as the other diseases.

Although DU-PAN-2 and 19-9 have been shown to detect unique epitopes, recently, Lan et al. (37) demonstrated that DU-PAN-2 and 19-9 epitopes can be coexpressed on the same mucin molecule. An ascites sample from a pancreatic adenocarcinoma patient expressing high levels of DU-PAN-2 (56,960 U/ml) and 19-9 (4098 U/ml) antigen units was applied to a DU-PAN-2 MAb-affinity column. All of the DU-PAN-2 antigen bonded to the column, whereas 31% of the 19-9 antigen activity passed through the column. Approximately 80% of the DU-PAN-2 and 49% of the 19-9 antigen activity were recovered after elution. These results suggest that 19-9 and DU-PAN-2 may be present on the same molecule but are not invariably coexpressed. That DU-PAN-2 molecules may show heterogeneous expression of the

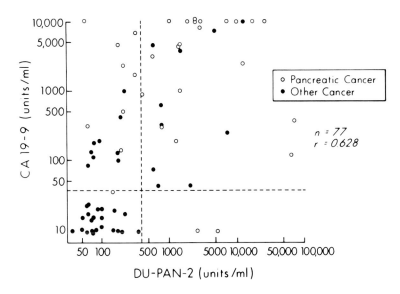

Figure 6   The relationship between individual serum levels of DU-PAN-2 and 19-9 in pancreatic and other cancer patients. The DU-PAN-2 levels were determined by competition RIA, as defined in Ref. 28. The 19-9 levels were determined by the RIA kit from Centocor, Malvern, Pennsylvania (*Source*: Ref. 30).

19-9 epitope was further suggested by immunoblotting experiments in which a panel of clinical samples containing high levels of DU-PAN-2 antigen were tested with DU-PAN-2 or 19-9 MAbs. The DU-PAN-2 antigen was demonstrated in bile, pancreatic juice, and serum from all six samples of the three body fluids tested, although migratory patterns were somewhat different. However, the 19-9 MAb immunostained only four of six samples tested (Figure 7). It was previously reported that the expression of 19-9 antigen was closely related to the presence of the Lewis gene that coded for the enzyme necessary for the biosynthesis of 19-9 epitope (38,39). Therefore, the absence of 19-9 antigens in two samples observed in the immunoblotting (Figure 7B) may be due to the patient's negative Lewis gene phenotype, Le (a⁻,b⁻). It is clear that every antigen revealed microheterogeneity in the blots.

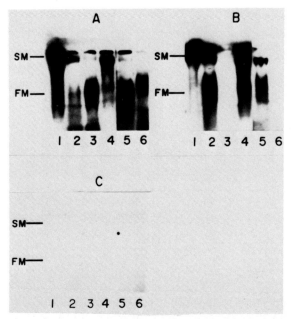

Figure 7   Immunoblotting of antigens from clinical samples selected for high DU-PAN-2 levels. Antigens from bile and pancreatic juice of pancreatic cancer patients (lanes 1 and 4), serum from a patient with hepatobiliary cancer (lane 2) and sera from pancreatic cancer patients (lanes 3, 5, and 6) were subjected to 1% agarose gel electrophoresis and immunoblotted with MAbs DU-PAN-2 (A), 1909 (B), and control antibodies (IgG1 and IgM) (C) (*Source*: Ref. 37).

DISCUSSION AND PERSPECTIVES

The first MAbs to human pancreatic adenocarcinoma were reported in 1982 (21). To date, there are more than a dozen reported MAbs. Of these, only a few have been sufficiently characterized to evaluate their clinical usefulness. Even so, from these studies we can begin to evaluate the potential successes and limitations of diagnostic procedures for pancreatic adenocarcinoma involving MAbs. The main potential applications of MAbs for the in vitro diagnosis of human pancreatic adenocarcinoma rests in certain immunohistochemical applications and in serum diagnostic tests using RIA or ELISA. Regarding immunohistological applications, we remain skeptical that any truly tumor-specific pancreatic adenocarcinoma antigens will be described.

Additionally, the problem of evaluating the serum assays, such as DU-PAN-2, 19-9, and other future markers, for early detection of pancreatic cancer is formidable because there are no known high-risk groups and screening of elderly patients with gastrointestinal complaints will require large numbers of patients surveyed over a long follow-up period.

Nevertheless, some of the MAb-defined tumor-associated antigens will undoubtedly prove useful in augmenting conventional morphological classification of benign and malignant pancreatic disease. Specifically, we foresee panels of antipancreatic MAbs being used in conjunction with panels of antibodies from other organ systems to diagnose, or rule out, pancreatic adenocarcinoma in certain difficult cases of chronic pancreatitis or distant metastases with no obvious primary tumor.

Considering serum diagnostic application, it is obvious that the most promising diagnostic tests that have yet been developed use antigenic epitopes that are expressed on large glycoprotein molecules in the serum (5). For pancreatic adenocarcinoma, thus far, these include DU-PAN-2 and CA 19-9 (28,40). These antigens have been amenable to the development of RIA and ELISA serum assays for a number of reasons, including (1) biochemical stability of the antigen; (2) the presence of multiple epitopes on each molecule; (3) the availability of sufficient quantities of high-titered antigen samples (e.g., ascites, serum, bile) to establish a standardized assay and to screen a large enough number of patient samples to draw meaningful conclusions; and (4) the antigen is actively secreted by normal ductal cells or tumor cells in organs that are well vascularized.

The initial working hypothesis for using these tumor markers in diagnostic applications was that serum concentrations would correspond to tumor burden. Accurate measurements that allow calculation of tumor burden are difficult to obtain from pancreatic cancer patients. Thus, this hypothesis has never been tested in a meaningful manner. Our DU-PAN-2 studies in benign and malignant liver disease suggest that other factors can often be proposed to explain elevated serum levels. These include enhanced expression and secretion of DU-PAN-2 antigen from nonmalignant ductal cells and decreased catabolism of the molecules in the liver. These other factors can be triggered by malignant and nonmalignant disease. As was initially hypothesized with malignant disease, the tumor itself may also secrete antigen that contributes to the serum concentration. The lack of animal and in vitro models of human ductal cell differentiation and transformation makes it difficult to establish the physiology of DU-PAN-2 and other secreted glycoprotein antigens.

The results obtained, to date, on serum assays with antimucin antibodies suggest that their clinical uses may include use of panels of MAbs for differential diagnosis and/or antigen monitoring during therapy. These applications will require better definition and characterization of the populations of mucin molecules associated with different malignancies and benign disease. Altered glycosylation of mucins in malignant disease can result in heterogeneous molecular populations that can express none, one, or several of the epitopes currently defined by the MAbs to mucinlike antigens.

Information gained from the serum marker studies of mucin antigens should also serve as a guideline for the identification of other potentially useful antigens for serum assays. Investigators could look for stable, secreted molecules and deemphasize somewhat the tissue specificity of the antigens being evaluated because tissue reactivity does not always correlate with serum concentration. Other potention candidates for diagnostic considerations may include glycolipids, growth factors that are secreted by pancreatic adenocarcinomas, or cellular oncogene products.

Finally, active immunization of humans with tumor cells, subcellular fractions, and soluble antigens as therapeutic modalities has provided useful information on the immunogenicity of human melanoma antigens (41). Similar studies in pancreatic cancer patients could provide data about which antigens of adenocarcinomas are immunogenic in man and perhaps indicate which molecular class or classes of antigens deserve further studies for diagnostic and/or therapeutic potential.

ACKNOWLEDGMENTS

The authors gratefully acknowledge and appreciate the efforts and skills of Teresa Hylton in the preparation and processing of this manuscript and the many technical contributions of Frank Tuck. Part of the work presented in this chapter was supported by grants CA 32672 and CA 4044 from the National Cancer Institute.

REFERENCES

1. F. V. Ona, N. Zamcheck, P. Dhar, T. Moore, and H. Z. Kupchik, *Cancer 31*:324 (1973).
2. F. B. Gelder, C. J. Reese, A. R. Moosa, T. Hall, and R. Hunter, *Cancer Res. 38*:313 (1978).
3. H. Koprowski, Z. Steplewski, K. Mitchell, M. Herlyn, D. Herlyn, and J. P. Fuhrer, *Somatic Cell Genet. 5*:957 (1979).
4. R. S. Metzger, M. T. Gaillard, S. J. Levine, F. L. Tuck, E. H. Bossen, and M. J. Borowitz, *Cancer Res. 42*:601 (1982).
5. H. G. Rittenhouse, G. L. Manderino, and G. M. Hass, *Lab. Med. 16*:556 (1985).
6. M. Nuti, Y. A. Teramoto, R. Mariani-Constantini, P. Horan Hand, D. Colcher, and J. Schlom, *Int. J. Cancer 29*:539 (1982).
7. R. S. Metzgar, D. M. Mahvi, M. J. Borowitz, M. S. Lan, W. C. Meyers, H. F. Seigler, and O. J. Finn, *Monoclonal Antibodies and Cancer Therapy*. Alan R. Liss, New York (1985), p. 63.
8. J. L. Magnani, B. Nilsson, M. Brockhaus, D. Zopf, Z. Steplewski, H. Koprowski, and V. Ginsburg, *J. Biol. Chem. 257*:14365 (1982).
9. E. Witebsky, N. R. Rose, and H. Nadel, *J. Immunol. 85*:568 (1960).
10. N. R. Rose, R. S. Metzgar, and E. Witebsky, *J. Immunol. 85*: 575 (1960).
11. R. S. Metzgar, *Nature 203*:660 (1964).
12. R. S. Metzgar, *J. Immunol 93*:176 (1964).
13. S. Githens, in *The Exocrine Pancreas: Biology, Pathobiology and Diseases* (V. L. W. Go et al., eds.), Raven Press, New York (1986), p. 21.
14. M. S. Lan, O. J. Finn, P. D. Fernsten, and R. S. Metzgar, *Cancer Res. 45*:305 (1985).
15. J. L. Magnani, Z. Steplewski, H. Koprowski, and V. Ginsburg, *Cancer Res. 43*:5489 (1983).
16. S. I. Hakomori, *Cancer Res. 45*:2405 (1985).
17. T. Feizi, *Nature 314*:53 (1985).
18. M. Yuan, S. H. Itzkowitz, A. Palekar, A. M. Shamsuddin, P. C. Phelps, B. F. Trump, and Y. S. Kim, *Cancer Res. 45*:4499 (1985).
19. C. Cordon-Cardo, K. O. Lloyd, J. Sakamoto, M. E. McGroarty, L. J. Old, and M. R. Melamed, *Int. J. Cancer 37*:667 (1986).

20. E. Uchida, Z. Steplewski, E. Mroczek, M. Buchler, D. Burnett, and P. M. Pour, *Int. J. Pancreatol.* *1*:213 (1986).
21. I. Parsa, A. L. Sutton, C. K. Chen, and C. Delbridge, *Cancer Lett.* *17*:217 (1982).
22. J. Chin and F. Miller, *Cancer Res.* *45*:1723 (1985).
23. W. H. Schmiegel, M. Kalthoff, R. Arndt, J. Gieseking, H. Greten, G. Kloppel, C. Kreiker, A. Ladak, V. Lampe, and S. Ulrich, *Cancer Res.* *45*:1402 (1985).
24. M. A. Hollingsworth and R. S. Metzgar, in *Monoclonal Antibodies in Cancer* (S. Sell and R. A. Reisfeld, eds.), Humana Press, Clifton, N.J. (1985).
25. S. Z. Yuan, J. J. L. Ho, M. Yuan, and Y. S. Kim, *Cancer Res.* *45*:6179 (1985).
26. B. F. Atkinson, C. S. Ernst, M. Herlyn, Z. Steplewski, H. F. Sears, and H. Koprowski, *Cancer Res.* *42*:4820 (1982).
27. S. A. Berson and R. S. Yalow, *J. Clin. Invest.* *38*:1996 (1959).
28. R. S. Metzgar, N. Rodriguez, O. J. Finn, M. S. Lan, V. N. Daasch, P. D. Fernsten, W. C. Meyers, W. F. Sindelar, R. S. Sandler, and H. F. Seigler, *Proc. Natl. Acad. Sci. USA 81*: 5242 (1984).
29. M. J. Borowitz, F. L. Tuck, W. F. Sindelar, P. D. Fernsten, and R. S. Metzgar, *J. Natl. Cancer Inst.* *72*:999 (1984).
30. N. Sawabu, D. Toya, Y. Takemori, N. Hattori, and M. Fukui, *Int. J. Cancer 37*:693 (1986).
31. A. E. Haviland, M. J. Borowitz, P. G. Killenherg, M. S. Lan, and R. S. Metzgar *Int. J. Cancer* (in press).
32. D. M. Mahvi, W. C. Meyers, R. C. Bast, H. F. Seigler, and R. S. Metzgar, *Ann. Surgery 202*:440 (1985).
33. E. Engvall, J. Johsson, and P. Perlmann, *Biochim. Biophys. Acta 251*:427 (1971).
34. I. Sakurabayashi, T. Kawai, T. Yamanaka et al., *Rinsho Byori* (*Journal of Clinical Pathology*) *34*:705 (1986) (in Japanese).
35. B. C. Del Villano and V. R. Zurawski, Jr., *Lab. Res. Methods Biol. Med. 8*:269 (1983).
36. V. Savarino, C. Mansi, V. Pugliese, G. B. Ferrara, V. Arcuri, and G. Celle, *Digestion 29*:1 (1984).
37. M. S. Lan, R. C. Bast, Jr., M. I. Colnaghi, R. C. Knapp, D. Colcher, J. Schlom, and R. S. Metzgar, *Int. J. Cancer 39*:68 (1987).

38. M. Brockhaus, M. Wysocka, J. L. Magnani, Z. Steplewski, H. Koprowski, and V. Ginsburg, *Vox Sang.* *48*:34 (1985).

39. E. F. Grollman, A. Kobata, and V. Ginsburg, *J. Clin. Invest.* *48*:1489 (1969).

40. B. C. Del Villano, S. Brennan, P. Brock, C. Bucher, V. Liu, M. McClure, B. Rake, S. Space, B. Westrick, H. Schoemaker, and V. R. Zurawski, Jr., *Clin. Chem.* *29*:549 (1983).

41. P. O. Livingston, L. J. Old, and H. F. Oettgen, *Monoclonal Antibodies and Cancer Therapy*. Alan R. Liss, New York (1985), p. 537.

8
Monoclonal Antibody Assays for Prostatic Tumor

Ming C. Wang, Carl S. Killian, Ching-Li Lee, and T. Ming Chu / Roswell Park Memorial Institute, Buffalo, New York

INTRODUCTION

According to the American Cancer Society's data (1), prostatic cancer is the second most common cancer in males (90,000 new cases in 1986) and is the third leading cause of male cancer death (26,100 in 1986) in the United States. In spite of these grim statistics, prostatic cancer is highly curable if it is detected and treated while the disease is still confined to the prostate (2,3). Therefore, assay of prostatic tumor markers in the serum or other body fluids for early detection of the cancer is of utmost importance in controlling this malignant disease. The assay of prostatic tumor markers also is of great value in evaluation of treatment efficacy, in monitoring progression of the disease and in the early prediction of the recurrence of the disease. Prostatic tumor markers are also a useful tool for differential diagnosis of metastasized tumor of unknown origin, which is crucial in determining the treatment mode.

Since the 1930s when Gutman and Gutman (4) discovered that the activity of acid phosphatase in the sera of patients with metastasized prostatic tumor is elevated compared with that in the sera of normal males, the search for prostatic markers has been the endeavor of many investigators (5-24). Antigenic markers, in particular, are the subject of many studies. Before the advent of hybridoma technology, polyclonal antisera, which are generated by immunizing animals with seminal plasma or the extracts of prostatic tumor, were used to identify the antigenic markers of prostatic tumor (5-7,9). Although a number of the markers have been identified with this approach, none is prostatic tumor-specific. It may be that prostatic tumor-specific antigens do exist, but they do not elicit, in the animal, an immune response strong enough for the production of the discernible amount of antibodies. With the development of hybridoma technology, many monoclonal antibodies (MAbs) have been generated in an attempt to probe prostatic tumor-specific antigens (15,16,18-21,25). This approach is based on the belief that MAbs are more suitable reagents than polyclonal antisera for detecting subtle antigenic changes associated with the malignant transformation. In addition, MAbs against established prostatic tumor markers, such as prostatic acid phosphatase (PAP) and prostate-specific antigen (PA), have been generated in an effort to improve the sensitivity and specificity of the diagnostic procedures exploiting these markers (26-31). In this chapter we shall review these recent developments in the immunodiagnosis of prostatic cancer.

PROSTATIC ACID PHOSPHATASE AS A TUMOR MARKER

Acid phosphatase has been used as a prostatic tumor marker since 1938 (4). As a diagnostic procedure, the conventional method of measuring catalytic activity of acid phosphatase in the serum has some drawbacks: It is not sensitive enough to efficiently detect early stage malignancy, and it cannot distinguish the elevated serum levels of acid phosphatase caused by prostatic cancer from those caused by other diseases (32). In 1964, Shulman et al. (33) reported that the antiserum from an animal immunized with prostatic fluid reacted only with the acid phosphatase of prostatic fluid and prostate but not with the extracts of nonprostatic tissues. Their observations suggested the feasibility of developing an immunoassay procedure specific for PAP. In 1974, Cooper and Foti (34) reported the first immunoassay procedure capable of detecting nanogram levels of PAP. Their procedure, a classic competitive-type radioimmunoassay (RIA) employing double antibody, was subsequently simplified to become a solid-phase RIA and was tested clinically (35). Their results showed that RIA of PAP is a far superior procedure for detecting prostatic cancer when compared with the conventional method of measuring acid phosphatase activity. In 1976, Chu et al. (36) reported a counterimmunoelectrophoresis procedure for detecting PAP in the serum. Their procedure has been subjected to a nationwide field trial, and the resultant data demonstrate the diagnostic superiority of this procedure over the conventional enzymatic method (37). Promising results of these pilot studies have aroused enthusiasm for using immunoassay of PAP as a diagnostic tool for prostatic cancer, and numerous studies for this have been carried out with various forms of immunoassay procedures (38-48). All of the studies used anti-PAP antiserum to trap PAP in the specimen. In recent years, anti-PAP MAbs have been used in place of polyclonal antibodies of animal serum origin, based on the considerations that MAbs can offer many advantages over polyclonal antisera (49). The procedures employing MAbs will be discussed in the following.

Diagnostic Utility of Assays Utilizing Monoclonal
Antibodies to Prostatic Acid Phosphatase

Enzyme Immunoassay

Currently there are two similar enzyme immunoassay (EIA) procedures employing MAbs. In the first method, developed by Lin
and coworkers (50), PAP in the specimen is reacted with anti-
PAP MAb (27) and the resultant immune complex is precipitated
by polyethylene glycol, washed, and the PAP activity determined.
A preliminary study involving 23 prostatic cancer patients showed
that 2 of 4 stage B, 3 of 13 stage C, and 12 of 16 stage D patients
had elevated concentration of PAP in the serum, whereas serum
PAP concentrations in 10 males and 17 nonprostatic cancer patients were all within the normal range ($\leqslant 2$ ng/ml). This procedure has not been compared with those employing polyclonal
antisera, and it has not been subjected to a large-scale clinical
trial. Therefore, whether or not it is superior to the procedures
employing polyclonal antisera remains to be determined.

A second EIA procedure, developed by Roche Diagnostics as
a kit, is similar to the one described above, but instead of using
polyethylene glycol as precipitant, second polyclonal antibody
reagents are used. Kaplan et al. (51) have clinically evaluated this
procedure together with the EIA using polyclonal anti-PAP antibody reagents, RIA, and conventional PAP enzyme activity measurement. Their data showed that the EIA, which employs MAb,
has the highest sensitivity, but lowest specificity among the assays
evaluated. Their results also indicated that the procedure employing MAb detected more early-stage prostatic cancer than did other
procedures. However, it should be emphasized that the procedures should be tested on specimens from more patients before
an unequivocal conclusion can be made.

Two-Site Immunoradiometric Assay

The two-site immunoradiometric assay procedure was developed
by Wang and his colleagues (52) of Hybritech, Inc. Two MAbs,
each recognizing a distinct antigenic determinant on PAP, are employed in this procedure. The first MAb immobilized on plastic
beads is for capturing PAP in the serum, while the second MAb
labeled with ^{125}I, is for tagging PAP to provide a quantitative
indicator. Davies and Gochman (53) have compared the clinical

merit of this procedure with those of the enzyme activity measurement and polyclonal antibody-based RIA. Their results showed that the MAb-based immunoradiometric procedure had diagnostic sensitivity and specificity slightly higher than those of the polyclonal antibody-based RIA. The greater sensitivity of the MAb-based procedure appears to be due to its capability to detect more early-stage cancer. In this study, the enzyme activity measurement appeared to be the least sensitive procedure to detecting prostatic cancer, but its specificity was comparable to that of the MAb-based immunoradiometric procedure and was even better than that of the RIA.

Two-Site Immunoenzymometric Assay

The two-site immunoenzymometric assay (IEMA), developed by Loor et al. (31) of Cetus Corp., is similar to that of the two-site immunoradiometric assay described previously, but instead of using ^{125}I as a label, horseradish peroxidase (HRP) is used. Thus, after incubation the enzymatic activity of HRP rather than radioactivity is measured. In a preliminary study, this procedure detected 33% of stage A, 50% of stage B, 45% of stage C, and 91% of stage D prostatic cancer cases, but none of 107 patients with nonprostatic cancer gave positive results (54). The study comparing this method with other PAP assay procedures has not been performed. A more extensive study involving more patients is certainly needed for assessing the clinical value of this method.

Enzyme-Amplified Monoclonal Immunoenzymometric Assay

The enzyme-amplified MAb IEMA reported by Most et al. (55) is a variation of the two-site IEMA. It differs in the way the activity of an enzymatic label (alkaline phosphatase) is determined. In this procedure, alkaline phosphatase-catalyzed hydrolysis of NADP to NAD, is coupled to the alcohol dehydrogenase-catalyzed reduction of NAD to NADH, which in turn is coupled to the diaphorase-catalyzed conversion of iodonitrotetrazolium to formazan. This enzyme-amplification system greatly increases the analytical sensitivity, enabling the procedure to detect PAP at a concentration of 0.05 ng/ml. With this procedure, the median value of serum PAP in 140 apparently healthy males was 0.7 ng/ml and the 95th percentile was 1.5 ng/ml. When the upper unit of normal was set at 2 ng/ml, only one of 140 (0.7%) healthy males showed serum levels of PAP exceeding this value. Of 204 patients referred for serum PAP measurements, an elevated level of PAP was found in 13 patients. These 13 patients did not have abnormal activity of serum acid phosphatase as determined by a conventional enzymatic method. Prostatic cancer was found in 10 of these 13 patients, including four cases of untreated, nonmetastatic cancer; the remainder of this group consisted of two patients with benign prostatic hypertrophy (BPH) and one patient with an undiagnosed condition. On the other hand, abnormal serum acid phosphatase activity measured by a conventional method was found in five patients with normal serum PAP concentration as determined by the enzyme-amplified immunoassay. Of these five patients, prostatic cancer was confirmed in two. In the report of Moss et al. (55) sufficient clinical data concerning those 204 patients entering the study were not provided; hence, it is impossible to assess the diagnostic specificity and sensitivity of the assay procedures. Nonetheless, it was clearly shown that the diagnostic sensitivity of the enzyme-amplified immunoassay was far superior to that of conventional enzyme activity measurements. It remains to be seen if this new immunoassay employing MAbs is better than other immunoassay procedures for PAP.

At this juncture, it is pertinent to discuss the question concerning the validity of measuring serum PAP concentration for screening general population for detection of prostate cancer. Watson and Tang (56) and Carroll (57) argued that PAP measurements would not be a useful tool for screening the general male population. This is because the prevalence of prostatic cancer is relatively low (most of the population do not have this malignancy in spite of the high incidence of prostatic cancer compared with other male cancers); even with a diagnostic specificity of 94-95% (i.e., false-positive rate of 5-6%), there will be many false-positive reactions and, consequently, a very low positive predictive rate, which renders PAP measurement impractical as a screening tool. As an example, Watson and Tang (56) have calculated that at a prevalence rate of 35:100,000 and with a diagnostic sensitivity of 70% and specificity of 94% as reported by Foti et al. (35), only one of 244 males with positive PAP results actually would have prostatic cancer. Such a low positive predictive rate is unacceptable for the test to be used alone in screening. This view has now been generally accepted.

Because PAP is not a prostatic tumor-specific antigen (7) and is not even qualitatively a prostate-specific enzyme (58-61), it is doubtful, even with the use of MAbs, that the diagnostic specificity of the PAP test could be upgraded to a level much higher than currently available. Thus, it appears that measurement of serum PAP concentrations in the general male population is of questionable clinical utility. However, a different view should also be considered. From the same data set used in the calculation by Watson and Tang (56), it can be estimated that the probability that a person with a positive test result actually has prostatic cancer is about 40 times that of a person with a negative result. Therefore, there also is a compelling reason to place individuals with positive test results under scrutiny, which may lead to the early detection of more cases of prostatic cancer. There is another reason for performing PAP tests on apparently healthy males. At present, the most common routine procedure for detecting prostatic cancer is digital rectal examination, which is fairly accurate and inexpensive (62). However, there have been cases in whom prostatic cancer was detected by PAP test but not by the rectal examination (46). Thus, PAP testing can apparently supplement the digital rectal examination in the detection of prostatic cancer.

In pondering the use of the PAP test as a screening procedure, a proposal by Cohen and Dix (63) deserves serious consideration. These investigators suggest that, instead of using interindividual reference ranges for determining abnormality, as has been done conventionally, the intraindividual reference range resulting from routine screening should be used to determine abnormality. Thus, routine screening should be initiated in middle-age when the prevalence of prostatic cancer is low; and any unusual deviation of the shape of the normal PAP-versus-age curve, shown by repeated testing, should then be taken as a sign of prostatic abnormality. Thus, an individual is considered to be normal as long as his serum PAP level is not consistently elevated above what is to be expected from his own normal curve, even though his serum PAP value may be above the conventionally adopted, statistically determined, interindividual upper-normal limit. Many false-positive results could thus be eliminated, resulting in improvement of the positive predictive rate. This proposal certainly warrants a trial.

Other Clinical Uses of Prostatic Acid Phosphatase Assays

The previous discussion has been focused on the use of the PAP
test as a diagnostic tool for early detection of prostatic cancer.
Another important aspect of the PAP test, namely its use in the
follow-up of the disease, should also be discussed. In fact, this is
now the most effective clinical use for PAP assays. Killian et al.
(64) used a quantitative counterimmunoelectrophoresis procedure
to examine the PAP levels in the sera of stage A_2 to D_1 prostatic
cancer patients, who had received definitive surgical or radiation
therapy before receiving either chemotherapy or no treatment at
all. They also examined the PAP levels in the sera of stage D_1
patients who were receiving chemotherapy, hormonal treatment,
or surgical treatment. They found that the PAP level in serum was
a useful indicator of disease recurrence and progression and was
a useful monitor of the treatment response. For comparison, they
also measured the serum acid phosphatase activity in the same
study and found that the enzyme activity measurement was inferior to the counterimmunoelectrophoresis method in predicting
recurrence, in following disease progression, and in assessing treatment. Similar conclusions were also reached by Vihko and coin-
vestigators (64) using an RIA and a conventional method of serum
acid phosphatase activity measurements.

Davies and Griffiths (66) measured PAP concentration in prostatic cancer patients' sera with an RIA and an EIA and found that
the PAP concentration in some patients returned to normal after
treatment, but the incidence of reduction in the concentration was
less with increasing severity of the disease. Cooper and collaborators (67) using an IEMA procedure, made a longitudinal study of
serum PAP in prostatic cancer patients who had been subjected to
hormonal manipulation. They found that the immunoassay of
PAP was a valuable indicator of treatment resposne and disease
progression. Similar observations were made by Moon et al. (68)
using an RIA procedure. However, Zweig and Ihde (69) reported
that although serum PAP concentrations decreased in patients
responding to hormonal therapy, the serum PAP concentrations
decrease in only a small number of patients responding to chemotherapy. Furthermore, they noted that there were cases in which
the PAP concentrations decreased in spite of progressing disease.
These investigators felt that PAP measurements cannot be relied
upon as the sole basis for clinical judgment when metastases are pres-

ent. On the other hand, they considered PAP measurements might be valuable in confirming clinical assessment.

All the work described was performed with a procedure employing polyclonal antiserum. In the work of Kaplan et al. (51) mentioned earlier, various procedures (enzyme activity, RIA, polyclonal EIA, and MAb EIA) also were compared relative to their utility in monitoring disease in patients who were receiving chemotherapy or radiation therapy. The results showed that the MAb EIA was the most sensitive, but least specific, method in detecting active disease. The reason for low clinical specificity of the MAb EIA method is unclear. In considering the merits of MAb-based assays versus those of polyclonal antibody-based assays, the question of whether or not the methods being compared are in optimal form should always be kept in mind. If one method is inferior to the other, then the question is whether poor quality of the immunologic reagent is responsible or whether the procedure has an inherent inferiority. So far, there are no reports with sufficient data for such a comparison.

Aside from the clinical value, PAP is a useful immunohistochemical marker for identification of metastasized tumor of unknown origin (70). Whether or not anti-PAP MAbs can actually offer advantages over polyclonal antibodies in immunohistochemical classification of tumors remains to be determined. Small qauntities of acid phosphatase, reactive with anti-PAP antibodies, have been found in a few normal and nonprostatic malignant tissues (58-61). Therefore, caution should be exercised in interpreting the results. Another clinical area on which anti-PAP MAbs have potential value is radioimaging of prostatic tumor. Goldenberg and DeLand (71) and Vihko and colleagues (72) have shown that radioisotope-labeled polyclonal anti-PAP antibodies (rabbit or goat) are of value in locating metastasized prostatic tumor in patients. Monoclonal antibody with its high specificity and ease of purification should provide advantages over polyclonal antibodies in radioimaging. Lee and his associates (73) have demonstrated that ^{125}I-labeled anti-PAP MAb is specifically taken up by human prostatic tumors grown in nude mice. This work points to the potential value of anti-PAP MAb in radioimaging of tumors in human patients. Whether MAbs are indeed better than polyclonal antibodies in locating disseminated prostatic tumor in the human body requires further studies.

PROSTATE-SPECIFIC ANTIGEN AS A TUMOR MARKER

Wang et al. in 1979 (7), reported the purification and partial
characterization of an antigen, which occurs in normal, benign
hypertrophic, and cancerous prostatic tissues, but not in other
normal or diseased tissues. The specificity of the antigen has subsequently been confirmed by other studies using polyclonal antiserum or MAbs (28,29,74-76). In the prostate, the antigen is
located in epithelial cells comprising the ductal element (28,29,
74,75). This antigen, called PA, is a glycoprotein existing in the
prostate gland and prostatic fluid (and hence seminal plasma)
(77,78) in many isomeric forms (77) that may have the same
protein moiety but with various amounts of carbohydrate. Purified PA has an isoelectric point of 6.9 and a molecular weight
of 33,000-34,000 as determined by molecular sieving and sodium
dodecyl sulfate-polyacrylamide electrophoresis (SDS-PAGE)
(77). Recently, from complete amino acid sequence data, the
molecular weight of the protein portion of PA has been determined to be 26,496 (80). Although the physicochemical properties of this antigen have been well characterized (79,80), its
biological function, if any, is unclear. Ban and coworkers (81)
and Watt et al. (80) have shown that PA has proteolytic activity
and Lilja (82) has reported that this proteolytic activity of PA
is related to liquefaction of semen clots.

Although PA is not a prostatic tumor-specific antigen, its
potential as a prostate tumor marker is suggested from the clinical
utility of PAP, which is not a prostatic tumor-specific antigen,
either. Shortly after the identification and purification of PA,
it was shown with rocket immunoelectrophoresis that some
prostatic cancer patients' sera contained PA (83). This observation led Kuriyama et al. (84) to develop a highly sensitive
IEMA method for examining serum levels of PA. By use of this
method, they found that normal male serum PA concentrations
ranged from less than 0.1 ng/ml to 2.6 ng/ml, whereas this antigen
was not detectable in female sera. With 1.8 ng/ml (mean + 2 SD)
as the upper limit of normal, an elevated PA concentration was detected in the sera of 63% of stage A, 79% of stage B, 77% of stage
C and 86% of stage D prostatic cancer patients. Abnormal levels
of serum PA were also seen in 68% of BPH patients. Other investigations (54,85-88) using commercially available assay kits have

confirmed the observation that PA levels are elevated in many BPH and prostate cancer patient's sera.

Earlier studies on the clinical usefulness of the PA test used the polyclonal antiPA antibodies exclusively. In recent years, MAb-based procedures for assay of PA have been developed and become commercially available. These procedures are discussed in the following:

Diagnostic Use of Assays with Monoclonal Antibodies to Prostate-Specific Antigen

Immunoradiometric Assay

This procedure developed by Hybritech Corp. is based on the same principle as that in the two-site immunoradiometric method for assaying PAP (see Sec. II). Siddall and collaborators (88) have used this method to examine PA concentrations in prostatic cancer patients' sera. They also used the immunoradiometric procedure to assay PAP in serum. Their data showed that the PA measurement was more sensitive than the PAP measurement in detecting prostatic cancer at all stages. When the operational limit of upper normal was set at 10 ng/ml, the serum PA level was found to be elevated in 43% of 91 untreated patients with non-metastatic prostatic cancer, whereas the serum PAP level was elevated in 17% of these patients. In 60 untreated patients with metastasized prostatic cancer, the elevation of serum PA and PAP levels were 92 and 65%, respectively. None of 10 BPH patients had serum PA levels above the upper limit of normal. These investigators also performed 2 to 4-year longitudinal studies on serum PA and PAP concentrations in patients and found that the changes in the serum PA concentration correlated with the clinical status better than did the changes in serum PAP concentrations. They also found that the elevated level of PA in serum at the time of first examination, with or without a concomitant elevated level of PAP in the serum, was of prognostic significance; i.e., if the initial level of PA was abnormal, the patient had high risk of disease progression within 3 years.

Immunoenzymometric Assay

Loor and his coworkers (54) have developed an MAb-based, two-site immunoenzymometric assay (IEMA) method for PA. This

procedure is identical to their IEMA method for assaying PAP (see
Sec. II). When 8 ng/ml was set as an operational upper limit of
normal, serum PA levels in 39% of stage A, 77% of stage B, 90% of
stage C, and 91% of stage D prostatic cancer patients exceeded the
upper limit of normal. Serum PA levels in 34% of BPH patients
also exceeded the upper limit. Compared with the results obtained with the polyclonal antibody-based procedure of Kuriyama
et al. (89) in which the operational upper limit of normal was set
at 7.5 ng/ml, this method was more sensitive in detecting prostatic
cancer at all stages. On the other hand, it was less specific because
it picked up more BPH cases. Data of Siddall et al. (88) using
MAb-based immunoradiometric procedures (see previous section),
also indicated that the MAb-based procedure was more sensitive
than the polyclonal antibody-based procedure of Kuriyama et al.
(89), it did not pick up BPH cases. However, it should be noted
that more rigorous evidence for the diagnostic superiority of a
MAb-based method should come from experiments in which an
MAb method is tested simultaneously with polyclonal antibody-
based method in an identical group of patients so that variation
of results caused by sampling and other factors can be eliminated.
    In both of the studies just cited (88,89), it was observed
that PA concentrations in the serum were in discordance with the
PAP concentrations. In some instances, the PA level in the serum
was elevated, whereas the PAP level was normal; in some other instances, the PA level remained normal but the PAP level was elevated. Thus, by concurrent measurement of PA and PAP concentrations in the serum, more cases of prostatic cancer could be detected. These results confirmed the previous observations by
Kuriyama et al. (89) and others (85,87) using polyclonal antibody-
based procedures.

Other Clinical Uses of Prostate-Specific Antigen Assays

Whether or not serum PA measurements can be used for screening
is debatable, as is the use of serum PAP measurements. The arguments for and against using PAP measurement as a screening test,
which have been disucssed in Sec. II, can also be applied here. The
most certain clinical usefulness of the PA test is in the monitoring
of disease. Killian and collaborators (90) have shown, with a polyclonal antibody-based procedure, a significant association between

serially measured PA levels and disease-free survival time. They found that the serum PA level was useful in predicting and confirming recurrence of disease. These investigators have also shown that PA is superior to PAP and alkaline phosphatase for prognostic reliability of disease progression (91). The usefulness of PA as a marker for monitoring prostatic cancer has also been reported by other investigators using polyclonal antibody-based procedures (85,87). As mentioned, Siddall et al. (88) using an MAb-based procedure also found PA measurement was useful in monitoring the course of disease and in providing valuable information for making clinical decisions. Thus far, studies comparing polyclonal antibody-based methods with MAb-based methods relative to their usefulness for monitoring prostatic cancer have not been performed. Therefore, it remains unknown whether or not MAb-based methods are superior to polyclonal antibody-based procedures in monitoring prostatic cancer.

Aside from being a useful prostatic tumor marker in the serum test discussed earlier, many studies using polyclonal anti-PA antibodies have shown that PA is a very useful immunohistochemical marker for prostatic tumor (74,92-108). Immunoenzymatic staining for PA has been shown to have potential value in the classification of metastasized tumor of unknown origin (74,93,95, 96,100-102,104,105). The staining characteristics of PA allows adenoid cystic carcinoma of the prostate to be distinguished from the usual acidinic adenocarcinomas of the prostate (109). Cytosarcoma phyllodes of the prostate has also been reported to give negative results in immunoperoxidase staining for PA (110), as do the urinary bladder tumors invading the prostate (74).

Data accumulated, so far, show that the staining of PA has diagnostic specificity of 100%, but the diagnostic sensitivity ranged from 70 to 100% in different laboratories. One factor that may contribue to the variation of the sensitivity data is the effect of hormonal treatment on the expression of PA by tumor cells. Grignon and Troster (111) compared the results of immunohistochemical staining before and after diethylstilbestrol therapy and found that in five of 11 patients in the posttreatment group, the staining with both PA and PAP was reduced. Their results suggested that the study, which consisted of many specimens from patients being treated with the hormone, resulted in data of lower sensitivity. Another factor that may account for the variation in the sensitivity data obtained by different investigators is, among others, the quality of the polyclonal antiserum used. The use of MAbs should overcome this problem. With hybridoma technology, it is possible to generate antibody of high quality in large quantities, and thus standardization of the antibody reagents and the ensurance of reproducible results are possible. Furthermore, use of MAbs in immunohistochemical staining results in lower background staining and, hence, in higher sensitivity in our experiments. Papsidero et al. (112) used anti-PA MAb (29) in the immunohistochemical studies of metastasized tumors of various origins. Their results showed that all of 25 prostatic tumor specimens obtained from various metastatic sites (breast, lymph nodes, liver, bone, bladder, bowel wall, and seminal vesicle) gave positive results, while none of 73 specimens of metastasized, nonprostatic tumor specimens from various sites showed positive staining.

In many immunohistochemical studies of PA (29,95,97,99, 100,103,105), observations have been made indicating variation in the percentage of cells stained and the intensity of staining from specimen to specimen; well-differentiated tumors tend to have a higher percentage of cells stained when compared with poorly differentiated tumors, and the intensity of the staining of well-differentiated tumors also tends to be stronger. Therefore, if the staining method employed is not sensitive enough, for example, because of poor quality of reagents, some tumor specimens with low PA concentrations may not be stained. Although in the study of Papsidero et al. (112), the MAb-based method gave 100% diagnostic sensitivity and specificity and, theoretically, the method employing MAb should be superior to the polyclonal antibody-based method, more studies are required to determine whether MAb-based procedures are indeed better than polyclonal antibody-based procedures.

An observation made by Chu et al. (113) is pertinent, with an important implication in the generation of human MAb. These investigators have found a PA-binding immunoglobulin (PABG) of the IgG class in the human serum. The level of this circulating PABG was elevated only in patients with an advanced stage of prostatic cancer. These data suggested that PABG is an autoantibody and that generation of human anti-PA MAb by fusing patients' B lymphocytes with myeloma cells is feasible (16).

Human anti-PA MAb, if it can be generated, will be of great value
in tumor imaging and other clinical applications.

OTHER MONOCLONAL ANTIBODY-DEFINED ANTIGENS
WITH POTENTIAL VALUE AS TUMOR MARKERS

In recent years, there have been a number of reports concerning
mouse MABs raised against intact cells of human prostatic tumor
lines or against membrane preparations of BPH or prostatic tumor
tissue (15,18-21,25,28,76,114-116). A human MAb reactive with
human prostate has also been reported (16). Among these antibodies are anti-PA and anti-PAP antibodies. It has not yet been
reported if the antigens recognized by these antibodies, except PA
and PAP, are released into the circulation and appear in the serum
as elevated levels in prostatic cancer patients. Even if these antigens are not released into the blood, some of them may still have
potential value as markers for immunohistochemical classification
of tumor. Some of these MAbs have been reviewed by Chu (19)
and Starling et al. (117). Here, we would like to discuss only
those MAbs with potential diagnostic value because of their specificity.

KR-P8

The MAb KR-P8, reported by Raynor et al. (20), was generated
against intact cells of a human prostatic tumor line, PC-3. The
antigen, called P8, recognized by KR-P8 antibody is a glycoprotein with molecular weight range of 48,000-75,000 (118). Antigen P8 is a secretory product of both normal and malignant
prostate epithelium and is present in urine and seminal plasma;
it is also present on the surface of 90% of cells of the PC-3 line
and of 67% of cells of another human prostate tumor line, DU-
145. The antigen is absent from the surface of normal peripheral
blood leukocytes, and the cells of a number of lymphoblastic
lines. Among clinical specimens examined, the antigen is present
in normal, BPH, and cancerous prostate tissue, but not in other
normal or malignant tissues. Thus, P8 antigen is, like PA, a prostatic organ site-specific antigen. Although P8 antigen has not been
detected in the sera of healthy males using an immunoblot assay
procedure, a more sensitive method may discern the antigen in the
sera. Whether or not the antigen is present in prostatic cancer pa-

tients' sera has not been reported, but such a possibility exists because P8 antigen is also detected in the metastasized prostatic tumor. The P8 antigen is biochemically and immunologically distinct from PA, but its secretory nature, its location in prostatic epithelium, and its specificity resemble those of PA, and it is likely that P8 antigen may also have diagnostic value.

PEQ 226

Leung and colleagues (25) recently reported this MAb raised against a membrane preparation of a human prostate tumor. It recognizes a membrane-associated protein with molecular weight of 100,000, and it does not react with PA or PAP. Immunohistochemical study revealed that this antibody reacted with normal prostate and eight of nine prostate tumor specimens. The antibody showed no significant activity toward 17 other normal tissues of various origin, including liver, kidney, and gastrointestinal tract. The antigen recognized by PEQ 226 antibody thus appears to be another prostatic organ site-specific antigen, similar to PA. Whether or not this antigen is released into blood or into other body fluids has not been reported.

Turp 27

Turp 27 is one of the MAbs obtained by Starling et al. (14) by injecting the membrane preparations of pooled specimens of BPH and cancerous prostatic tissues into mice. The antigen defined by Turp 27 antibody occurs in BPH and malignant prostatic tissue as well as, in reduced concentration, in normal prostatic tissues. By use of RIA, it has been shown that this antibody does not react with the membranes of nonprostatic tissues. The staining of tissue specimens with immunoperoxidase has revealed that the antibody does not react with various normal or cancerous nonprostatic tissues, except those tissues from normal breast. The antibody is not reactive with cancerous breast tissues, but in three of the six normal breast specimens they examined, several cells within a few normal ducts were stained. Presence of the antigen in a few cells of breast tissue may not pose a serious problem in interpreting the data should the antigen recognized by Turp 27 antibody be used as a marker of prostatic tumor, which occurs only in males. Should the observation that there is a reduced concentration of this antigen in normal prostate tissue be confirmed and the antigen be a secretory product of prostate tumors, the antigen theoretically would be a more specific tumor marker than are PA, PAP, and P8 antigen.

83.21

Monoclonal antibody 83.21 was also prepared by Starling's group (119,120). This antibody was raised against the cells of a human prostatic tumor line, DU-145, and is directed against a membrane glycoprotein with molecular weight of 180,000 (121). It binds to the cells of two human prostatic tumor lines (PC-3 and DU-145), three human bladder tumor lines (T-24, 639V, and 647V), and a cytomegalovirus-transformed human embryonic lung line; but it does not bind to the cells of 38 normal or malignant human cell lines. With the immunoperoxidase-staining technique, the antibody has been shown to react with 6 of 7 undifferentiated, 4 of 5 poorly differentiated, 1 of 3 moderately differentiated, but none of 4 well-differentiated primary prostatic tumor specimens. The antibody also reacted with one of four undifferentiated and none of two well-differentiated, metastasized prostatic tumor specimens. The most striking feature of this antibody is that it does not react with normal prostatic and BPH tissues. This antibody was reactive also with one of four primary cancerous bladder specimens examined, but it was not reactive with two benign bladder tumors and three normal bladder specimens examined. Immunoperoxidase staining of 15 other primary adenocarcinoma specimens obtained from lung, colon, liver, breast, melanoma, pancreas, and kidney revealed the absence of antigen recognized by 83.21 antibody in these specimens. Of 30 normal tissue specimens (from lung, breast, heart, spleen, liver, colon, pancreas, testes, vas differens, and bladder) examined by immunoperoxidase staining, none gave positive results; but positive staining was seen in proximal convoluted tubules of two normal kidney specimens. Although the antigen recognized by 83.21 antibody is not strictly prostatic tumor-specific, its absence in most of the tissues, including normal prostatic and BPH tissues, endows it with a potential usefulness in the diagnosis of prostatic cancer. Should the antigen defined by 83.21 antibody be used as a prostatic tumor marker, it would be most useful when employed in conjunction with other tumor markers.

CONCLUSION

In recent years a number of MAb-based methods for assaying the
two most common prostatic tumor markers, PA and PAP, have
been developed. Whether or not these procedures are superior to
those employing polyclonal antibodies or antisera still remain to
be determined; more data are needed to draw unequivocal conclusions. The PA and PAP are not prostatic tumor-specific antigens,
and as can be expected when they serve as markers in the assay for
detecting prostatic cancer, a substantial number of false-positive
results are observed. The use of MAb antibody may alleviate the
problem, but cannot eliminate it totally. An ideal assay method
for the detection of cancer should be the one with absolute specificity as well as sensitivity; therefore, a positive test will indicate
the presence of a cancer, and a negative result the absence of cancer. Such a procedure requires marker reagents that are specific
for the particular type of neoplasm to be detected. For prostatic
cancer, such markers have not been found, despite the effort of
extensive investigations. Many MAbs have been generated against
prostatic tumor but none are prostatic tumor-specific. Some of
these antibodies such as anti-PA and anti-PAP MAbs are of disease-
monitoring value. Whether or not the antibodies now available
will be of clinical value in early detection of prostatic cancer remains to be seen.

ACKNOWLEDGMENT

Our work described was supported by NIH grants CA-15437 and
CA-34536. The authors thank Joan Ogledzinski for secretarial
assistance in preparation of this paper.

REFERENCES

1. American Cancer Society, *Cancer Facts and Figures* (1986).
2. J. D. Schmidt and J. Pollen, in *Prostatic Cancer* (G. P. Murphy,
    ed.), PSG Publishing Co., Littleton, Mass. (1979), p. 129.
3. M. A. Bagshaw, in *Prostatic Cancer* (G. P. Murphy, ed.), PSG
    Publishing Co., Littleton, Mass. (1979), p. 151.
4. A. B. Gutman and E. D. Gutman, *J. Clin. Invest. 17*:473
    (1938).

5. R. H. Flock, V. C. Urich, C. A. Patel, and J. M. Opitz, *J. Urol.* *84*:134 (1960).

6. R. J. Ablin, *Cancer 29*:1570 (1972).

7. M. C. Wang, L. A. Valenzuela, G. P. Murphy, and T. M. Chu, *Invest. Urol. 17*:159 (1979).

8. J. Muntzing and T. Nilsson, *Scand. J. Urol. Nephrol. 6*:107 (1972).

9. C. W. Moncure, C. L. Johnston, Jr., W. E. Koontz, Jr., and M. J. V. Smith, *Cancer Treat. Rep. 59*:105 (1975).

10. G. E. Brannen, D. M. Gomolka, and D. S. Coffey, *Cancer Treat. Rep. 59*:127 (1975).

11. L. E. Broder, B. S. Weinstraub, S. W. Rosen, M. H. Cohen, and F. Tejada, *Cancer 40*:211 (1977).

12. U. Dunzendorfer, N. Katopodis, A. M. Dnistrian, C. C. Stock, M. K. Schwartz, and W. F. Whitmore, Jr., *Invest Urol. 19*:194 (1981).

13. E. J. Zampella, E. L. Bradley, and T. G. Pretlow, *Cancer 49*: 384 (1982).

14. J. E. Pontes, *J. Urol. 130*:1037 (1982).

15. A. M. Carroll, M. Zalutsky, S. Schatten, A. Bhan, L. L. Perry, C. Sobotka, B. Benacerraf, and M. I. Greene, *Clin. Immunol. Immunopathol. 33*:268 (1984).

16. D. H. Lowe, H. H. Handley, J. Schmidt, I. Royston, and M. C. Glassey, *J. Urol. 132*:780 (1984).

17. M. Hall, S. S. Mickey, A. S. Wenger, and L. M. Silverman, *Clin. Chem. 31*:1689 (1985).

18. J. J. Rusthoven, J. B. Robinson, A. Kolin, and P. H. Pinkerton, *Cancer 56*:289 (1985).

19. T. M. Chu, in *Monoclonal Antibodies in Cancer* (S. Sell and R. A. Reisfeld, eds.), The Humana Press, Clifton, N. J. (1985), p. 309.

20. R. H. Raynor, T. Mohanakumar, C. W. Moncure, and T. A. Hazra, *J. Urol. 134*:384 (1985).

21. J. Lindren, M. Blaszczyk, B. Atkinson, Z. Steplewski, and H. Koprowski, *Cancer Immunol. Immunother. 22*:1 (1986).

22. V. M. Doctor, A. R. Sheth, M. N. Simha, N. J. Arbratti, J. P. Aaveri, and N. A. Sheth, *Br. J. Cancer 53*:547 (1986).

23. M. Kuriyama, T. Tekeuchi, I. Shinoda, M. Okano, and T. Nishiura, *Prostate 8*:301 (1986).

24. J. Guevara, Jr., B. H. Herbert, A. K. Raymond, and J. G. Batsakis, *Cancer Res. 46*:3599 (1986).

25. J. Leung, M. Stone, J. Koda, S. Hochschwender, C. Halverson, R. Bartholomew, *6th Int. Congr. Immunol.* p. 516 (1986) (abstract).
26. H. S. Lilleheji, B. K. Choe, and N. R. Rose, *Mol. Immunol. 19*: 1119 (1982).
27. C. L. Lee, C. Y. Li, Y. H. Jou, G. P. Murphy, and T. M. Chu, *Ann. N.Y. Acad. Sci. 390*:52 (1982).
28. A. E. Frankel, R. V. Rouse, M. C. Wang, T. M. Chu, and L. A. Herzenberg, *Cancer Res. 42*:3714 (1982).
29. L. D. Papsidero, G. A. Croghan, M. C. Wang, M. Kuriyama, E. A. Johnson, L. A. Vlanezuela, and T. M. Chu, *Hycridoma 2*: 139 (1982).
30. J. F. Myrtle, W. Schakelford, R. M. Bartholomew, and J. Wampler, *Clin. Chem. 29*:1216 (1983) (abstract).
31. R. M. Loor, D. Buck, T. M'Timkulu, S. K. DeWitt, D. Lippman, R. Loffland, B. Fendly, and N. Jung, *Hybridoma 4*:77 (1985) (abstr.).
32. L. T. Yam, *Am. J. Med. 56*:604 (1974).
33. S. Shulman, L. Mamrod, M. J. Gonder, and W. A. Soanes, *J. Immunol. 93*:474 (1964).
34. J. F. Cooper and A. Foti, *Invest. Urol. 12*:98 (1974).
35. A. G. Foti, J. F. Cooper, H. Herschman, and R. R. Malvaez, *N. Engl. J. Med. 297*:1357 (1977).
36. T. M. Chu, M. C. Wang, W. W. Scott, R. P. Gibbons, D. E. Johnson, J. D. Schmidt, S. A. Loening, G. R. Prout, and G. P. Murphy, *Invest. Urol. 15*:319 (1978).
37. Z. Wajsman, T. M. Chu, J. Saroff, N. Slack, and G. P. Murphy, *Urology 13*:8 (1979).
38. Y. Ban, M. C. Wang, and T. M. Chu, *Urol. Clin. N. Am. 11*:269 (1984).
39. W. Hengst, M. Fisher, and H. Sparwasser, *Tumor Diag. 4*:197 (1980).
40. S. Dass, N. L. Bowen, and K. D. Bagshawe, *Clin. Chem. 26*: 1583 (1980).
41. P. Vihko, A. Kostama, O. Janne, E. Sajanti, and R. Vihko, *Clin. Chem. 26*:1544 (1980).
42. K. Gericke, K. P. Kohse, G. Pfleiderer, S. H. Fluchter, and K. H. Bichler, *Clin Chem. 28*:596 (1982).
43. G. P. DeVries and G. T. B. Sanders, *Am. J. Clin. Pathol. 78*: 189 (1982).

44. A. L. Babson, *Clin. Chem. 30*:1254 (1984).
45. J. L. Carson, J. M. Eisenberg, L. M. Shaw, H. L. Kundel, and
    K. A. Soper. *J. Am. Med. Assoc. 253*:665 (1985).
46. P. Vihko, M. Kontturi, O. Lukkarinen, J. Ervasti, and R.
    Vihko, *Cancer 56*:173 (1985).
47. J. Fleischmann, W. J. Catalona, W. R. Fair, W. D. W. Heston,
    and M. Menon, *J. Urol. 129*:312 (1983).
48. J. Griffiths, D. F. Rippe, and P. R. Panfili, *Clin. Chem. 28*:183
    (1982).
49. E. D. Sevier, G. S. David, J. Martinis, W. J. Desmond, R. M.
    Bartholomew, and R. Wang, *Clin. Chem. 27*:1797 (1981).
50. M. F. Lin, C. L. Lee, and T. M. Chu, *Clin. Chim. Acta 10*:
    263 (1983).
51. L. A. Kaplan, I. W. Chen, M. Sperling, B. Bracken, and E. A.
    Stein, *Am. J. Clin. Pathol. 84*:334 (1985).
52. R. Wang, W. F. Bermudez, R. L. Saunders, W. A. Present,
    R. M. Bartholomew, and T. Adams, *Clin. Chem. 27*:1063
    (1981) (abstr.).
53. S. N. Davies and N. Gochman, *Am. J. Clin. Pathol. 79*:114
    (1983).
54. R. M. Loor, T. M'Timkulu, N. Jung, S. D. DeWitt, R. Loffland,
    M. S. Soloway, and P. Guinan, *J. Clin. Immunoassay 9*:153
    (1986).
55. D. W. Mostt, C. H. Self, K. B. Whitaker, E. Bailyes, K. Siddle,
    A. Johannsson, C. J. Stanley, and E. H. Cooper, *Clin. Chim.
    Acta 152*:85 (1985).
56. R. A. Watson and D. B. Tang, *N. Engl. J. Med. 303*:497
    (1980).
57. B. J. Carroll, *N. Engl. J. Med. 298*:912 (1978).
58. B. K. Choe, E. J. Pontes, N. R. Rose, and M. D. Henderson,
    Invest. Urol. 15:312 (1978).
59. J. W. Wojcieszyn, M. C.Wang, C. L. Lee, G. P. Murphy, and
    T. M. Chu, *J. Appl. Biochem. 1*:223 (1979).
60. L. T. Yam, A. J. Janckila, C. Y. Li, and W. K. Lam, *Invest.
    Urol. 19*:34 (1981).
61. O. L. Podhajcer, J. E. Filmus, and J. Mordoh, *Mol. Cell. Bio-
    chem. 66*:39 (1985).
62. P. Guinan, I. Bush, V. Ray, R. Vieth, R. Rao, and R. Bhatti,
    N. Engl. J. Med. 303:499 (1980).
63. P. Cohen and D. Dix, *Clin. Chem. 30*:171 (1984).

64. C. S. Killian, F. P. Vargas, N. H. Slack, G. P. Murphy, and
    T. M. Chu, *Ann. N.Y. Acad. Sci. 390*:122 (1982).
65. P. Vihko, M. Kontturi, O. Lukkarinen, and R. Vihko, *J. Urol.
    133*:797 (1985).
66. S. N. Davies and J. C. Griffiths, *Clin. Chim. Acta 122*:29
    (1982).
67. E. H. Cooper, N. B. Pidcock, D. Daponte, R. W. Glashan, E.
    Rowe, and M. R. G. Robinson, *Eur. Urol. 9*:17 (1983).
68. T. D. Moon, R. L. Vessella, M. Eickhoff, and P. H. Lange,
    Urology 22:16 (1983).
69. N. H. Zweig and D. C. Ihde, *Cancer Res. 45*:3945 (1985).
70. M. Nadji and A. R. Morales, *Ann. N.Y. Acad. Sci. 390*:133
    (1982).
71. D. M. Goldenberg and F. H. DeLand, *Urol. Clin. N. Am. 11*:
    277 (1984).
72. P. Vihko, J. Heikkila, M. Kontturi, L. Wahlberg, and R. Vihko,
    Ann. Clin. Res. 16:51 (1984).
73. C. L. Lee, E. Kawinski, J. Horoszewicz, and T. M. Chu, *J.
    Tumor Marker Oncol. 1*:47 (1986).
74. M. Nadji, S. Z. Tabei, A. Castro, T. M. Chu, G. P. Murphy,
    M. C. Wang, and A. R. Morales, *Cancer 48*:1229 (1981).
75. L. D. Papsidero, M. Kuriyama, M. C. Wang, J. Horoszewicz,
    S. S. Leong, L. Valenzuela, G. P. Murphy, and T. M. Chu,
    J. Natl. Cancer Inst. 66:37 (1981).
76. M. P. W. Gallee, C. C. J. van Vroonhoven, H. A. H. M. van der
    Korput, T. H. van der Kwast, F. J. W. ten Kate, J. C. Romijn,
    and J. Trapman, *Prostate 9*:33 (1986).
77. M. C. Wang, M. Kuriyama, L. D. Papsidero, R. M. Loor, L. A.
    Valenzuela, G. P. Murphy, and T. M. Chu, *Methods Cancer
    Res. 19*:179 (1982).
78. M. C. Wang, L. A. Valenzuela, G. P. Murphy, and T. M. Chu,
    Oncology 39:1 (1982).
79. M. C. Wang, R. M. Loor, S. L. Li, and T. M. Chu, *IRCS Med.
    Sci. 11*:327 (1983).
80. K. W. K. Watt, P. J. Lee, T. M'Timkulu, W. P. Chan, and R. M.
    Loor, *Proc. Natl. Acad. Sci. 83*:3166 (1986).
81. Y. Ban, M. C. Wang, K. W. K. Watt, R. Loor, and T. M. Chu,
    Biochem. Biophys. Res. Comm. 123:482 (1984).
82. H. Lilja, *J. Clin. Invest. 76*:1899 (1985).

83. L. D. Papsidero, M. C. Wang, L. A. Valenzuela, G. P. Murphy, and T. M. Chu, *Cancer Res. 40*:2428 (1980).
84. M. Kuriyama, M. C. Wang, L. D. Papsidero, C. S. Killian, T. Shimano, L. Valenzuela, T. Nishiura, G. P. Murphy, and T. M. Chu, *Cancer Res. 40*:4568 (1980).
85. R. J. Liedtke and J. D. Batjer, *Clin. Chem. 30*:649 (1984).
86. A. Larson, A. Fritjofsson, B. J. Norlen, J. S. Gronowitz, and R. G. Ronquist, *Scand. J. Clin. Lab. Invest. 45*:81 (1985).
87. A. Ruibal, J. Morote, G. Encabo, J. Genolla, and J. A. de Torres, *Int. Oncodev. Biol. Med.*, 13th Annual Meeting, (1985) (abstr.).
88. J. K. Siddall, E. H. Cooper, D. W. W. Newling, M. R. G. Robinson, and P. Whelan, *Eur. Urol. 12*:123 (1986).
89. M. Kuriyama, M. C. Wang, C. L. Lee, C. S. Killian, L. D. Papsidero, H. Injai, R. M. Loor, M. F. Lin, T. Nishiura, N. H. Slack, G. P. Murphy, and T. M. Chu, *J. Natl. Cancer Inst. 68*:99 (1982).
90. C. S. Killian, N. Yang, L. M. Emrich, F. P. Vargas, M. Kuriyama, M. C. Wang, N. Slack, L. D. Papsidero, G. P. Murphy, T. M. Chu, and the Investigators of the National Prostatic Cancer Project, *Cancer Res. 45*:886 (1985).
91. C. S. Killian, L. J. Emrich, F. P. Vargas, N. Yang, R. Priore, G. P. Murphy, and T. M. Chu, *J. Natl. Cancer Inst. 76*:179 (1986).
92. B. S. Stein, R. P. Patersen, S. Vangore, and A. R. Kendall, *Am. J. Surg. Pathol. 6*:553 (1982).
93. E. P. Allhoff, J. H. Proppe, C. M. Chapman, C. W. Lin, and G. R. Prout, Jr., *J. Urol. 129*:315 (1983).
94. D. M. Purnell, B. M. Heatfield, and B. F. Trump, *Cancer Res.*, *44*:285 (1984).
95. B. S. Stein, S. Vangore, and R. P. Paterson, *Urology 24*:146 (1984).
96. M. Ghazizadeh, S. Kagawa, K. Maebayashi, K. Iizumi, and K. Kurokawa, *Urol. Int. 39*:9 (1984).
97. D. W. Ellis, S. Leffers, J. S. Davies, and A. B. P. Ng, *Am. J. Clin. Pathol. 81*:279 (1984).
98. N. Azumi, H. Shibuya, and M. Ishikura, *Am. J. Surg. Pathol. 8*:545 (1984).
99. J. I. Epstein and J. C. Eggleston, *Human Pathol. 15*:853 (1984).

100. M. S. Bentz, C. Cohen, L. R. Budgeon, and L. Demers, *Urology*, *23*:75 (1984).
101. D. T. Tell, J. M. Khoury, H. G. Taylor, and S. P. Veasey, *J. Am. Med. Assoc.* *253*:3574 (1985).
102. M. M. Walther, V. Nassar, R. C. Harruff, B. B. Mann, Jr., D. P. Finnerty, and K. O. Hewen-Lowe, *J. Urol.* *134*:769 (1985).
103. M. C. Mathieu and J. M. Caillaud, *Bull. Cancer* *72*:27 (1985).
104. J. Steffens, W. Friedman, and H. Lobeck, *Eur. Urol.* *11*:91 (1985).
105. H. Svanholm, *Microbiol. Immunol. Scand. Sec. A.* *94*:7 (1986).
106. H. Ito, K. Yamaguchi, H. Sumiya, O. Matzuzaki, and J. Shimazaki, *Eur. Urol.* *12*:49 (1986).
107. N. T. Shah, S. E. Tuttle, S. L. Strobel, and L. Ghandi, *J. Surg. Oncol.* *29*:265 (1985).
108. J. I. Epstein and J. N. Woodruff, *Cancer* *57*:111 (1986).
109. F. P. Kuhajda and R. B. Mann, *Am. J. Clin. Pathol.* *81*;257 (1984).
110. C. Manivel, B. V. Shenoy, M. R. Wick, and L. P. Dehner, *Arch. Pathol. Lab. Med.* *110*:534 (1986).
111. D. Grignon and M. Troster, *Prostate* *7*:195 (1985).
112. L. D. Papsidero, G. A. Croghan, J. Asirwatham, J. Gaeta, P. Abenoza, L. Englander, and L. Valenzuela, *Am. J. Pathol.* *121*:451 (1985).
113. T. M. Chu, M. Kuriyama, E. Johnson, L. D. Paisidero, C. S. Killian, G. P. Murphy, and M. C. Wang, *Transplant. Proc. 16*: 481 (1984).
114. J. J. Starling, S. M. Sieg, M. L. Beckett, P. R. Wirth, Z. Wahab, P. F. Schellhammer, L. E. Ladaga, S. Poleskic, and G. Wright, Jr., *Cancer Res.* *46*:367 (1986).
115. J. S. Horoszewicz, S. S. Leong, E. Kawinski, and T. M. Chu, *14th Int. Cancer Cong.* (Budapest), 151 (1986).
116. S. S. Leong, J. S. Horoszewicz, and E. A. Mirand, *14th Int. Cancer Cong.* (Budapest), 702 (1986).
117. J. J. Starling, M. L. Beckett, G. L. Wright, Jr., in *Monoclonal Antibodies and Cancer* (C. L. Wright, Jr., ed.), Marcel Dekker, New York (1984), p. 253.
118. R. H. Raynor, T. A. Hazra, C. W. Moncure, and T. Mohanakumar, *Prostate* *9*:21 (1986).

119. J. J. Starling, S. M. Sieg, M. L. Beckett, P. F. Schellhammer, L. E. Ladaga, and G. L. Wright, Jr., *Cancer Res. 42*:3084 (1982).
120. G. L. Wright, Jr., M. L. Beckett, J. J. Starlung, P. F. Shell-hammer, S. M. Sieg, L. E. Lladaga, and S. Poleskic, *Cancer Res. 43*:5509 (1983).
121. J. J. Starling and G. L. Wright, Jr., *Cancer Res. 45*:804 (1985).

9

CA 19-9, a Monoclonal Antibody-Defined Marker for Gastrointestinal Malignancy

Vincent R. Zurawski, Jr. / Centocor, Malvern, Pennsylvania, and Harvard Medical School, Boston, Massachusetts

INTRODUCTION

Attempts to apply monoclonal antibody (MAb) technology to the solution of problems in cancer diagnosis and therapy have been prodigious in the last 10 years. Remarkably, despite these vast efforts, precise clinical applications of MAbs to these problems have only recently begun to emerge.

The development of diagnostic applications for MAbs with real clinical utility is one of the important goals of clinicians and researchers alike who produce and experiment with antibodies directed at tumor-associated antigenic determinants. Construction of an immunoassay is only a first step toward this goal. More important is the clinical testing of the assay that will delineate application(s) that can provide the physician with new information with which he can act on behalf of his patient.

This chapter will review the development of a particular MAb designated 19-9 and the attempts to characterize the determinant and antigen(s) to which the 19-9 antibody binds. It will also review the development of a diagnostic blood test that utilizes the antibody and the current status of the investigations that have attempted to identify a clinical utility for this test, particularly among patients with gastrointestinal malignancy.

THE 19-9 ANTIBODY

The 19-9 antibody is synthesized by a cloned murine hybridoma designated 1116NS 19-9, which was produced by Koprowski and his colleagues (1). This hybrid cell line was produced using the method of Kohler and Milstein (2) with spleen cells from a mouse immunized with cells from a colorectal carcinoma cell line designated SW1116 (3). These spleen cells that were fused with the 653 variant of the P3 × 63 AG8 myeloma cell line described by Kearney et al. (4). The 19-9 antibody is an IgG_1 (1). By use of a radioimmunoassay (RIA) the antibody was found to bind to five of eight colorectal carcinoma cell lines tested but not to several other epithelial and nonepithelial cancer cell lines nor to carcinoembryonic antigen (CEA) (1).

No further characterization of the biochemical characteristics of the antibody or amino acid sequence analyses have been attempted. Clones of the hybridoma that synthesize the 19-9 antibody have been in the author's laboratory for approximately 7 years and have remained stable producers of antibody for all of that time.

THE CA 19-9 ANTIGENIC DETERMINANT AND ANTIGEN

Because the potential clinical value of the 19-9 antibody was recognized relatively quickly, efforts were made to characterize the nature of the epitope and antigen(s) to which the antibody binds. It had been observed that the binding of 19-9 antibody to

SW1116 cells could be prevented by treatment of these cells with neuraminidase but not with ficin, which suggested that the CA 19-9 determinant might reside on a ganglioside. Indeed, Magnani et al. (5) first characterized the epitope, which has been designated CA 19-9 (6), as the carbohydrate portion of a monosialoganglioside. This ganglioside was also found in lipid extracts of colonic, gastric, and pancreatic adenocarcinomas obtained from treatment of frozen tissue specimens (5). The structural analysis of this carbohydrate identified it as a sialylated lacto-N-fucopentaose II (Figure 1) (7).

Recently, using a microsomal preparation from SW1116 cells, Hansson and Zopf (8) have reported on the biosynthetic pathway involved in the synthesis of the carbohydrate illustrated in Figure 1. It appears that the biosynthesis proceeds via the addition of a sialic acid to a type I Lewis blood group precursor chain followed by addition of a fucose residue to the chain in the presence of the Lewis fucosyltransferase rather than via addition of a sialic acid to a completed Le[a] blood group structure in which the fucose would already be present on the precursor chain. This result indicates that glycosylation in tumor cells and perhaps in other specialized epithelial cells may proceed by many different pathways, depending upon the differentiation state of the cell.

Koprowski and coworkers (9) also observed apparent immunoreactivity of the 19-9 antibody with a substance in the serum of patients with colon carcinoma; however, very little of this substance could be extracted from such sera using organic solvents. In fact, this serum antigen was reported to be a mucinlike protein by Magnani et al. (10). Recent work by Klug et al. has confirmed this observation (11). Moreover, the CA 19-9-containing glycoprotein was also purified from SW1116 cell supernates by this group, indicating that this colon carcinoma cell line could synthesize and shed the glycoprotein as well as the ganglioside described by Magnani and coworkers.

Klug et al. (11) also devised a purification scheme that allowed for a more complete biochemical characterization of the glycoprotein than had been reported. The protein was isolated from a very high-molecular-weight glycoprotein complex. In purified form it was found to be a single molecular species with an apparent molecular mass of 210 kD. Amino acid and carbohydrate compositions of the purified CA 19-9 antibody glycoprotein are

NeuNAcα 2−3Galβ 1−3GlcN Acβ 1−3Galβ 1−4Glc

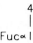

Figure 1   Structure of the oligosaccharide designated CA 19-9 to which the 19-9 MAb binds. The sugar residues are presented using standard abbreviations: NeuNAc, *N*-acetyl-neuraminic acid (sialic acid); Fuc, fucose; GalNAc, *N*-acetyl-galactoseamine; GlcNAc, *N*-acetyl-glucosamine; Gal, galactose; Glu, glucose. The presence of the Fuc and NeuNAc residues are essential for 19-9 binding to the oligosaccharide. (*Source*: Ref. 7)

presented in Tables 1 and 2. Both *O*- and *N*-linked oligosaccharides have been found associated with the CA 19-9-containing protein (N. LeDonne, unpublished observations). Hanisch and coworkers (12,13) were also able to identify high-molecular-weight glycoproteins containing CA 19-9 determinants in both human seminal plasma and milk. Furthermore, Kalthoff et al. (14) have found CA 19-9-containing glycoproteins in the pancreatic juice of individuals with both malignant and nonmalignant pancreatic disease and in apparently healthy subjects, suggesting that these proteins may be physiologic exocrine pancreatic secretion products.

Table 1   Carbohydrate Composition of the CA 19-9-Containing Glycoprotein Isolated from SW1116 Cells

Sugar[a]	Molar ratio[b]
Fucose	4.1
Mannose	1.0
Galactose	11.8
N-acetyl-galactosamine	2.5
N-acetyl-glucosamine	4.9
N-acetyl-neuraminic acid	5.1

[a]Composition was determined using trimethylsilyl derivatives of individual sugars.
[b]Molar ratios were computed with mannose set at 1.0.
Source: Modified from Ref. 11, with permission.

Table 2 Amino Acid Composition of the CA 19-9-Containing Glycoprotein Isolated from SW1116 Cells

Residue	Mole %	Residue	Mole %
Asp	5.1	Pro	7.3
Glu	9.8	Tyr	2.5
cmCys[a]	0.0	Val	5.1
Ser	19.7	Met	0.9
Gly	8.4	Ile	3.4
His	1.5	Leu	5.6
Arg	5.5	Phe	2.7
Thr	8.8	Lys	4.1
Ala	7.5		

[a]Below the limits of detection.
Source: From Ref. 11, with permission.

The author has also observed in human saliva elevated levels of CA 19-9 that were associated with high-molecular-weight glycoproteins. Thus, the presence of CA 19-9-containing glycoprotein in at least four such sites supports the likelihood that the CA 19-9 determinant may be a component of several normal exocrine products found in the body.

TISSUE DISTRIBUTION OF CA 19-9

Numerous reports have appeared that describe the distribution of antigens containing the CA 19-9 determinant in normal adult, fetal, and malignant tissues (15-25). The first of these reports (15) focused on the distribution of CA 19-9 in malignant tissue by using an immunoperoxidase assay on fixed, paraffin-embedded tumors. Most colon tumors (59%) were found to express CA 19-9. Focal areas of staining were observed in six of 40 positively stained specimens, whereas most tumor cells stained in the remaining 34. Moreover, 86% of pancreatic and 89% of gastric adenocarcinoma specimens stained in a strongly diffuse manner. Whenever patient sera contained elevated CA 19-9 levels, tumors were found to be expressing the determinant. In addition, however, it was also noticed that some cells of the columnar epithelium that line the ducts of the pancreas, liver, and gallbladder stained positive along with those of the gastric epithelium (15). Hirohashi et al. (20) observed focal expression of CA 19-9 in 62% of gastric carcinoma specimens and only in those containing the Le[a] blood group antigen. This group also observed some staining of normal gastric mucosa specimens, particularly, those that were metaplastic. These data also support the notion that antigens containing the CA 19-9 determinant can be normal secretion products of these exocrine epithelia. The CA 19-9 determinant was also observed in other normal tissue types by Arends et al. (19) and Bara et al. (23).

Atkinson et al. (15) also observed the presence of CA 19-9 in some other nongastrointestinal tumors, e.g., of the lung, bladder, thyroid, and ovary, but only infrequently among breast carcinomas. Charpin et al. (16) observed the presence of CA 19-9 in ovarian tumors as well, including 27% of serous tumors, 76% of mucinous tumors, and in ovarian tumors of other histopathological types.

Arends and coworkers (17,19) attempted to assess the correlation of the presence or absence of CA 19-9 in colorectal carcinomas to localization, stage, grade, and histopathological type of the cancers and, also, directly to survival of patients with colorectal carcinomas (21). Although an apparent trend toward more aggressive tumors was noted in patients in whom tumor cells were uniformly positive for CA 19-9, this trend did not reach statistically significant levels. This group concluded that the presence or absence of CA 19-9 in colonic adenocarcinomas was not likely to provide a sensitive independent assessment of patient prognosis. Olding et al. (22) found CA 19-9 in dysplastic areas of noncancerous colonic epithelium in patients with chronic ulcerative colitis, but the results were not clearly correlated to the degree of dysplasia. Consequently, the usefulness of immunoperoxidase staining of tissue with the 19-9 antibody to help in the discrimination between benign and precancerous lesions is also doubtful.

Thus, the distribution of CA 19-9 in tissue has provided further evidence that the determinant can be associated with normal exocrine epithelial cells and with the secretory products of these cells, consistent with studies on the CA 19-9-containing antigens. Moreover, numerous epithelial malignancies, particularly those of the gastrointestinal tract, express CA 19-9. This expression and shedding of CA 19-9-containing antigen by tumor cells into surrounding vascular beds probably explains why elevated CA 19-9 levels are found in the sera of some tumor patients.

CA 19-9 IN SERA

Introduction

Koprowski and his colleagues (9,26) were the first to observe the presence of a substance, which inhibited the binding of the 19-9 MAb to target cells, in the blood of colorectal, gastric, and pancreatic carcinoma patients. By using the same inhibition radioimmunoassay Sears et al. (27) showed that the levels of this substance measured at different times in the same patient with colorectal cancer varied. These results prompted development of a more convenient immunoradiometric assay (IRMA) described by Del Villano et al. (6) that uses the 19-9 antibody. The 19-9 IRMA is a solid-phase assay that utilizes 0.25-in. polystyrene balls coated with 19-9 antibody as a solid phase and radioiodinated 19-9 antibody as a tracer in a "forward-sandwich" format with two incubations of 3 hr each (6).

The clinical testing of any diagnostic immunoassay must follow a pattern similar to the one illustrated in Table 3. The first step in such testing involves the determination and distribution of serum levels for the antigen in question in patients with several diseases, both malignant and nonmalignant, and in individuals who are apparently healthy. Attempts to correlate regression and progression of disease with decreases or increases, respectively, of the serum antigen level must also be accomplished. Then the specific clinical usefulness of an assay can be evaluated for monitoring the clinical course of a disease or to characterizing a patient, either in a differential diagnostic or prognostic way. Finally, testing of an assay for help in early detection of a disease might be contemplated. Comparative evaluation of an assay with other assays might also be performed to determine the value of a panel of such assays for a particular application.

Table 3   Steps in the Evaluation of an In Vitro Diagnostic Test for Cancer

Distribution of values
    sensitivity in patient populations
    specificity in patient and control populations
Correlation of changes in values with regression and progression of disease
Definition of clinical utility
    monitoring of cancer patients
    classification of patients
        prognosis
        differential diagnosis
    early detection of cancer
    screening asymptomatic individuals
Use of diagnostic tests in panels for patient evaluation

Distribution of Serum CA 19-9 Levels

Several studies have been completed that describe the distribution of serum CA 19-9 levels in different populations. These studies have relied on the CA 19-9 IRMA to determine these levels. Del Villano et al. (6) and Del Villano and Zurawski (28) presented data that indicated that serum CA 19-9 levels were frequently elevated in patients with pancreatic, hepatobiliary, gastric, and primary hepatocellular carcinoma. Levels were less often elevated in patients with cancer of the large bowel, particularly in patients with early-stage disease. Serum CA 19-9 levels were much less often elevated in patients with cancers of the breast, lung, or other nongastrointestinal sites. Among patients with nonmalignant disorders, it appeared that CA 19-9 elevations could also occur in a significant number of patients with obstructive jaundice or with liver disease leading to a high degree of cirrhosis or necrosis of that organ (28). In contrast, CA 19-9 levels were very infrequently elevated in normal blood donors (6,28). More recently, it has also been shown that serum CA 19-9 levels were not frequently elevated in individuals who smoke cigarettes (29). Ritts et al. (30) confirmed all these results in a rigorous study using samples from the National Cancer Institute Serum Bank.

    Conclusions drawn from these studies were (1) that elevations of serum CA 19-9 appear to occur most frequently in patients with epithelial malignancies of the upper gastrointestinal tract and appendate organs, and (2) that CA 19-9 levels are less frequently elevated in patients with malignancies of the large bowel, except in advanced disease. Moreover, the relatively high specificity of the test for malignancy indicated that further development of the test as a laboratory adjunct for evaluating patients with, or suspected of having, pancreatic adenocarcinoma might be of clinical value. Also, the elevations occurring in patients with advanced colorectal cancer indicated that it might be important to evaluate the utility of monitoring this group of patients using serum CA 19-9 levels. Similar results and conclusions have been presented by others (31-43). In all of these studies, emphasis has been placed most frequently on the potential for using serum CA 19-9 levels in evaluating patients with pancreatic adenocarcinoma or tumors of the upper gastrointestinal tract.

These investigations have helped define the apparent specificity and sensitivity of the CA 19-9 IRMA among several populations, but the clinical usefulness of a diagnostic laboratory test hinges on the ability of the clinician to use the data provided by that test in a decision-making process. Therefore, further investigations aimed at specific clinical uses of the immunoassay have been undertaken by several groups. Potential advantages of measuring serum CA 19-9 levels preoperatively and longitudinally following surgery among patients with colorectal, ovarian, and pancreatic cancer have received the most attention.

Colorectal Cancer

The CA 19-9 levels were first observed to be elevated in the sera of colorectal cancer patients by Koprowski et al. (9). These results were confirmed by Ritts et al. (30) and Kuusela et al. (33), but less than one-half of patients with advanced disease and a much smaller fraction of those with localized disease were found to have elevated CA 19-9 levels. Sears et al. (27) first proposed the CA 19-9 levels might be of value in monitoring the clinical course of patients with colorectal carcinoma. In that study, however, a number of questions remained to be answered concerning the clinical usefulness of the test in this application. In particular, the relative sensitivity of the CA 19-9 IRMA compared with the CEA assay and the overall correlation of sustained elevations in CA 19-9 or increasing levels and decreasing levels with progression or regression of disease, respectively, were not clarified. Consequently, studies aimed at further elucidation of these questions have been completed (44-48).

A conclusion drawn from all of these investigations was that, although there may be individual patients in whom CA 19-9 levels are elevated or increasing—potentially placing individuals in this group at risk for clinical recurrence—the numbers of such patients are relatively small. Consequently, use of the CA 19-9 IRMA alone to monitor the clinical course in colorectal cancer patients is less valuable than the use of CEA levels alone. Some gains may acrue by using both assays together, however. A typical summary of the data presented in these investigations is shown in Table 4. More work will be required to determine if the CA 19-9 and CEA pair of assays will provide clinically useful information for monitoring patients or predicting patient outcomes.

Ovarian Cancer

Charpin et al. (16) presented immunoperoxidase-staining data on frozen sections of ovarian tumors that clearly demonstrated the presence of CA 19-9 on epithelial ovarian cancers of all histopathological types, with 76% of mucinous tumor specimens and 27% of serous tumor specimens staining positively. Consequently, a number of investigators have explored the potential clinical use of the CA 19-9 IRMA in evaluating patients with ovarian carcinoma. Kremer et al. (49) have shown that serum CA 19-9 levels were elevated in approximately 25% of serous ovarian carcinomas, in agreement with the 17% reported by Bast et al. (50). In the latter investigation, fewer than 5% of the patients studied had mucinous tumors. In cases of serous tumors where CA 19-9 levels are elevated, typically, CA 125 levels (51) are also elevated and at higher levels (Figure 2).

In four additional studies (52–56), serum elevations of CA 19-9 were observed in a fraction of ovarian cancer patients. In three of these studies (52,53,56), decreases in CA 19-9 levels were observed accompanying regression of disease associated with therapeutic procedures. In the study of Bast et al. (50), however, only a 33% overall correlation was observed in monitoring the clinical course of ovarian cancer, contrasted to a 94% correlation for CA 125, which led this group to conclude that the CA 19-9 IRMA would be of marginal value when compared with the CA 125

Table 4   Distribution of Paired CA 19-9 and CEA Assay Values in Patients with Colorectal Carcinoma

CA 19-9[a]	CEA[a] Normal (< 5.0)	Elevated (> 5.0)	Total
Normal (< 37.0)	50	74	124
Elevated (≥ 37.0)	7	89	96
Total	57	163	220

[a]For CEA, 5.0 ng/ml was used as a reference value, and for CA 19-9, 37 U/ml was used as a reference value to discriminate elevated from nonelevated samples.
Source: From Ref. 48, with permission.

immunoassay for monitoring patients with nonmucinous epithelial ovarian cancer. This conclusion is generally supported by all of the other studies. An area that remains to be explored, however, is the possible use of serum CA 19-9 levels in monitoring or otherwise evaluating patients with mucinous tumors. These tumors are less likely to have elevated CA 125 levels, particularly in the early stage (57).

Pancreatic Cancer

Because the sensitivity of the assay for pancreatic adenocarcinoma was high, Del Villano et al. (6) and Ritts et al. (30) proposed, early on in the evaluation of the CA 19-9 IRMA, that clinical applications of the assay for this disorder might be the most important to explore. It was also recognized by these investigators that pancreatic carcinoma is discovered nearly always in an advanced stage and that survival time of patients is usually less than 1 year. Consequently, any testing of clinical applications of the CA 19-9 IRMA in this disease would be limited. Nonetheless, clinical investigations have proceeded.

Klapdor et al. (36) found that among 33 patients with pancreatic adenocarcinoma, 27 (82%) had preoperative serum CA 19-9 levels of 37 U/ml or higher compared with none of 56 healthy controls and only one of 21 patients with chronic pancreatitis. This group was the first to make the specific proposal,

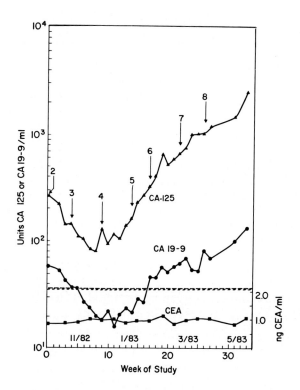

Figure 2 Serum CA 19-9, CA 125, and CEA levels followed longitudinally in a patient with ovarian carcinoma. The typically higher elevations of CA 125 relative to those of CA 19-9 or CEA can be observed. (*Source*: From Ref. 50, with permission.)

therefore, that the CA 19-9 IRMA might be a useful diagnostic tool in the differential diagnosis of exocrine pancreatic cancer from chronic pancreatitis. Moreover, they followed a small group of patients who had undergone resections of pancreatic carcinomas and showed that serum CA 19-9 levels decreased in the days following their resections. Consequently, they suggested that the assay might also have value in monitoring patients being treated for the disease.

More recently, Steinberg and coworkers (58) have reported on a well-characterized group of patients with pancreatic adenocarcinoma, nonmalignant pancreatic disorders, and other abdominal diseases selected to mimic signs and symptoms of patients with pancreatic cancer. In their study, preoperative serum CA 19-9 levels were determined for 37 patients with biopsy-proven adenocarcinoma of the pancreas, 23 of whom had unresectable disease, and 157 control patients. They found that by using a reference value of 75 U/ml, rather than one of 37 U/ml, a higher specificity of the CA 19-9 for malignant disease was achieved (Table 5). At the higher reference value, the sensitivity of the test for detecting pancreatic malignancy was 86.5%—78.6% for resectable and 91.3% for nonresectable disease—with a specificity of 93.5% (58). In addition, it was noted in this study that the concomitant use of CA 19-9 and CEA together—at reference values of 75 U/ml and 5 mg/ml, respectively—could improve the specificity of cancer detection to 99.1%, but with an expected loss of sensitivity to 38.8%. Thus, the use of the CA 19-9 IRMA as a differential diagnostic tool was also supported by this work.

Several other groups have reported similar findings that have led to some consensus on the notion that the CA 19-9 IRMA might be used as a differential diagnostic tool (44,59-68). Conditions must be applied to such use, however. Serum CA 19-9 levels are more often elevated in patients with acute pancreatitis than in patients in whom chronic pancreatitis is present, even above the 75 U/ml reference value (59,63). Moreover, some particularly high serum CA 19-9 levels have been observed in patients with obstructive jaundice or advanced cirrhosis (28). In fact, DelFavero et al. (67) have observed a correlation between serum bilirubin and CA 19-9 levels in patients with both pancreatic and extrapancreatic disease.

Consequently, as with any laboratory test, the use of other clinical, radiological, and laboratory tests together with the serum CA 19-9 level provides the best information on which to base diagnostic proposals. Satake et al. (6) have, for example, discussed the use of the assay together with serum elastase, other pancreatic enzymes, and CEA. Sakahara et al. (66) explored the correlation between CA 19-9 levels and computerized tomography (CT) findings in patients with chronic pancreatitis and pancreatic adenocarcinoma. In their study, CA 19-9 results alone were appar-

Table 5 Comparison of Sensitivity and Specificity Data for CA 19-9 Alone and the Combination of CA 19-9 and CEA[a]

	CA 19-9		CA 19-9 + CEA
	≥ 37 U/ml	≥ 75 U/ml	≥75 U/ml + ≥ 5 ng/ml
Sensitivity			
CAP	33/37 (89.2)	32/37 (86.5)	12/31 (38.8)

	CA 19-9		CA 19-9 + CEA
	<37 U/ml	<75 U/ml	<75 U/ml + < 5 ng/ml
Specificity			
BP	39/48 (81.3)	45/48 (93.8)	19/19 (100)
NPAP	33/34 (97.1)	33/34 (97.1)	30/30 (100)
BJ	47/58 (81.0)	51/58 (87.9)	57/58 (98.3)
M	7/7 (100)	7/7 (100)	3/3 (100)
Total	126/147 (85.7)	136/147 (93.5)	109/110 (99.1)

[a] Abbreviations used in the table are: CAP, cancer of pancreas; BP, benign pancreatic disease; NPAP, nonpancreatic abdominal pain; BJ, benign jaundice; M, malabsorption on a nonpancreatic basis. Numbers in parentheses are percentages.

Source: Reproduced in modified form from Ref. 58 with permission.

ently useful in the differential diagnosis of chronic pancreatitis from pancreatic carcinoma, with good correlation to CT results using a 37 U/ml reference value. Elevated CA 19-9 levels were found in 44 of 55 (80%) patients with pancreatic carcinoma and only two of 22 (9%) with chronic pancreatitis. If a reference value of 100 U/ml was used, no patients with nonmalignant disease had elevated values, and 69% still had elevations in the cancer group. There also was some correlation of the size of the tumor with serum CA 19-9 levels. In tumors less than 3 cm in diameter, elevations occurred in only one of eight (13%) patients. Interestingly, of the 55 tumor patients, six had normal CT scans, all but one of which also had serum CA 19-9 levels less than 37 U/ml. In that single case patient, the CA 19-9 level was 52 U/ml. This patient had a 1.7-cm malignant mass that was totally resected. This data suggests that in a limited number of patients, because localized pancreatic enlargement can occur in patients with chronic pancreatitis, CA 19-9 findings may be able to augment the results of CT scans. Moreover, taken together, abnormal CT scans and positive CA 19-9 levels appear to be highly predictive of the presence of pancreatic malignancy.

Tatsuta et al. have published results very similar (62) to those of Sakahara and coworkers. Serum CA 19-9 elevations occurred most frequently in patients with tumors larger than 3 cm and in those in the head of the pancreas. In addition, they found that CA 19-9 levels in pancreatic juice were more highly elevated in patients with malignant versus nonmalignant pancreatic disease; however, CA 19-9 levels in pancreatic fluid were of little value in discriminating between patients with pancreatolithiasis and pancreatic tumors, as comparable levels were noted in both diseases. This is not surprising because CA 19-9 is found in the epithelial cells lining the ducts of the normal pancreas (15). Nonetheless, the clinical use of CA 19-9 levels measured in pancreatic juices probably deserves further investigation.

The use of the CA 19-9 assay in monitoring patients with pancreatic carcinoma has also been explored by Takami et al. (68). They observed a trend toward correlation between rising and falling CA 19-9 levels and the progression of disease and apparent response to therapy, respectively. However, the clinical utility of this observation remains a question because of the highly aggressive nature of pancreatic carcinoma. On the other hand, as better therapeutic regimens are developed, or if disease can be discovered earlier, this monitoring application may prove to be of clinical value. Tempero et al. (69), for example, have attempted to use the assay to follow the clinical course of patients treated with MAb therapy.

Other Malignancies

Most clinical investigations of the CA 19-9 IRMA have centered on its potential use as a diagnostic tool for pancreatic, colorectal, and ovarian cancer patients. There have been a few other possible uses suggested, however, that are worth mentioning. Ritts et al. (30) implied that the greatest usefulness of the assay may be for tumors in the upper abdomen. Subsequently, Ritts has also observed significant elevations of serum CA 19-9 levels in patients with hepatobiliary carcinoma and advanced gastric carcinoma (R. E. Ritts, Jr., personal communication). Therefore, not surprisingly, it was proposed that the assay may have some value in the differential diagnosis of peptic ulcers from gastric cancer (70). This potential application has remained largely unexplored to date, however, and represents an area for future investigation.

There may also be some value in using the CA 19-9 assay to follow the treatment of liver metastasis. For example, even the most obvious application of the assay to colorectal carcinoma may be to follow treatment of liver metastases as new chemotherapeutic, immunotherapeutic, or surgical procedures are developed to treat these lesions (45). The CA 19-9 and CEA assays will need to be compared, however, to assess which will be more effective in this application.

Other Applications

As with other assays that define tumor-associated but not tumor-specific markers, CA 19-9 levels have been found elevated in a small fraction of numerous nonmalignant conditions and in a larger fraction of a limited number of such conditions (28). Duffy et al. (71) reported that elevations occur very frequently in patients with cystic fibrosis. This result should not interfere with the use of the assay among tumor patients because cystic fibrosis patients are nearly always children at much lower risk for gastrointestinal malignancy; however, Roberts et al. (72) suggested that these elevations may have potential value in the diagnosis of cystic fibrosis patients. This potential application of the assay probably does merit some further exploration. No other applications for the assay in patients with other nonmalignant disorders have been proposed.

CONCLUSIONS

The 19-9 antibody was one of the first MAbs produced that was directed against an apparently tumor-associated antigen. Initial optimism regarding the specificity of the determinant to which the antibody binds has been somewhat dampened. Nonetheless, it appears that the antibody will be a useful tool for research and perhaps for clinical applications.

The CA 19-9 immunoassay, for example, has received much attention by clinical investigators as a potential tumor marker for gastrointestinal malignancy. Interestingly, although the 19-9 MAb was originally prepared from spleen cells of a mouse immunized with a colorectal carcinoma cell line, it appears that serum CA 19-9 levels are most frequently elevated in the sera of patients with epithelial malignancies of the gastrointestinal tract and appendates in the upper abdomen. In particular, a high frequency of CA 19-9 elevations have been found in patients with pancreatic adenocarcinoma. In contrast, elevations have been infrequent in patients with chronic pancreatitis, particularly when a 75 U/ml or 100 U/ml, rather than a 37 U/ml, reference value has been used. Therefore, numerous studies have suggested that a most likely clinical use of the CA 19-9 immunoassay would be in the differential diagnosis of chronic pancreatitis from pancreatic carcinoma. Limitations of this application with respect to size and location of the tumor and correlation of CA 19-9 levels with CT scans, fine-needle biopsy results, and other laboratory or radiographic analyses deserve further exploration. The abundant information already available on this potential application, however, suggests that it may be one of the most important to be proposed for this immunoassay. Of course, the precise clinical benefit of this application to the physician and patient alike still must be adequately defined; however, because any diagnostic decision relies on the synthesis of much clinical, radiographic, and laboratory information, the addition of another piece of such information obtained at relatively low cost and with seemingly high predictive value should ultimately be of use to the clinician.

Radiolabeled 19-9 antibody has also been used as a radioimmunoscintigraphic tool for the diagnostic imaging of recurrent tumors of the large bowel (73), a clinical application that has not been reviewed in this chapter. This application will certainly receive more attention in the future, as will others of both the 19-9 antibody and the CA 19-9 immunoassay. Moreover, Steplewski et al. (74) have reported the successful establishment of a cell line that synthesizes a class-switched 19-9 antibody with an IgG_{2a} isotype. This new antibody may have some potential as a therapeutic agent for certain malignancies. Such explorations continue to provoke excitement over the incredible potential of even a single MAb and dramatically underscore the great future for the entire field of clinical applications for MAbs.

ACKNOWLEDGMENT

The author would like to thank Ms. Darnella Resetar for her help in preparing the manuscript.

REFERENCES

1. H. Koprowski, Z. Steplewski, K. Mitchell, M. Herlyn, D. Herlyn, and P. Fuhrer, *Somatic Cell Genet. 5*:957 (1979).
2. G. Kohler and C. Milstein, *Nature 256*:495 (1975).
3. A. Leibovitz, J. C. Stinson, W. B. McCombs, III, C. E. McCoy, K. C. Mazur, and N. D. Mabry, *Cancer Res. 36*:4562 (1976).
4. J. F. Kearney, A. Radbruch, B. Leisegang, and K. Rajewski, *J. Immunol. 123*:1548 (1979).
5. J. L. Magnani, M. Brockhaus, D. F. Smith, V. Ginsburg, M. Blaszczyk, K. F. Mitchell, Z. Steplewski, and H. Koprowski, *Science 212*:55 (1981).
6. B. C. Del Villano, S. Brennan, P. Brock, C. Bucher, V. Liu, M. McClure, B. Rake, S. Space, B. Westrick, H. Schoemaker, and V. R. Zurawski, Jr., *Clin. Chem. 29*:549 (1983).
7. J. L. Magnani, B. Nilsson, M. Brockhaus, D. Zopf, Z. Steplewski, H. Koprowski, and V. Ginsburg, *J. Biol. Chem. 257*:14365 (1982).
8. G. C. Hansson and D. Zopf, *J. Biol. Chem. 260*:9388 (1985).

9. H. Koprowski, D. Herlyn, Z. Steplewski, and H. F. Sears, *Science* 212:53 (1981).

10. J. L. Magnani, Z. Steplewski, H. Koprowski, and V. Ginsburg, *Cancer Res.* 43:5489 (1983).

11. T. L. Klug, N. C. LeDonne, Jr., T. F. Greber, and V. R. Zurawski, Jr., *Cancer Res.* (in press).

12. F. G. Hanisch, G. Uhlenbruck, and C. Dienst, *Eur. J. Biochem.* 144:467 (1984).

13. F. G. Hanisch, G. Uhlenbruck, C. Dienst, M. Stottrop, and E. Hippauf, *Eur. J. Biochem.* 149:323 (1985).

14. H. Kalthoff, C. Kreiker, W. H. Schmiegel, H. Greten, and H. G. Thiele, *Cancer Res.* 46:3605 (1986).

15. B. F. Atkinson, C. S. Ernst, M. Herlyn, Z. Steplewski, H. F. Sears, and H. Koprowski, *Cancer Res.* 42:4820 (1982).

16. C. Charpin, A. K. Bhan, V. R. Zurawski, Jr., and R. E. Scully, *Int. J. Gynecol. Pathol.* 1:231 (1982).

17. J. W. Arends, T. Wiggers, B. Schutte, C. T. Thijs, C. Verstinjnen, J. Hilgers, G. H. Blijham, and F. T. Bosman, *Int. J. Cancer* 32:289 (1983).

18. H. Raux, F. Labbe, M. C. Fondaneche, H. Koprowski, and P. Burtin, *Int. J. Cancer* 32:315 (1983).

19. J. W. Arends, C. Verstynen, F. T. Bosman, J. Hilgers, and Z. Steplewski, *Hybridoma* 2:219 (1983).

20. S. Hirohashi, Y. Shimosato, Y. Ino, Y. Tome, N. Watanabe, T. Hirota, and M. Itabashi, *Gann* 75:540 (1984).

21. J. W. Arends, T. Wiggers, C. Verstijnen, J. Hilgers, and F. T. Bosman, *Int. J. Cancer* 34:193 (1984).

22. L. B. Olding, C. Ahren, J. Thurin, D. A. Karlsson, C. Svalander, and H. Koprowski, *Int. J. Cancer* 36:131 (1985).

23. J. Bara, E. H. Zabaleta, R. Mollicone, M. Nap, and P. Burtin, *Am. J. Clin. Pathol.* 85:152 (1986).

24. E. C. Gong, S. Hirohashi, Y. Shimosato, M. Watanabe, Y. Ino, S. Teshima, and S. Kodaira, *J. Natl. Cancer Inst.* 75:447 (1985).

25. K. Iwase, K. Kato, A. Nagasaka, K. Miura, K. Kawase, S. Miyakawa, T. Tei, S. Ohtani, M. Inagaki, S. Shinoda, A. Nakai, T. Ohyama, Y. Horigushi, H. Nakano, and M. Itoh, *Gastroenterology* 91:576 (1986).

26. M. Herlyn, H. F. Sears, Z. Steplewski, and H. Koprowski, *J. Clin. Immunol.* 2:135 (1982).

27. H. F. Sears, M. Herlyn, B. Del Villano, Z. Steplewski, and H. Koprowski, *J. Clin. Immunol. 2*:135 (1982).

28. B. C. Del Villano and V. R. Zurawski, Jr., *Immunodiagnostics*, Vol. 8 (J. Hyun and R. Aloisi, (eds.), Alan R. Liss, New York (1983), p. 269.

29. P. J. Green, S. K. Ballis, P. Westkaemper, H. G. Schwartz, T. L. Klug, and V. R. Zurawski, Jr., *J. Natl. Cancer Inst. 77*: 337 (1986).

30. R. E. Ritts, B. C. Del Villano, V. L. M. Go, R. B. Herberman, T. L. Klug, and V. R. Zurawski, Jr., *Int. J. Cancer 33*:339 (1984).

31. Y. Ariyoshi, M. Kuwabara, M. T. Suchi, K. Ota, and M. Fukushima, *Igaku No Ayumi 125*:918 (1983).

32. H. Jalanko, P. Kuusela, P. Roberts, P. Sipponen, C. Haglund, and O. Makela, *J. Clin. Pathol. 37*:218 (1984).

33. P. Kuusela, H. Jalanko, P. Roberts, P. Sipponen, J. P. Mecklin, R. Pitkanen, and O. Makela, *Br. J. Cancer 49*:135 (1984).

34. R. Souchon, M. F. Souchon, J. Boese-Landgraf, U. Baer, K. Koppenhagen, M. Matthes, and R. Fitzner, *Cancer Detect. Prev. 8*:101 (1985).

35. R. Yoshikawa, K. Nishida, M. Tanigawa, K. Fukumoto, and M. Kondo, *Digestion 31*:67 (1985).

36. R. Klapdor, U. Lehmann, M. Bahlo, H. Greten, H. V. Ackerrn, M. Dallek, and W. H. Schreiber, *Tumor Diagn. Ther. 4*:197 (1983).

37. R. Klapdor, U. Klapdor, M. Bahlo, and H. Greten, *Tumor Diagn. Ther. 5*:161 (1984).

38. M. Okura, N. Itakura, T. Sakishima, H. Tajiri, and H. Ozaki, *Shokaki Geka 2*:221 (1984).

39. H. J. Staab, A. Hornung, F. A. Anderer, and G. Kieninger, *Dtsch. Med. Wochenschr. 109*:1141 (1984).

40. G. Mennini, C. Zanna, G. Silecchia, et al., *Chir. Gastroenterol. 18*:397 (1984).

41. F. Safi, M. Buchler, B. Schenkluhn, and H. G. Beger, *Dtsch. Med. Wochenschr. 109*:1869 (1984).

42. M. K. Gupta, R. Arciaga, L. Bocci, R. Tubbs, R. Bukowski, and S. D. Deodhar, *Cancer 56*:277 (1985).

43. Y. Ariyoshi, M. Kuwabara, H. Akatsuka, K. Koto, and T. Suchi, *Igaku No Ayumi 130*:129 (1984).

44. H. J. Staab, T. Brummendorf, A. Hornung, F. A. Anderer, and G. Kieninger, *Klin. Wochenschr. 63*:106 (1985).

45. H. Sears, J. W. Shen, M. Herlyn, B. Atkinson, P. F. Engstrom, and H. Koprowski, *Am. J. Clin. Oncol.* 8:108 (1985).
46. J. J. Szymendera, M. P. Nowacki, I. Kozlowicz-Gudzinska, and M. Kowalska, *Dis. Colon Rectum.* 28:895 (1985).
47. Y. Moriya, S. Watanabe, K. Hojo, and Y. Koyama, *Nippon Daicho Komonbyo Gakkai Zasshi* 38:640 (1985).
48. B. H. Novis, E. Gluck, P. Thomas, G. D. Steele, V. R. Zurawski, Jr., R. Stewart, P. T. Lavin, and N. Zamcheck, *J. Clin. Oncol.* 4:987 (1986).
49. M. Kremer, J. F. Chatal, C. Curtet, and J. Y. Doulliard, *Int. Soc. Oncodev. Biol. Med., 11th Annual Meeting*, Stockholm, September 11-13 (1983) (abstr.).
50. R. C. Bast, Jr., T. L. Klug, E. Schaetzl, P. Lavin, J. M. Niloff, T. F. Greber, V. R. Zurawski, Jr., and R. C. Knapp, *Am. J. Obstet. Gynecol.* 149:553 (1984).
51. R. C. Bast, Jr., T. L. Klug, E. St. John, E. Jenison, J. M. Niloff, H. Lazarus, R. S. Berkowitz, T. Leavitt, C. T. Griffiths, L. Parker, V. R. Zurawski, Jr., and R. C. Knapp, *N. Engl. J. Med.* 309:883 (1983).
52. M. Inoue, J. Saitoh, Y. Abe, Y. Inoue, G. Ueda, and O. Tanizawa, *Acta Obst. Gynaecol.* 37:2411 (1985).
53. P. A. Canney, P. M. Wiliinson, R. D. James, and M. Moore, *Br. J. Cancer* 52:131 (1985).
54. T. Miyoshi, H. Nishimura, N. Ookura, H. Moriasaki, H. Kobayashi, T. Tasaki, H. Ushijima, and M. Yakushiji, *Igaki Kenkyu* 54:796 (1984).
55. S. Negishi et al., *Gan No Rinsho* 6:655 (1985).
56. T. Noda, S. Saitoh, Y. Ando, A. Nakanishi, C. Maruya, S. Yoh, K. Hino, Y. Kiyozuka, and M. Ichijo, *J. Jpn. Soc. Cancer Ther.* 20:797 (1985).
57. V. R. Zurawski, Jr., R. C. Knapp, N. Einhorn, P. Kenemans, R. Mortel, K. Ohmi, R. C. Bast, Jr., R. E. Ritts, Jr., and G. Malkasian, *Gynecol. Oncol.* (in press).
58. W. M. Steinberg, R. Gelfand, K. K. Anderson, J. Glen, S. H. Kurtzman, W. F. Sindelar, and P. P. Toskes, *Gastroenterology* 90:343 (1986).
59. G. Heptner, S. Domschke, M. U. Schneider, and W. Domschke, *Dtsch. Med. Wochenschr.* 110:624 (1985).
60. A. Malesci, M. A. Tommasini, P. Bocchie, Z. Zerbi, E. Beretta, M. Vecchim, and V. DiCarlo, *Ric. Clin. Lab.* 14:303 (1984).

61. K. Satake, G. Kanazawa, I. Kho, Y.-S. Chung, and K. Ume-
    yama, *Am. J. Gastroenterol. 80*:630 (1985).
62. M. Tatsuta, H. Yamamura, H. Iishi, M. Ichii, S. Noguchi, R.
    Yamamoto, and S. Okuda, *Cancer 56*:2669 (1985).
63. K. Satake, G. Kanazawa, I. Kho, Y.-S. Chung, and K. Ume-
    yama, *J. Surg. Oncol. 29*:15 (1985).
64. W. H. Schmiegel, C. Kreiker, W. Eberl, R. Arndt, M. Classen,
    H. Greten, K. Jessen, H. Kalthoff, N. Soehendra, and H.-G.
    Thiele, *Gut 26*:456 (1985).
65. R. Farini, C. Fabris, P. Bonvicini, A. Piccoli, G. DelFavero,
    R. Venturini, A. Panucci, and R. Naccarato, *Eur. J. Cancer
    Clin. Oncol. 21*:429 (1985).
66. H. Sakahara, K. Endo, K. Nakajima, T. Nakashima, M. Koi-
    zumi, H. Ohta, A. Hidaka, S. Kohno, Y. Nakano, A. Naito,
    T. Suzuki, and K. Torizuka, *Cancer 57*:1324 (1986).
67. G. DelFavero, C. Fabris, M. Plebani, A. Panucci, A. Piccoli,
    L. Perobelli, S. Pedrazzoli, U. Baccaglini, A. Burlina, and
    R. Naccarato, *Cancer 57*:1576 (1986).
68. H. Takami, S. Hishinuma, J. Shintoku, Y. Ogata, and O. Abe,
    Gan No Rinsho 31:631 (1985).
69. M. A. Tempero, P. M. Pour, E. Uchida, D. Herlyn, and Z.
    Steplewski, *Hybridoma 5*:S133 (1986).
70. A. Ruibal, G. Encabo, R. Gefaell, E. Martinez-Miralles,
    J. M. Fort, and J. Fernandez-Llamazares, *Bull. Cancer 70*:
    438 (1983).
71. M. J. Duffy, F. O'Sullivan, T. J. McDonnell, and M. X. Fitz-
    gerald, *Clin. Chem. 31*:1245 (1985).
72. D. D. Roberts, D. L. Monsein, R. C. Frates, Jr., M. S. Cher-
    nick, and V. Ginsburg, *Arch. Biochem. Biophys. 244* (1986).
73. J.-F. Chatal, J.-C. Saccavini, P. Fumoleau, J.-Y. Douillard,
    C. Curtet, M. Kremer, B. LeMevel, and H. Koprowski, *J.
    Nucl. Med. 25*:307 (1984).
74. Z. Steplewski, G. Spira, M. Blaszczyk, M. D. Lubeck, A. Rad-
    bruch, H. Illges, D. Herlyn, K. Rajewsky, and M. Scharff,
    Proc. Natl. Acad. Sci. USA 82:8653 (1985).

10
Application of Monoclonal Antibodies to Carcinoembryonic Antigen

Diane Logan and Abraham Fuks / McGill Cancer Centre, McGill University, Montreal, Quebec, Canada

INTRODUCTION

Carcinoembryonic antigen (CEA) was discovered in adenocarcinomas of the colon by Gold and Freedman in 1965 (1). It was termed an oncofetal antigen because it was present in tumors derived from endodermal cells of human digestive epithelium and in the embryonic gut, but it was absent from normal adult tissues (2). Carcinoembryonic antigen is a glycoprotein with a molecular weight of 180,000 (3) and consists of a single polypeptide chain and multiple carbohydrate side chains, with an average carbohydrate content of 50-60% (4). It is a relatively hydrophilic molecule (5) that may be purified by perchloric acid or aqueous extraction (6).

Since its original discovery, CEA has been detected in the sera of patients with a wide variety of malignant and nonmalignant disease states (7-9). Carcinoembryonic antigen has also been isolated from various biological fluids including washings of normal colons (10), gastric juice (11), amniotic fluid (12), plasma of the umbilical cord (13), and saliva (14). In tumor-bearing patients with elevated serum CEA levels, the CEA is rapidly cleared from the serum within 2-14 days (15) after resection of the tumor. It is metabolized primarily via the liver (16).

Because CEA was detected in the sera of tumor-bearing patients, immunoassays were developed with the aim of using the assay as a screening test for malignancy. Thomson et al. (17), in 1969, developed the first immunoassay for CEA using polyclonal anti-CEA sera. Subsequently, Hoffmann-LaRoche and Abbott Laboratories both released commercial CEA assays using polyclonal anti-CEA sera. However, Hansen et al. (7) demonstrated that the serum CEA level, as determined by a polyclonal immunoassay, was not useful as a screening test for colonic carcinoma because elevated serum CEA levels could be detected in a variety of malignant and nonmalignant chronic inflammatory conditions such as pancreatitis, ulcerative colitis, cirrhosis of the liver, and emphysema. Furthermore, elevated serum CEA levels were detected in otherwise healthy people who smoke by Alexander et al. (18).

The role of the polyclonal CEA immunoassay in clinical medicine has since been delineated by Beatty et al. (8,9) as well as by other investigators (19-30). In patients with colon carcinoma, peroperative CEA values correlate with the stage of disease and are indicative of prognosis. Although high preoperative levels do not correlate well with the extent of local disease, they do suggest the presence of metastatic disease, particularly in patients who have a persistent postoperative elevation. Serum CEA levels may also be used in the postoperative follow-up for monitoring the recurrence of disease, elevated CEA levels may precede the clinical detection of a recurrence by 3-19 months. However, colonic carcinomas that are not well differentiated may not be readily monitored by CEA levels, unless they are positive for CEA immunohistologically, because elevated serum CEA levels do not occur when the tumor tissue staining result is negative for CEA (31). Serum CEA levels may also be used to monitor the recurrence of disease in noncolonic carcinomas and to monitor the response to chemotherapeutic interventions. However, not all carcinomas within a specific histological type are positive for CEA, and thus, a normal CEA level is not of value per se in determining the status of a disease. In those patients in whom the CEA level is elevated, it is useful as an adjunct to other clinical assessment measurements. Finally, a serum CEA level may rise because of hepatotoxicity induced by chemotherapeutic agents, as reported by Savrin et al. (32), and this may decrease the usefulness of the serum CEA level in monitoring the response to chemotherapy.

Because the serum CEA level was found to be elevated in a number of malignant and nonmalignant disease states, investigators studied CEA or CEA-reactive substances from many tissues to further define the CEA molecule and to determine if the CEA molecule from each source was biochemically or immunologically identical. This led to the delineation of a family of molecules that demonstrated immunological or biochemical similarities to the material originally defined as CEA.

CARCINOEMBRYONIC ANTIGEN AND CARCINO–EMBRYONIC ANTIGENLIKE SUBSTANCES

Von Kleist et al. isolated from normal colon, lung, and spleen tissues a substance they termed nonspecific cross-reacting antigen (NCA) (33) by virtue of its reactivity with antisera prepared against CEA. It has also been detected in the cytoplasm of granulocytes (34). A number of related species have since been defined with molecular weights of 60,000-110,000. The first 24 amino acid residues from the NH2-terminus of NCA (35) are identical to CEA except for the substitution of alanine for valine at position 21 in the CEA sequence. Also, methionine is present in NCA but not in CEA. Immunological studies have revealed that some of the antigenic determinant of NCA are distinct from CEA in addition to those that are shared.

Other CEA-like substances also have been described. Kupchik et al. (36) isolated an antigen immunologically identical with CEA from the serum and the liver of a patient with cirrhosis of the liver. A substance from bile designated as BGP1, which is immunologically distinct from NCA and CEA, was isolated by Svenberg (37). Another CEA-like substance, designated NCA2, was isolated from meconium and normal adult feces and has also been found to be present in the cytoplasm and mucus of gastrointestinal tissues by Burtin et al. (38).

Carcinoembryonic antigenlike substances from various tumors have been isolated and compared with CEA. An NCA-like substance from hepatic metastases of colonic carcinoma, with a molecular weight of 110,000, was isolated by Kessler et al. (39). Immunolgical studies revealed it was more closely related to NCA than to CEA. De Young and Ashman (40) isolated CEA-like substances from hepatic metastases of colon, gastric, and lung carcinomas. Although the molecular weights were similar, the carbohydrate contents varied.

Carcinoembryonic antigen or CEA-like substances have also been isolated from pancreatic, breast, prostatic, and ovarian carcinomas (41-45). Most were immunologically distinct from the original colonic carcinoma CEA.

Thus, it appears that CEA is not a single molecule but, rather, represents a family of molecules whose definition could be clarified by the determination of the overlapping sets of antigenic determinants. Also, further studies of the colonic CEA and CEA-like substances for antigenic determinants specific to the different molecules were necessary if immunoassays and immunohistopathological analyses were to be more clinically useful.

ANTIGENIC DETERMINANTS OF CARCINOEMBRYONIC ANTIGEN AND CARCINOEMBRYONIC ANTIGENLIKE SUBSTANCES

Sundblad et al. (46) analyzed CEA from hepatic deposits of metastatic colonic adenocarcinoma with rabbit anti-CEA sera. They concluded that there were approximately 15 sites recognized by such antisera, of which 10 sites were CEA-specific and five sites were shared by NCA.

Further studies of the CEA antigenic determinants or epitopes have been greatly aided by the use of monoclonal antibody (MAb) technology (47) because MAbs recognize a single antigenic determinant, whereas polyclonal antisera concurrently recognize many epitopes.

Haskell et al. (48), using seven MAbs, concluded that there were five distinct epitopes on CEA. Two epitopes were overlapping, one epitope was shared by NCA, and one epitope was recognized by two MAbs with different affinities.

Hedin et al. (49) evaluated eight anti-CEA MAbs and also concluded that there were five epitopes, which resided in the protein. Because there was no binding to reduced and alkylated CEA, the epitopes had to be conformational epitopes because these treatments disrupt the secondary and tertiary structures of the molecule. The fact that these MAbs reacted with CEA after Smith degradation, which removes 50% of the carbohydrate, also suggested that the epitopes resided in the protein.

Haggarty et al. (50) analyzed a library of 18 anti-CEA MAbs. The antibodies were classified into nine groups by an additive-binding assay and a solid-phase competitive inhibition assay. Five of the nine groups contained one MAb each. One group had four MAbs that recognized the same antigenic determinant. The other three groups had more than one MAb in each group; further studies revealed that they did not all bind precisely to the same epitope even though they were grouped together by competitive inhibition assays. Seven MAbs cross-reacted with NCA. Five of the MAb groups recognized conformational determinants, for they did not react with reduced and alkylated CEA. Some MAbs reacted with purified CEA but not with the CEA on the surface of HCT-8R cells, although most recognized both antigens. This suggested that some of the CEA-specific MAbs recognized epitopes that were either in the membrane-bound portion of CEA or that the membrane caused steric hindrance. Binding of MAbs was also studied on CEA fragments, and groups of MAbs reacted with different subsets. Some MAbs reacted with all of the fragments, suggesting that they recognized a repetitive epitope. It was postulated that this could be a carbohydrate determinant, because this is usually the most common repetitive sequence of a glycoprotein and the site was still recognized after reduction.

Blaszczyk et al. (51) reported one MAb that appeared to recognize a carbohydrate determinant.

Nichols et al. (52) studied the reactivity of eight purified CEA preparations from hepatic metastases of colonic adenocarcinoma with six MAbs directed to carbohydrate sturctures. One MAb directed at a Y determinant on carbohydrate structures, reacted with all specimens tested, wheras one MAb, directed at a dimeric X carbohydrate structure, reacted with only two CEA preparations. The authors concluded that the CEA molecule was closely associated with a specific carbohydrate chain terminting in a Y structure.

Thus, the original CEA appears to belong to a heterologous family of antigens with overlapping of antigenic determinants. There may be as many as 15 antigenic determinants present on CEA. Some are repetitive and could be either a peptide or carbohydrate epitope. Five antigenic determinants are in the peptide sequence and are conformational. Five antigenic determinants are shared with NCA. Carbohydrate determinants are probably also present. Certainly, some of the antigenic determinants are shared by the CEA molecules from different carcinomas, others may be unique. Whether or not such differences are entirely in the peptide sequence remains to be elucidated. A workshop to compare the MAb anti-CEA reagents from different laboratories is currently being organized. Attempts to clone the CEA gene, and thus determine its entire structure, are also on-going. The use of MAbs is important if immunoassays, immunohistological evaluation and in vivo radioimmunolocalization studies are to be sufficiently sensitive and specific to be of value, especially in the clinical setting, for the early detection of specific carcinomas, for the diagnosis of sites of origin of the carcinoma unknown primary syndrome, for delineation of the presence and extent of metastatic disease, and for the follow-up to treatment.

IMMUNOASSAYS

Both Hoffmann-LaRoche and Abbott Laboratories have released polyclonal anti-CEA immunoassays. However, Hansen et al. (7) and other investigators (8,9,18) demonstrated that elevated serum CEA levels occur in many malignant and nonmalignant disease states. Subsequently, many other assay designs, including solid phase assays were developed as attempts were made to overcome both the cumbersome liquid-phase method and the interassay variability. Assay variability was also a potential problem because the polyclonal anti-CEA sera recognized many antigenic determinants, and the titer and perhaps antibody specificity used in the assay varied with each bleeding to procure the sera.

Köhler and Milstein's (47) method of hybridoma formation and the resultant production of MAbs provided an avenue for increasing the specificity and reproducibility of the CEA assay technique. Indeed, if the MAb were to be unique for the CEA of a specific carcinoma, then the specificity of the immunoassay would be enhanced and the cross-reactivity eliminated.

Several investigators have reported on the application of MAbs to CEA immunoassays.

Kupchik et al. (53) reported the use of an MAb on an affinity column to purify radiolabeled CEA for use in the polyclonal CEA immunoassays. A 2.5-fold increase in the sensitivity of a double-antibody, solid-phase assay was observed when this affinity-purified radiolabeled CEA was used as a tracer. Direct use of the MAb in the immunoassay was not possible, however, because the desired sensitivity could not be obtained.

Buchegger et al. (54) examined 380 serum samples from 167 patients with malignant or nonmalignant disease states and 134 samples from healthy smokers and nonsmokers. The assay was a solid-phase, sandwich enzyme-linked immunosorbent assay (ELISA) on polystyrene beads. That is, beads coated with polyclonal goat anti-CEA serum were exposed to heat-treated patient serum samples and then to mouse anti-CEA MAbs, followed by a goat antimouse antibody conjugated to alkaline phosphatase. Then the values obtained on the same samples with the traditional polyclonal liquid-phase competitive inhibition assay, as described by Thomson et al. (17) and modified by Mach et al. (55), were compared. An excellent correlation between the two assay values was noted with a coefficient of correlation of 0.88 for colorectal carcinoma, 0.83 for breast and gastric carcinoma, and 0.86 for cirrhosis of the liver, and 0.92 for normal patients. For patients with sequential CEA level determinations, the monoclonal enzyme immunoassay (M-EIA) was as accurate as the conventional assay in predicting recurrence. However, the M-EIA was not superior to the conventional assay for discriminating between malignant and nonmalignant disease states or between various types of carcinoma.

In a second study (56), this same group reported on the use of three MAbs specific for three different epitopes on CEA in an M-EIA on 196 serum samples from patients with various carcinomas, cirrhosis of the liver and healthy blood donors, both smokers and nonsmokers. Polystyrene beads coated with two of the MAbs were exposed to heat-treated serum samples and then exposed to a third MAB, that had been conjugated to alkaline phosphatase. Assay sensitivity was 0.6 ng/ml. Again, the results were compared with values obtained by a traditional liquid-phase competitive inhibition RIA. Good correlation occurred between the two assays with correlation coefficients of 0.95 for colorectal carcinoma, 0.93 for breast and lung carcinoma, and 0.88 for normal donors and for those with nonmalignant disease. Unfortunately, the numbers of slightly elevated CEA levels in nonmalignant disease states were not reduced with the M-EIA.

Hedin et al. (57) reported on an M-EIA that was a solid-phase sandwich type assay. A murine MAb, bound through cyanogen bromide to a nitrocellulose disk, was exposed to heat-treated serum and then to a second MAb conjugated to galacto-sidase. The two MAbs recognized two different epitope sites on CEA. Specificity was increased because the first MAb did not react with either NCA1 or BGP1, and it was only weakly reactive with NCA2. The second MAb reacted with CEA and NCA2. Five commercially available CEA assays (CEA Roche Test Kit—Z-gel assay; CEA EIA test kit from Hoffmann-LaRoche which uses one MAb, Abbott CEA RIA; Serono Diagnostic CEA kit; and Phadebas CEA PRIST) were compared with the MAb assay in the study. The commercial CEA assays were unable to differentiate between CEA and NCA2. No normal tissues, except colon tissue reacted with the MAbs used in the immunoassay of this study. Sensitivity was 0.5 ng/ml. One hundred eighty samples from patients with malignant and nonmalignant disease states and normal individuals were examined with the M-EIA and a conventional radioimmunoassay (Phadebas CEA PRIST, Pharmacia). Increased specificity for carcinoma was noted primarily because of a decrease in the CEA values in the sera of patients with nonmalignant disease states. With 3 ng/ml as the upper limit of normal, five of 40 nonmalignant disease samples gave positive results with RIA and none of 40 samples gave positive results with the M-EIA. In nonmalignant liver disease, using an upper limit for normal of 5 ng/ml, 26 of 45 (58%) samples gave positive results with the RIA and two of 45 (4%) gave positive results with the M-EIA. In ulcerative colitis, again using an upper limit for normal of 5 ng/ml, five of 25 samples gave positive results with the RIA and none of 25 gave positive results with the M-EIA. When the upper limit of normal was lowered to 3 ng/

ml, 20 of 25 of these sera samples gave positive results with the
RIA while seven of 25 gave positive results with the M-EIA. There
were no differences in the actual CEA values for sera of patients
with malignant disease states obtained by both assays, and the correlation coefficient was 0.95.

Herlyn et al. (58) reported on an RIA using a solid-phase sandwich assay. Polystyrene beads coated with a MAb were exposed
to serum samples and then to a radiolabeled MAb. Fourteen
MAbs from different research centers were examined and grouped
into six groups by additive-binding assays, immunoprecipitation of
radiolabeled colorectal cell lines, and competitive-binding assays.
With various combinations of the MAbs, the authors tested the
sera of 311 patients and normal donors. A lower false-positive
rate, when compared with the conventional Roche CEA assay,
was noted in several combinations. Of 115 healthy donors, none
had elevated serum CEA levels with four of the six MAb combinations tested, and up to 9% of the results were positive with the
other two MAb combinations. Between 1.4 and 4.4% of sera
from cases of inflammatory and benign diseases of the gastrointestinal tract gave positive results. Between 56 and 75% of the
cases of advanced gastrointestinal tumors gave positive results,
depending upon the MAb combinations used. In each combination, the primary MAb belonged to group 1 or 2. Group 1 had
only one MAb that recognized only a 180,000 molecular weight
molecule; group 2 had five MAbs, and each recognized both a
180,000- and a 160,000-molecular weight molecule. Whereas
the other four groups recognized various combinations of molecules with molecular weights of 180,000, 160,000, and 40,000,
all four groups recognized a 50,000 molecular weight species.
They concluded that a double-determinant immunoassay with a
panel of MAbs could improve upon the conventional CEA assays
by reducing the false-positivity rate.

Certainly, the use of MAbs in immunoassays appears to have
the potential of improving the discrimination of the immunoassay for malignant disease versus nonmalignant disease detection.
The report of Hedin et al. (57) demonstrates that the use of
MAbs can reduce the false-positive rate for normal sera as well
as for sera from patients with cirrhosis of the liver and ulcerative colitis. The report by Herlyn and coworkers (58) reveals
that MAbs in various combinations can reduce the false-positive

rate, if the appropriate antibodies are selected by trial and error,
and that the percentage of sera of patients with advanced gastrointestinal malignancies with elevated serum CEA levels varies with
the MAb combinations chosen. Most of these assays are now only
for investigational use. Those commercial assays currently available are not yet entirely specific for malignancy. As new MAbs
are produced and selected for their specificities for the CEA or
CEA-like substances of various carcinomas, immunoassays may
become available that are specific for malignancy and perhaps for
the subsets of malignant disease.

IMMUNOHISTOLOGY

The role of anti-CEA antibodies in the immunohistochemical
analysis of tissue specimens also has been carefully examined.
    Specimens may be examined by an immunofluorescent or an
immunoperoxidase method. The immunofluorescent method is
used on freshly frozen tissues specimens and has the disadvan-
tage that it requires either performance soon after a specimen is
obtained or special storage to preserve the specimen for later
examination. The immunoperoxidase method is generally applied
to paraffin-embedded tissue specimens, and although it requires
more manipulation of the tissue specimen, it has the advantage
that it may be applied at any time to a tissue specimen taken
from large banks of pathological specimens.
    In either method, antibodies to the antigen of interest are
incubated with the tissue section and then with an antibody to
the species from which the first antibody was obtained. This
second antibody is conjugated to a fluorescent tag or to peroxidase. If the antibody is conjugated to an enzyme such as peroxidase then a substrate for the enzyme is added and a colored
product is obtained. When the enzyme is peroxidase, the endogenous peroxidase activity of the cells must be inactivated to
prevent background staining. This may be accomplished by the
use of periodic acid solution and 3,3'-diaminobenzidine tetrahy-
drochloride or hydrogen peroxide before the application of the
antibodies. Staining procedures are further classified as direct or
indirect. In direct staining the antibody specific for the antigen
is conjugated to the fluorescent tag or enzyme. In the indirect
staining the second antibody directed to the species producing the

first antibody is conjugated to the fluorescent tag or the enzyme.

The detection of CEA in immunohistological specimens was first described by Gold et al (59) on colonic tumor specimens, and since then many studies have been reported.

The role of polyclonal anti-CEA sera in the immunohistological evaluation of colorectal carcinoma was delineated by O'Brien et al. (60). By use of polyclonal rabbit anti-CEA sera previously absorbed with normal tissue extracts, they demonstrated (1) that CEA could be detected in normal colon, (2) that poorly differentiated colorectal carcinoma contained much less CEA than well-differentiated colorectal carcinomas, (3) that positive staining in the presence of carcinoma in neoplastic polyps is not a reliable diagnostic criterion for malignancy, (4) that failure to demonstrate CEA in a gland-forming carcinoma makes a diagnosis of colorectal carcinoma unlikely, and (5) that lymph node micrometastases from colorectal carcinoma are as easily detected by routine staining as they are by positive staining for CEA.

Furthermore, the role of polyclonal anti-CEA sera in the immunohistological analysis of other tissues has been evaluated. Denk et al. (61) reported a study of CEA in various carcinomas using polyclonal rabbit anti-CEA and indirect immunofluorescence on 64 tissue specimens. In colonic carcinoma the intensity of the staining varied with the degree of differentiation; well-differentiated colonic carcinomas stained the most intensely. In gastric and pancreatic carcinoma, similar but less intense staining was noted. Carcinoembryonic antigen was not detected in hepatic carcinoma, lymphosarcoma of the stomach, lung carcinomas (well-differentiated adenocarcinoma, squamous or anaplastic types), breast carcinoma (anaplastic and papillary types), ovarian (cystadenocarcinoma types), or squamous anal carcinoma.

Lung carcinomas and transitional cell carcinomas have also been examined with polyclonal anti-CEA sera (62,63) and variable percentages of various histological types and degrees of differentiation have been stained.

The aforementioned studies demonstrate why polyclonal anti-CEA sera are not useful for the immunohistological evaluation of tissue specimens in the carcinoma unknown primary syndrome to determine its site of origin and for the examination of

lymph nodes for the presence of occult metastatic disease. Polyclonal anti-CEA reacts with tissue specimens of many noncolonic,
as well as colonic, carcinomas and frequently reacts weakly, or not
at all, with poorly differentiated tissues. Hence, further studies
were undertaken with MAbs, that might offer an increase in specificity.

Tsutsumi et al. (64) examined pancreatic carcinoma and normal pancreatic tissue using a peroxidase-antiperoxidase (PAP)
indirect immunoperoxidase method with polyclonal antibodies and
anti-CEA MAbs. For polyclonal sera they used conventional rabbit anti-CEA sera, rabbit anti-CEA sera absorbed with spleen extracts, and rabbit anti-NCA sera. The murine MAbs were commercially obtained preparations. Positive staining occurred with all six
antibodies on normal colonic and gastric tissues. In gastric and
colonic carcinomas, staining occurred with all of the antibodies,
except the anti-NCA antibody, which reacted more intensely with
normal (especially gastric) tissue. When comparing frozen sections with paraffin sections, it was noted that the intensity of the
staining decreased in the paraffin sections, especially in normal
tissue. No CEA, or only a very small amount of CEA or CEA-like
substance, was detected in the normal pancreas. A small quantity
of NCA or CEA-like substances containing epitopes shared by
NCA were detected in the pancreatic ducts, especially in frozen
sections.The NCA or CEA-like substances sharing NCA epitopes
were detected in the duct cells of hyperplastic pancreatic tissue
and in the cells of pancreatic carcinoma. Hence, it appeared that
NCA or NCA-like determinants were detected in normal or hyperplastic pancreatic tissue, whereas NCA and CEA determinants
were detected in pancreatic carcinoma.

Hockey et al. (65) examined gastric carcinoma primary tumors
and metastases with a murine MAb to CEA known to react with
colonic, gastric, and some ductal mammary carcinomas. The MAb
did not react with normal tissues or NCA from the lung. Ninety-
two percent of 119 primary tumors stained positively while 83%
of metastases from 81 tumors stained positively. In two patients,
metastatic disease was detected in lymph nodes previously reported as negative for metastatic disease by routine morphological
study. Sixty patients with two or more metastatic lesions were
available for disease evaluation; 20% of the secondaries were non-

concordant for positive staining. Thus, the CEA status of a single lesion does not enable confident prediction of positivity in other metastases.

Yachi et al. (66) evaluated four anti-CEA MAbs that recognized four different epitopes. With the PAP immunoperoxidase method, three of four MAbs stained normal colon tissue, whereas the other MAb reacted only with fetal stomach and gastric and colonic carcinomas. This MAb tended to react mainly with moderately or poorly differentiated adenocarcinoma lesions. It was suggested that this reagent might recognize a carbohydrate determinant.

Nap et al. (67) examined 56 benign breast lesions and 92 malignant breast lesions. They used a PAP indirect immunoperoxidase method with polyclonal goat anti-CEA sera, polyclonal rabbit anti-CEA sera, polyclonal anti-NCA sera, and murine anti-CEA MAbs. The polyclonal anti-CEA were examined for reactivity with, and without, prior absorption with normal tissues. With unabsorbed anti-CEA sera, breast carcinoma, benign inflammatory breast lesions, and fibroadenomas, all stained positively for CEA. With an anti-CEA MAb, benign breast lesions and fibroadenoma lesions were negative for CEA, whereas only 42% of the breast carcinomas stained positively for CEA. With an MAb to NCA, 48% of breast carcinomas, 84% of benign breast lesions, and 50% of fibroadenomas stained positively. The results with unabsorbed polyclonal anti-CEA sera and anti-NCA MAb were not identical, and it was postulated that NCA was not the only antigen responsible for false-positive reactions.

Jothy et al. (68) compared the reactivity of nine MAbs with polyclonal rabbit anti-CEA for reactivity in various malignant and nonmalignant tissue specimens by the PAP indirect immunoperoxidase method. Two MAbs—D14 and B18—were found to have a high degree of specificity for colonic carcinoma and did not stain normal colonic tissues. These two MAbs did not stain most other noncolonic adenocarcinomas. On paraffin sections, D14 did not significantly stain normal colonic epithelium, whereas D14 reacted with both normal and neoplastic components on frozen sections, suggesting that the region recognized by D14 is more sensitive to the fixation procedure in normal tissue than in neoplastic tissue. Specifically, D14 stained 100% of colonic carcinomas, independently of their location or degree of differentiation, and stained only 8% of carcinomas of nondigestive organs. Antibody B18 reacted with 100% of colonic carcinomas and with 21% of carcinomas from nondigestive carcinomas. Metastatic deposits of colonic carcinoma were also positive. Both D14 and B18 also reacted with a subset of gastric, pancreatic, and hepatocellular carcinomas. Antibodies D14 and B18 did react weakly with breast carcinomas, but only when a very high antibody concentration was used. As noted by other authors of various studies, the polyclonal rabbit anti-CEA sera, previously absorbed with normal human serum and human liver and kidney powder, reacted with carcinomas from different digestive and nondigestive organs as well as with normal colonic epithelium. Other MAbs tested in this study had variable degrees of staining, but none were as specific as D14 and B18. Liquid-phase RIAs and competitive immunoenzymatic assays confirmed that D14 and B18 recognized different epitopes of CEA. Antibody D14 reacted with an epitope that is conformationally and sterically distinct from B18. Antibody B18 reacted with an epitope that is not conformationally dependent and is present on CEA fragments. Also, the B18-recognized epitope was shared by NCA, whereas D14 recognized an epitope unique to CEA. It was concluded that these two MAbs could be particularly useful probes for immunohistochemical studies to distinguish colonic carcinomas from other types of carcinomas. Their use to identify "premalignant" lesions remains to be investigated.

In conclusion, the use of MAbs has improved immunohistological evaluation. Polyclonal anti-CEA sera react with many different histological types of carcinoma in variable degrees, and many poorly differentiated specimens do not stain positively. Normal or benign lesions also stained positively in many instances. Monoclonal antibodies increased specificity for malignant tissue versus normal tissue, as has been demonstrated by Tsutsumi et al. (64), Hockey et al. (65), Yachi et al. (66) and Nap et al. (67). Also, Yachi and coworkers (66) demonstrated that the detection of CEA in moderately or poorly differentiated histologic sections was possible. Finally, Jothy and collaborators (68) have demonstrated that MAbs may also react preferentially with only one type of carcinoma.

IN VIVO RADIOIMMUNOLOCALIZATION

Since Quinones et al. (69) first demonstrated in 1971 the binding of ^{125}I-labeled rabbit IgG anti-hCG (human chorionic gonadotropin) to human choriocarcinoma grafts in golden hamsters, investigations have been launched to assess the efficacy of anti-CEA antibodies in the detection of primary and metastatic carcinomas.

In nude mice with grafted colonic carcinomas, Mach et al. (70) demonstrated the binding of affinity-purified ^{131}I-labeled goat anti-CEA antibodies. However, when the same antisera was used on the mice with different donor grafts, a great variance in the uptake of the anti-CEA sera was noted. Similar findings were noted by Goldenberg et al. (71).

The first study in humans was performed by Goldenberg et al. (72) using purified ^{131}I-labeled anti-CEA in 18 patients. Almost all of the CEA-producing tumors were detected and no false-positive results were obtained.

Mach et al. (73) compared the uptake of ^{131}I-labeled purified goat anti-CEA and ^{125}I-labeled purified goat IgG for uptake in tumors and adjacent tissues in patients about to undergo resection for carcinoma. The uptake of anti-CEA/IgG was 5:1. Measurements of the radioactivity in the resected specimens revealed that the percentage of uptake by the tumor was minute compared with the total injected dose.

The heterogeneity of the polyclonal anti-CEA sera for various CEA, or CEA-like substance, antigenic determinants on carcinomas, normal tissue and inflammatory disease states resulted in uptake of labeled antibodies in many malignant and nonmalignant tissues, and thus, further studies have used MAbs because of their enhanced specificity and fixed titer.

Mach et al. (74) examined 28 patients with ^{131}I-labeled anti-CEA MAb. Twenty-six patients had colonic carcinoma and two patients had pancreatic carcinoma. Patients were scanned at 24, 38, 48, and 72 hr postinjection. Fourteen of 28 patients had a radioactive spot corresponding to the tumor site at 36-48 hr after injection, six of 28 patients had doubtful sites of uptake, and eight of 28 patients were negative for uptake. In one of the patients illustrated, a seven- to ten-fold greater uptake of the MAb was noted in the tumor than in the surrounding tissue.

Nonspecific uptake by the reticuloendotheial system has been a major problem in many studies. The nonspecific uptake is particularly a problem in the liver, which is a frequent site of metastatic disease. Some of the nonspecific background can be eliminated by using MAbs that do not cross-react with normal tissue. However, complexes of antibody and CEA have been demonstrated in the circulation (75) after the injection of radiolabeled antibodies, and the Fc portion of the antibody in these complexes facilitates the uptake of these complexes by the reticuloendothelial system. Furthermore, when antibodies bind to CEA on any cell, the complexes may cross-link and become internalized, and the subsequent rapid degradation and excretion of the radiolabel results in a loss of the ability to detect the binding (76). For these reasons attention has been focused on the use of MAb fragments.

Mach et al. (77) demonstrated a decrease in the nonspecific uptake in the liver with the use of ^{131}I-labled $F(ab')_2$. Tumor detection occurred in 38% of their patients, but because the number of patients was small, no conclusions could be drawn about the efficacy of $F(ab')_2$ fragments over intact antibody.

Which radioactive isotope is the one of choice is not clear. Iodine-131 is poorly detected by gamma-counters and delivers a high radiation dose to the patient. Iodine-123 is more readily detected by gamma-counters and delivers a lower radiation dose but has a short half-life of 13 hr. Indium-111 is well detected, delivers a lower dose of radiation to patients, and has a reasonable half-life. However, it requires careful coupling to the antibody to preserve the antibody affinity. Indium may also be preferable because dehalogenation of iodine occurs in vivo, which results in lower specific activity.

Delaloye et al. (78) reported a retrospective study investigating the use of ^{123}I-labeled Fab or $F(ab')_2$ fragments from anti-CEA MAbs. They evaluated 31 patients with primary, recurrent or metastatic colorectal carcinoma after they had noted that nude mice with human colon carcinoma grafts, when injected with ^{131}I-labeled $F(ab')_2$ or Fab fragments of anti-CEA MAbs, had markedly higher (3.5- to 11.7-fold) tumor/normal tissue localization ratios than with intact MAbs. They chose to use emission-computerized tomography (ECT) because in a previous study they had noted increased sensitivity with this third-generation technology. They chose ^{123}I as the label because the signal/noise ratio with the ^{131}I-labeled fragments was not high; they attributed the low signal to the ^{131}I and to the fact that they had used a low-affinity MAb. For this study of the comparison of Fab and F(ab')$_2$ fragment uptake, they used a new MAb specifically selected for its high affinity (5.8 $\times$ 10^9 M^{-1}) and its specificity. Fourteen patients were injected with ^{123}I-labeled F(ab')$_2$ and 17 patients with ^{123}I-labeled Fab fragments. Scanning by ECT at 1, 6, 24, and 48 hr was performed. Collectively, 86% of the tumor sites were detected. The F(ab')$_2$ detected 81%, whereas the Fab fragment detected 89% of the lesions. The quality of tumor images was superior with the Fab fragment because of earlier tumor uptake and less background in the spleen and liver. It was noted also that although nine patients had elevated serum CEA levels, visualization was still possible. Three of the tumors visualized weighed only 3-5 g. In one patient with two pulmonary metastases and a large liver metastatic lesion, none of the lesions were detected, even though the serum CEA level was 2500 ng/ml. Another patient had two pulmonary lesions, and both were detected.

Oredipe et al. (79) studied the application of a hand-held probe for the radioimmunodetection of anti-CEA MAbs to human colorectal carcinoma. They injected SW1116 human colorectal cancer cells complexed with an ^{125}I-labeled anti-CEA MAb at various concentrations subserosally into fresh autopsy colon specimens. They observed a linear relationship between the number of cells injected and the number of counts detected by the hand-held probe. They could detect 6.25 $\times$ 10^5 cells, which represents a lesion of less than 1 mm^3. They noted that such a lesion would not be palpated or detected by external scintigraphy.

Weinstein et al. (80) reported the use of MAbs for the detection of tumor by injecting the MAb into the tissue and allowing the antibody to be taken up by the lymphatic system in guinea pigs. They found by external scinitigraphy that lymph node metastases as small as 0.003 g were detectable.

Uptake ratios for MAbs could vary widely because an MAb recognizes only one epitope, and thus, the degree of uptake is proportional to the density of that epitope on the cell surface, the affinity of the antibody for the antigenic determinant, and the catabolism of the antibody in the circulation and in the cell. Therefore, some authors have suggested the use of multiple MAbs directed to known epitopes to increase the specificity. Results of such studies have yet to be reported.

In conclusion, the use of MAbs for in vivo detection of tumors and their metastases would be most useful in the clinical setting. At present, the use of radiolabeled MAbs is on only an investigational basis. Whether the use of whole molecules or the use of Fab or F(ab')$_2$ is the most efficacious method of detection remains to be determined. Also, whether MAbs should be injected intravenously, or subcutaneously requires further investigation and the result will probably be dependent upon the site to be examined. The use of the hand-held probe to detect the presence of disease, particularly in the intraoperative evaluation of disease, is an interesting concept that also requires further evaluation.

FUTURE PROSPECTS

Anti-CEA MAbs have been useful for delineating CEA as a family of molecules. The use of anti-CEA MAbs may also improve the clinical usefulness of immunoassays, immunohistochemical analyses, and in vivo radioimmunolocalization, as previously outlined.

However, whether or not MAbs will be found that are specific for neoplasms or for their subsets has yet to be determined. Most studies reported by various investigators, to date, have used murine MAbs. These antibody libararies recognize from five to nine epitopes on the CEA molecule. Rabbit antisera studies have suggested that at least 15 antigenic determinants exist. This difference may well be species-specific. Accordingly, human MAbs would be of particular interest. A few reports in the literature have demonstrated the presence of antibodies recognizing CEA in the serum of tumor-bearing patients. If further studies reveal that human antibodies recognize antigenic determinants that differ from murine antibodies, then human MAbs warrant particular attention. Of particular interest would be antibodies directed to carbohydrate determinants because carbohydrate structure production is often abnormal in neoplasms and could be specific for a particular subset of neoplasms. Also, such human monoclonal reagents might be more useful for in vivo administration for localization and, perhaps in the near future, for immunotherapy of tumors.

REFERENCES

1. P. Gold and S. O. Freedman, *J. Exp. Med. 121*:439 (1965).
2. P. Gold and S. O. Freedman, *J. Exp. Med. 122*:467 (1965).
3. H. S. Slayter and J. E. Coligan, *Biochemistry 14*:2323 (1975).
4. J. Krupey, P. Gold, and S. O. Freedman, *J. Exp. Med. 128*: 387 (1968).
5. C. Banjo, J. Shuster, and P. Gold, *Cancer Res. 34*:2114 (1974).
6. M. J. Krantz, L. Laferte, and N. Ariel, in *Methods in Enzymology* (J. J. Langane and H. Van Vurakin, eds.), Vol. 84, Academic Press, New York (1982).
7. H. J. Hansen, J. J. Snyder, E. Miller, J. P. Vandevoorde, O. N. Miller, L. R. Hines, and J. J. Burns, *Human Pathol. 5*:139 (1974).
8. J. D. Beatty and J. J. Terz, *Prog. Clin. Cancer 8*:9 (1982).
9. J. D. Beatty, C. Romero, P. W. Brown, W. Lawrence, Jr., and J. J. Terz, *Arch. Surg. 114*:563 (1979).
10. M. L. Egan, D. G. Pritchard, C. Todd, and V. L. W. Go, *Cancer Res. 37*:2638 (1977).
11. M. Vuento, E. Engmall, M. Seppala, and E. Ruoslahti, *Int. J. Cancer 18*:156 (1976).
12. H. Gadler, B. Wahren, J. Lindsten, K. Bremme, and E. Malmqvist, *Acta Med. Scand. 201*:411 (1977).
13. P. B. Dent, J. Chiavetta, S. Leefer, R. Richards, and W. E. Rawls, *Cancer 42*:224 (1978).
14. F. Martin and J. Devant, *J. Natl. Cancer Inst. 50*:1375 (1973).
15. P. Dhar, T. Moore, N. Zamchek, and H. Kupchik, *J. Am. Med. Assoc. 221*:31 (1972).
16. J. Shuster, M. Silverman, and P. Gold, *Cancer Res 33*:65 (1973).
17. D. M. P. Thomson, J. Krupey, S. O. Freedman, and P. Gold, *Proc. Natl. Acad. Sci. USA 64*:161 (1969).
18. J. C. Alexander, Jr., N. A. Silverman, and P. B. Chretien, *J. Am. Med. Assoc. 235*:1975 (1976).
19. K. J. Cullen, D. P. Stevens, M. A. Frost, and I. R. Mackay, *Aust. N. Z. J. Med. 6*:279 (1976).
20. M.Koch and T. A. McPherson, *Cancer 48*:1242 (1981).

21. H. Staab, F. A. Anderer, A. Brummendorf, A. Hornung, and R. Fischer, *Br. J. Cancer 45*:718 (1982).

22. E. te Velde, J. P. Persijn, R. E. Ballieux, and J. Faber, *Cancer 49*:1866 (1982).

23. P. Braun, G. Hildebrand, J. Izbicki, and G. Leyendecker, *Arch. Gynecol. 230*:263 (1981).

24. H. Tate, *Br. J. Cancer 46*:323 (1982).

25. L. Gunderson and H. Sosen, *Cancer 34*:1278 (1974).

26. E. W. Martin, M. Cooperman, G. King, L. Rinker, L. C. Carey, and J. P. Minton, *Am. J. Surg. 137*:167 (1979).

27. A. T. Ichiki, S. Krauss, K. L. Israelsen, T. Sonoda, and I. R. Collmann, *Oncology 38*:27 (1981).

28. H. C. Falkson, G. Flakson, M. S. Purtugal, J. J. Van Der Watt, and H. S. Schoeman, *Cancer 49*:1859 (1982).

29. K. E. Stall and E. W. Martin, Jr., *J. Reprod. Med. 26*:73 (1981).

30. R. H. Goslin, A. T. Skarin, and N. Zamcheck, *J. Am. Med. Assoc. 246*:2173 (1981).

31. R. Goslin, M. J. O'Brien, G. Steele, R. Mayer, R. Wilson, J. M. Corson, and N. Zamcheck, *Am. J. Med. 71*:246 (1981).

32. R. A. Savrin and E. W. Martin, Jr., *Cancer 47*:481 (1981).

33. S. von Kleist, G. Chavanel, and P. Burtin, *Proc. Natl. Acad. Sci. USA 69*:2492 (1972).

34. M. Border, S. Knobel, and F. Martin, *Eur. J. Cancer 11*:783 (1975).

35. E. Engvall, J. E. Shively, and H. Wrann, *Proc. Natl. Acad. Sci. USA 75*:1670 (1978).

36. H. Z. Kupchik and N. Zamcheck, *Gastroenterology 63*:95 (1972).

37. T. Svenberg, *Int. J. Cancer 17*:588 (1976).

38. P. Burtin, G. Chavanel, and H. Hirsch-Marie, *J. Immunol. 111*:1926 (1973).

39. M. J. Kessler, J. E. Shively, D. G. Pritchard, and C. W. Todd, *Cancer Res. 38*:1041 (1978).

40. N. J. DeYoung and L. K. Ashman, *Aust. J. Exp. Biol. Med. Sci. 56*:321 (1978).

41. S. R. Harvey, R. N. Girota, T. Nemotot, F. Ciani, and T. M. Chu, *Cancer Res. 36*:3486 (1976).

42. S. E. Chism, N. L. Warner, J. V. Wells, P. Crewther, S. Hunt, J. J. Marchalonis, and H. H. Fudenberg, *Cancer Res. 37*:3100 (1977).

43. T. M. Chu, E. D. Holyoke, and H. O. Douglass, *Cancer Res.* *37*:1525 (1977).
44. R. D. Williams, D. L. Bronson, A. D. Myl, J. P. Vandevoorde, and A. Y. Elliot, *Cancer Res.* *39*:2447 (1979).
45. R. Hill, B. Daunter, S. K. Khoo, and E. V. Mackay, *Mol. Immunol.* *18*:647 (1981).
46. G. Sundblad, S. Hammarstrom, and E. Engvall, *Protides Biol. Fluids* *24*:435 (1976).
47. G. Köhler and C. Milstein, *Nature* *256*:495 (1975).
48. C. M. Haskell, F. Buchegger, M. Schreyer, S. Carrel, and J.-P. Mach, *Cancer Res.* *43*:3857 (1983).
49. A. Hedin, S. Hammarstrom, and A. Larsson, *Mol. Immunol.* *19*:1641 (1982).
50. A. Haggarty, C. Legler, M. J. Krantz, and A. Fuks, *Cancer Res.* *46*:300 (1986).
51. M. Blaszczyk, K. Y. Pak, M. Herlyn, J. Lindgren, S. Pessano, Z. Steplewski, and H. Koprowski, *Cancer Res.* *44*:245 (1984).
52. E. Nichols, R. Kannagi, S. Hakomori, M. Krantz, and A. Fuks, *J. Immunol.* *135*:1911 (1985).
53. H. Z. Kupchik, V. R. Zurawski, Jr., J. G. R. Hurrell, N. Zamcheck, and P. H. Black, *Cancer Res.* *41*:3306 (1981).
54. F. Buchegger, M. Phan, D. Rivier, S. Carrel, R. S. Acolla, and J.-P. Mach, *J. Immunol. Methods* *49*:129 (1982).
55. J.-P-. Mach, P. Jaeger, M. M. Bertholet, C. H. Ruegsegger, R. N. Loosli, and J. Pettavel, *Lancet* *2*:535 (1974).
56. F. Buchegger, C. Mettraux, R. S. Acolla, S. Carrel, and J.-P. Mach, *Immunol. Lett.* *5*:85 (1982).
57. A. Hedin, L. Carlsson, A. Berglund, and S. Hammarstrom, *Proc. Natl. Acad. Sci. USA* *80*:3470 (1983).
58. M. Herlyn, M. Blasezczyk, H. F. Sears, H. Verrill, J. Lindgren, D. Colcher, Z. Steplewski, J. Schlom, and H. Koprowski, *Hybridoma* *2*:329 (1983).
59. P. Gold, M. Gold, and S. O. Freedman, *Cancer Res.* *28*:1331 (1968).
60. M. J. O'Brien, N. Zamcheck, B. Burke, S. E. Kirkham, C. A. Saravis, and L. S. Gottlieb, *Am. J. Clin. Pathol.* *75*:283 (1981).
61. H. Denk, G. Tappeines, R. Eckerstorer, and J. H. Holzner, *Int. J. Cancer* *10*:262 (1972).

62. N. C. J. Sun, T. D. Edgington, C. L. Carpentier, W. Mcaffee, R. Terry, and J. Bateman, *Cancer 52*:1632 (1983).

63. G. Jautzke and E. Altenaehr, *Cancer 50*:2052 (1982).

64. Y. Tsutsumi, N. Nagura, and K. Watanabe, *Am. J. Clin. Pathol. 82*:535 (1984).

65. M. S. Hockey, H. J. Stokes, H. Thompson, C. S. Woodhouse, F. MacDonald, J. W. L. Fielding, and C. H. J. Ford, *Br. J. Cancer 49*:129 (1984).

66. A. Yachi, K. Imai, H. Fujita, Y. Moriya, M. Tanda, T. Endo, M. Tsujisaki, and M. Kasaharada, *J. Immunol. 132*:2998 (1984).

67. M. Nap, H. Keuning, P. Burtin, J. W. Oosterhuis,and G. Fleuren, *Am. J. Clin. Pathol. 82*:526 (1984).

68. S. Jothy, S. A. Brazinsky, M. Chin-A-Loy, A. Haggarty, M. J. Krantz, M. Cheung, and A. Fuks, *Lab. Invest.54*:108 (1986).

69. J. Quinones, G. Mizejewski, and W. H. Beierwalter, *J. Nucl. Med. 12*:69 (1971).

70. J.-P. Mach, S. Carrel, C. Merenda, B. Sordat, and J. C. Cerottini, *Nature 248*:704 (1974).

71. D. M. Goldenberg, D. F. Preston, F. J. Primus, and H. J. Hansen, *Cancer Res. 34*:1 (1974).

72. D. M. Goldenberg, F. Deland, E. Kim, S. Bennett, J. J. Primus, J. R. van Nagell, N. Estes, P. DeSimone, and P. Rayburn, *N. Engl. J. Med. 298*:1384 (1978).

73. J.-P. Mach, S. L. Carrel, M. Forni, J. Ritschard, A. Donath, and P. Alberto, *N. Engl. J. Med. 303*:5 (1980).

74. J.-P. Mach, F. Buchegger, M. Forni, J. Ritschard, C. Buche, J. D. Lumroso, M. Schreyer, C. Girartdet, R. S. Acollo, and S. Carrel, *Immunology Today 2*:233 (1981).

75. F. J. Primus, S. J. Bennett, E. E. Kim, F. H. Deland, M. C. Zahn, and D. M. Goldenberg, *Cancer Res. 40*:497 (1980).

76. T. W. Chatenoud and J. F. Bach, *Immunol. Today 5*:20 (1984).

77. J.-P. Mach, M. Forni, J. Ritschard, F. Buchegger, S. Carrel, S. Widgren, A. Donath, and P. Alberto, *Oncodev. Biol. Med. 1*:49 (1980).

78. B. Delaloye, A. Bischof-Delaloye, F. Buchegger, V. von Fliedner, J.-P. Grob, J.-C. Volant, J. Pettavel, and J.-P. Mach, *J. Clin. Invest. 77*:301 (1986).

79. O. A. Oredipe, R. F. Barth, S. E. Tuttle, D. P. Houchens,
     M. O. Thurston, G. H. Hinkle, C. M. Mojzisik, D. Adams, I.
     Sautins, P. O'Dwyer, E. A. Miller, S. Jewell, D. Bucci, J.
     Ridihalgh, Z. Steplewski, and E. W. Martin, Jr., *Proc. Am
     Assoc. Cancer Res. 27*: March (1986), pg. 335-abstract 1331.

80. J. N. Weinstein, M. A. Steller, D. G. Covell, O. D. Holton,
     III, A.M. Keenan, S. M. Sieber, and R. J. Parker, *Cancer
     Treat. Rep. 68*:257 (1984).

11
Monoclonal Antibody Assays for Placental Alkaline Phosphatase

Derek F. Tucker / Imperial Cancer Research Fund, London, England

Anthony Milford Ward / Royal Hallamshire Hospital, Sheffield, England

INTRODUCTION

Alkaline phosphatases (EC 3.1.3.1.) are classified by their hydrolase and transferase activity on a variety of phosphate substrates and by common features such as peculiarly high pH optima (pH 10-10.5), dependence on zinc and magnesium ions, and a dimeric structure with monomer molecular weights between 40,000 and 70,000 (1). These enzymes are assumed to have physiological importance because they are present in nearly all living organisms, exhibit a considerable degree of conservation of active sites (2), and are frequently expressed in plasma membranes, focal points of many transport phenomena. Although resolution of the exact function(s) of alkaline phosphatases (APs) remains elusive, the serum elevations occurring in hepatobiliary and bone diseases that were first recognized more than four decades ago, have maintained their diagnostic value in clinical practice today. Knowledge of human APs advanced with the introduction of techniques of isoenzyme analysis, from which it became clear that several distinct forms exist and that their characterization and specific measurement might similarly provide the means to monitor several other disease states. Such studies led to three main forms of AP isoenzymes being distinguished, which were named for the tissues in which they predominate. There is general acceptance that at least three structural gene foci encode the protein moieties of these different glycoprotein enzymes. One codes for placental alkaline phosphatase (PLAP), at least one for the intestinal form (adult and fetal), and at least one for the tissue unspecific enzymes (liver-bone-kidney type) (3,4). More recent studies have provided evidence for a fourth locus that is closely related to the PLAP locus but controls the expression of PLAP-like enzyme in testis (5). The PLAP group of enzymes are distinguishable from other tissue APs by their thermostability, their electrophoretic, immunochemical, and enzymatic properties, and their exceptional genetic polymorphism (6,7). The interest in APs as potential biochemical markers of cancer dates back 17 years to the discovery of a closely related (8,9) circulating PLAP in a patient (Regan) with an oat-cell carcinoma of the lung (10). The latter "Regan" enzyme is one of the more frequent tumor variant forms and appears to be closely similar to the placental-type AP found in trace amounts in normal lung, cervix, and ovarian tissues (11-13). The other common tumor-associated form of heat stable APs are the "Nagao" or PLAP-like enzymes (14,15). These have trace expressed counterparts in normal testis (12,16) and characteristically differ from PLAP in their marked sensitivity to noncompetitive inhibition by L-leucine (14). Since their discovery, the occurrence of PLAP and PLAP-like APs in human tumor sera and tissues of diverse types has been well documented. The reported prevalence of elevated levels of these enzymes varies from 10-15% in patients with carcinoma of the lung, breast, and colon, whereas higher frequencies have been claimed in gynecological tumors (20-30%) and seminomas (50-70%) (reviewed in 17,18). The more reliable previous methods of placental-type isoenzyme assay have relied on their extreme resistance to heating as a major distinguishing feature or have been based on polyclonal antisera (6,19). Both types of assay have inherent difficulties in that they lack complete specificity for PLAP and the capacity to differentiate PLAP from PLAP-like AP. In recent times the developments in hybridoma technology have enabled the production of monoclonal antibodies (MAbs) that not only eliminate cross-reactivity with other nonplacental forms of AP but also permit discrimination within the PLAP isoenzyme group. The present purpose is to review the extent to which the use of such reagents, capable of recognizing structural or conformation changes at the level of single antigen epitopes, has fulfilled expectations of providing more specific assays for malignant disease.

MONOCLONAL ANTIBODIES TO PLACENTAL ALKALINE PHOSPHATASE

As part of the intense activity stimulated by the advent of MAb technology, there has recently been a resurgence of interest in the production of PLAP-specific reagents. The properties of such MAbs, that have been evaluated and that have shown early promise in tumor marker applications are summarized in Table 1. These MAbs were all produced in a similar manner, namely by primary immunization of mice with either purified trophoblast plasma membranes or allelic variants of PLAP derived from term placentas (20-25).

QUANTITATION OF SERUM PLACENTAL ALKALINE PHOSPHATASE USING MONOCLONAL ANTIBODIES

A number of sensitive assays of generally comparable precision have been developed for the specific estimation of circulating PLAP (Table 2). Of the nine assay systems listed, two have been correctly described as classic enzyme and radioimmunoassays (28, 22). However, the remaining seven detection systems have been variously termed enzyme (27), endogenous enzyme (22), enzyme-antigen (29), and amplified enzyme-linked immunoassay (31), as well as immunolocalization of enzyme activity (30), and immuno-

Table 1   Monoclonal Antibodies Used for Placental Alkaline Phosphatase
Assay of Potential Clinical Utility

MAb	Immunoglobulin type	Specificity	Ref.
H317	IgG1	Most PLAP phenotypes but not PLAP-like AP isoenzymes	20
NDOG2	IgG2b	Most PLAP phenotypes (and PLAP-like AP isoenzymes?)	21
E6	IgG2b	Three most abundant PLAP phenotypes PP(2),[a] PP(3),[a] PP(1)[a]: previously termed F, I, S	22
H17E2	IgG1	All major PLAP phenotypes plus testicular type PLAP-like APs	23
IQ(Bio) anti-PLAP	—	Presumed similar to H17E2	24
H7	IgG2a	Common PLAP phenotypes plus all phenotypes of testicular PLAP-like enzymes	25

[a]Donald and Robson nomenclature (26).

enzymometric assay (32).   All of the latter assays are essentially
based on the enzyme-antigen immunoassay principle, in which
the MAbs are bound directly or by a rabbit antimouse IgG bridge
to a solid phase, and the intrinsic enzymatic activity of the "captured" PLAP is measured at the detection step.   Therefore, for
consistency, assays developed using this principle have all been
considered to be immune-assisted enzyme immunoassays (IAEA)
and are referred to as such in Table 2.

The successful clinical exploitation of PLAP seroassay depends
upon several requirements common to other tumor marker systems.   In addition to sufficiently high frequency of PLAP elevations in neoplastic disease, to good proportionality of these elevations with the tumor mass, and to consistent marker recognition
before treatment and during follow-up, the absence of nonspecific elevations in healthy individuals is also of special importance.
As noted previously (33), the establishment of a normal range or

Table 2   Monoclonal Antibody Assays for Serum Placental Alkaline Phosphatase

Assay format	Sensitivity/ normal limits	Coefficient of variation (%)	Ref.
Microtitre plates			
H317 IAEA[a]	Lower limit of detection, 0.1 U/L (±0.07 µg/L)	Interassay 9.5	27
NDOG2 IAEA[a]	Upper limit of normal, 0.28 U/L	Not given	28
NDOG2 EIA[b]	Not given	Not given	28
E6 IAEA[a]	Lower limit of detection, 0.02 U/L;	Interassay 6.7	29
	upper limit of normal, 0.1 U/L	Interassay 3.8	
H17E2 IAEA[a]	Lower limit of detection, 0.14 OD (±0.04 U/L)	Interassay 11.0	30
IQ(Bio)AELIA[c]	Lower limit of detection, 0.06 U/L; upper limit of normal, 1.0 U/L	Interassay ± 6	31
Other solid-phase assays			
E6 IAEA[a]	Lower limit of detection, 0.12 U/L	Interassay 5.1-11.4 Intraassay 4.1-7.9	22
E6 RIA[d]	Comparable with E6 IAEA	—	22
H7 IAEA[a]	Lower limit of detection, 0.05 µg/L	Interassay 6.9-12.5 Intraassay 3.4-8.3	32

[a]Immune-assisted enzyme assay.
[b]Enzyme immunoassay.
[c]Amplified enzyme-linked immunoassay.
[d]Radioimmunoassay.

upper limit of normal has not been a major priority, but the
limited data available, particularly histograms of normal populations, indicates that in some individuals high levels of circulating
PLAP are present (34-37). Monoclonal antibody immunoassays
have similarly detected elevations in a variable proportion of apparently normal and nonmalignant disease populations (Table 3).
Evidence is presented, and discussed later, for believing that
smoking is responsible for most of these unexplained normal elevations, and also the reason why the highest frequencies have been
detected with assays using MAbs that recognize both PLAP and
PLAP-like enzymes (30,31). The best estimate of basal values for
a healthy reference population is that obtained recently by H7
IAEA (32). It was possible with this assay both to determine the
whole distribution of normal values and to characterize the antigen as PLAP-like enzyme by use of amino acid and peptide inhib-
itors. The upper limit of normality, as defined by this assay, was
2.5 μg/L. The tissues contributing to this normal basal level remain to be resolved, but possible sources include lung, testis,
thymus, cervix, and endometrium, in which trace expression of
PLAP-like enzymes has been described (11,12,42-44). The immunohistochemical detection of PLAP using MAbs has been reported for a variety of other normal, benign, and malignant tissues. How this relates to the tissue extract concentration of
PLAP, where this has also been determined, is shown in Table 4.
Positive immunoreactive staining has been confined to a small
number of the normal tissues tested (46,48), of which normal
lung extracts contain the highest concentrations of PLAP. Among
the different malignancies examined, benign and malignant ovarian, breast, endometrium, and especially testicular tumors, have
the highest proportion of positive staining. The high reactivity of
testicular tumors confirms previous findings with polyclonal
antibodies (49,50) and direct enzyme histochemistry (51). A
panel of six MAbs was used to define the expression of PLAP in
four of seven seminomas, three of seven embryonal carcinomas,
and one yolk sac carcinoma, and PLAP-like AP in two additional
seminomas and four embryonal carcinoma-containing tumors (52).
In the studies in Table 4, a much higher proportion of positive
values were generally obtained with tissue extracts than with sera.
Although total AP activity in tumor tissues was significantly higher
than in normal tissues, there was heterogeneity of expression of

Table 3 Serum Placental Alkaline Phosphatase Levels in Normal Controls and Nonmalignant Disease Populations

Assay	Source	No.	Range (U/L)	98th percentile	No. positive (%)	Ref.
H317 IAEA	"healthy" normals	120	—	0.1 U/L (0.07 µg/L)	0(0)	27
H317 IAEA	Patients with no known ovarian disease	12	—	0.1 U/L	0(0)	38
E6 IAEA	"Healthy" normals	—	0.02-0.12	0.05 U/L	—	29
E6 IAEA	Hospital population	1650	0.02-3.73	0.1 U/L	21(1.3)	29
E6 IAEA	Normals and nonmalignant disease patients	102	0.18-0.33	0.175 U/L	3(0.03)	39
E6 IAEA	Patients with liver disease on chronic dialysis	47	—	0.1 U/L	0(0)	40
		50	—	0.1 U/L	2(4)	
H17E2 IAEA	"Healthy" normals	213	0.07-0.5	—	35(16.4)	30
H17E2 IAEA	Patients with nonmalignant testicular disease	32	—	—	2(6.3)	41
IQ(Bio) AELIA	Normals and nonmalignant disease patients	81	—	1 U/L	7(9)	31
H7 IAEA	"Healthy" normals	253	—	2.5 µg/L	0(0)	32

Table 4 PLAP Levels and Immunohistochemical Staining of Normal, Benign, and Malignant Tissues

Tissue type	No.	PLAP tissue content (mU/g)	PLAP reactive staining No. positive (%)	MAb detection system	Ref.
Normal					
ovary	6	<0.3-32.4[a]	—	H317	38
ovary	10	<0.2-1.1	1/5 (20)	E6	29,45
lung	14	>1-~200	3/6 (50)	E6, NDOG2	29,46
breast	2	<1	—	E6	29
stomach	6	<1-~3	—	E6	29
cervix	2	—	2/2 (100)		46
thymus	1	—	1/1 (100)		46
fallopian tube	3	—	3/3 (100)	NDOG2	46
endometrium	22	—	21/22 (96)		44
Benign					
ovary	8	<0.3-10[a]	4/12 (33.3)	H317	38
ovary	3	2.3-7.9	2/3 (66.6)	E6	45
	44	—	11/44 (25)	NDOG2	28
Malignant					
ovary	6	1.2-53.6[a]	6/19 (31.6)	H317	38
ovary	35	<1-557	11/12 (91.7)	E6	29,45
	56	—	36/56 (64.3)	NDOG2	28
lung and bronchial	21	<1-~60	—	E6	29,39
breast	7	0.5-4.2[a]	5/7 (71.4)	H317	47
breast	158	<1-63.1	—	E6	29,39
	16	<1-70	—	E6	29
stomach	8	—	8/12 (66.6)	NDOG2	44
endometrium	8	—	7/7 (100)		
seminona, testis	7	—	7/7 (100)		
malignant teratoma, testis	7	—	7/7 (100)	H17E2	48
mixed tumor, testis	2	—	2/2 (100)		

[a]U/kg net weight.

PLAP. Although levels of PLAP were, therefore, not necessarily higher in malignant than in benign tumors, the degree of immuno-chemical staining was broadly correlated with the tissue content of PLAP. Finally, histochemical detection of alkaline phosphatase activity demonstrated a similar distribution to that seen with immunohistochemical localization of PLAP.

The reported incidence of elevated serum PLAP levels as detected by MAb assay in testicular and in the more common non-germ-cell tumors is presented in Table 5 and Table 6. The 54-100% positive detection rate in pure seminoma, or mixed tumors containing seminomatous elements, contrasts with the 5.2-25% positivity observed in breast, respiratory tract, and cervical cancers. On the other hand, the detection in ovarian cancer of usually between 30 and 50% positive sera, represents a potentially significant proportion of patients expressing the PLAP marker. Possibly because of selection problems, more ovarian cancer test sera came from patients whose tumors were of the serous histo-logical type. Of these 68 sera, 26 were positive compared with

Table 5 Serum Placental Alkaline Phosphatase Levels in Testicular Germ Cell Tumors

Tumor type	Assay	No.	Range (U/L)	No. positve (%)	Ref.
Seminoma		16	0.14-3.2	14 (88)	30
Mixed seminoma and teratoma	H17E2 IAEA	13	0.14-2.5	7 (54)	30
Malignant teratoma		21	0.14-1.3	7 (33)	30
Seminoma	H17E2 IAEA	16	0.14-3.2	15 (94)	53
Seminoma		11	0.17-2.8	11 (100)	54
Mixed tumor	H17E2 IAEA	6	0.38[a]		54
Malignant teratoma		9	0.13[a]		54
Seminoma	IQ(Bio) AELIA	35	1.7[b]	21 (60)	31
Nonseminoma		10	0.4[b]	1 (10)	31

[a]Mean value.
[b]Median value.

Table 6   Serum Placental Alkaline Phosphatase Levels in Non-Germ-Cell
Malignancies[a]

Cancer type	Assay	No.	Range	No. positive (%)	Ref.
Ovarian	H317 IAEA	65	—	23 (35)	27
		67	—	23 (34)	38
	NDOG2 IAEA	20	<0.25-4.54 U/L		28
	NDOG2 EIA	20	0.65-68.19 μg/ml		28
	E6 IAEA	10	—	4 (40)	29
		17	—	1 (5.9)	39
		20	—	9 (45)	40
		14	0.2-1.36 U/L	7 (50)	45
	H17E2 IAEA	38	0.17-1.4 U/L	8 (21.1)	55
		32	0.2-3.2 U/L	16 (50)	56
Cervical	H317 IAEA	16	—	4 (25)	27
	E6 IAEA	21	—	1 (4.8)	39
Breast	E6 IAEA	34	—	2 (5.9)	29
		286	—	15 (5.2)	39
Bronchial	E6 IAEA	18	—	4 (22.2)	29
Lung and					
bronchial		133	0.18-1.89 U/L	15 (11.2)	39

[a]In the references given, positive PLAP readings are also reported in single
endometrial, colon, gastric, pharyngeal, and pancreatic cancers, and in acute
myeloid leukemia and Hodgkin's disease.

nine of 21 and eight of 20 samples from patients with mucinous
and endometrioid carcinomas, respectively (Table 7).

CLINICAL APPLICATIONS OF PLACENTAL
ALKALINE PHOSPHATASE SEROASSAY

Testicular Cancer

The overall results of treatment of testicular cancer have improved
dramatically over the past decade (57). This improvement, at least
in part, is due to the development of marker systems that allow
for regular and precise assessment of tumor burden. The traditional marker systems utilizing α-fetoprotein (AFP) and the β-sub-
unit of human chorionic gonadotrophin (β-HCG) are best suited to

Table 7 Serum Placental Alkaline Phosphatase Levels in Relation to Ovarian Tumor Subtype and Stage

Tumor classification		Incidence positive sera	IAEA assay	Ref.
Type	Stage			
Malignant tumors				
papillary serous cystadeno-carcinoma	I—IV	26/68	H317,E6,H17E2	38,45,55,56
mucinous cysta-denocarcinoma	I—IV	9/21	H317,H17E2	38,55,56
endometrioid carcinoma	Ia—IV	8/20	H317,E6,H17E2	38,45,55,56
mesonephroid carcinoma	?—III	0/4	H317,H17E2	38,55
granulosa cell carcinoma	?—IV	2/5	H317,E6	38,45
mixed Mullerian tumor	?—IIa	0/2	E6,H17E2	45,55
carcinoma, unclassified	I—IV	8/23	H317,E6,H17E2	38,45,55,56
Benign tumors				
serous cysta-denoma	—	1/9	H317	38
serous cysta-denofibroma	—	0/2	E6	45
mucinous cysta-denoma	—	3/7	H317	38
endometrioma	—	0/2	H317	38

the management of nonseminomatous germ cell tumors, and it is here that the major advances in therapy have been experienced (58). The seminomatous tumors are, for the most part, exquisitely radiosensitive, but the small proportion that prove resistant to this treatment modality have been presented problems in management because they have been relatively silent in terms of the traditional markers for germ cell malignancy.

α-Fetoprotein is associated with yolk sac differentiation, either in the pure form as a yolk sac tumor or as constituent elements within embryonal carcinoma or teratoma. The β-subunit of HCG is similarly associated with specific cellular characteristics within the tumor, either as the pure choriocarcinoma or in those tumors that contain syncytiotrophoblast (59). Because of the relative frequency of these two cell types throughout the spectrum of non-seminomatous germ cell tumors, serum positivity for AFP or β-HCG may be encountered in approximately 90% of cases. Many other markers have been described for this group of tumors, including pregnancy-specific β-glycoprotein (SPI) (60), human placental lactogen (HPL), lactic dehydrogenase (LDH) (61), and carcinoembryonic antigen (CEA). Pregnancy-specific β-glyco-protein and HPL are essentially similar in cellular origin to β-HCG and rarely add information not yielded by that marker in the clinical management of the patient. Lactic dehydrogenase appears to be of relatively little value, except in the patient with large, bulk disease, and CEA is of value only in the pure embryonal carcinoma and in the rare Sertoli cell and interstitial tumors of testis.

Seminomatous tumors of testis are universally negative for AFP, and only those with a syncytiotrophoblastic element express β-HCG (59). The proportion of seminomas that show serum marker positivity, with traditional marker assays systems, is limited to about 10-15% (62). The H17E2 reactive PLAP, after making due allowance for smoking habit, is reported to be elevated in 80-90% of cases (41,63). Somewhat lower proportions are seen in other assay systems (31). Even allowing for the different reactivity of some MAbs, the addition of a PLAP assay to the traditional marker profile of AFP and β-HCG makes a radical change in the status of all testicular tumors.

A number of studies of PLAP in testicular tumors at presentation have been published (see Table 5). All show clear distinction between seminoma and normal controls. The levels recorded in nonseminomatous germ cell tumors are not significantly different from the control populations. Longitudinal studies of PLAP in the monitoring mode also have been reported with encouraging results. Levels correlate closely with clinical status and give accurate assessment of increasing tumor burden. Insufficient data is now available to allow kinetic marker elimination studies such as those used for AFP in yolk sac or endodermal sinus tumors (64).

Ovarian Cancer

Experience with PLAP assays in ovarian cancer is more limited, and the resultant picture is less clear. Unlike the testis, most ovarian cancers are of epithelial origin, and PLAP elevations have been reported in a proportion of all tumor types (see Table 7). The one malignant germ cell tumor with any significant frequency, dysgerminoma, does show consistent elevations of PLAP, which may prove to be of diagnostic and monitoring importance (65).

ELEVATED SERUM PLACENTAL ALKALINE PHOSPHATASE ACTIVITY IN SMOKERS

The data from various sources that demonstrate that cigarette smoking causes a significant elevation of serum PLAP levels is summarized in Table 8. Such high PLAP values occurring in normal individuals complicates the monitoring of tumor activity by PLAP measurements, especially in its application to the detection of early stage and recurrent disease. For example, in the longitudinal study of breast cancer patients (see Table 8), PLAP levels measured by polyclonal antibody RIA were found to be elevated in 34% of patients with benign, primary, and metastatic disease and who smoked, compared with 5% of nonsmoking women (66). Evidence for smoking being the cause was provided by the fall to normal levels within 2 months in a patient who ceased smoking after a myocardial infarction. The RIA results also suggested that the smoking-induced enzyme was immunologically related to the placental form of enzyme. Systematic studies using the substrate naphthol-ASNX-phosphate, in a very sensitive fluorometric assay for heat-stable alkaline phosphatase, also had shown significant elevations of PLAP in saliva and sputum as well as in serum. Increases in mean serum PLAP levels of six to seven times those of nonsmokers were observed (67), with some smokers exhibiting levels tenfold greater than the upper limit of nonsmokers. In a group of 285 patients with a variety of malignancies, 85% of the abnormal PLAP values fell within the range of 48 healthy smokers (68). Hence, these authors felt that PLAP would be only useful as a tumor marker in nonsmoking patients. They also demonstrated by enzyme neutralization experiments with rabbit anti-PLAP antibody that the enzyme inhibition curves with the smoking-induced serum enzyme and PLAP were similar. Even with the use of MAbs

Table 8 Fluorometric, Polyclonal, and Monoclonal Antibody Assay Systems Detecting Elevated Serum Placental Alkaline Phosphatase in Smokers

Assay	Study group	Mean PLAP values		PLAP normal upper limit	Ref.
		Nonsmokers (No.)	Smokers (No.)		
Polyclonal antibody RIA	Normal controls	0.55 ng/ml (28)	2.58 ng/ml (13)	2.14 ng/ml	66
	Breast cancer patients (benign, primary, and metastatic disease)	0.42-0.66 ng/ml (182)	1.44-1.90 ng/ml (46)		66
Fluorometric (for heat-stable AP)	Normal controls	0.068 U/L (51)	0.44 U/L (25)		67
		0.057 U/L (98)	0.378 U/L (65)		33
		0.063 U/L (82)	0.47 U/L (48)		68
	Patients with a variety of malignancies (No. = 285)	0.15 U/L (69)[a]	—	0.15 U/L	68
IQ(Bio) AELIA	Normals and patients with nonmalignant disease	0.055 U/L (34)[b]	0.52 U/L (47)[b]	0.1 U/L	31

H317 and H17E2 IAEA				
Normal controls (No. = 28) H317 assay	0.1 U/L (12)	0.1 U/L (16)	0.1 U/L	69
H17E2 assay	—	0.1 U/L (8)[a]		69
Patients with inflammatory lung disease (No. = 11) H317 assay	0.1 U/L (11)	—		69
H17E2 assay	0.1 U/L (4)[a]	—		69
H17E2 IAEA				
Normal controls (No. = 286)	—	—	0.08 U/L (35)[a]	30
Patients with testicular cancer in remission				
all germ cell tumors	0.10 U/L (70)	0.15 U/L (39)		54
seminoma only	0.05 U/L (40)	0.14 U/L (22)		54
Seminoma patients after 1-year follow-up				
orchidectomy only	0.05 U/L (10)[b]	0.29 U/L (5)[b]		70
orchidectomy and chemotherapy	0.02 U/L (7)[b]	0.36 U/L (4)[b]		70

[a]Number exceeding normal upper limit.
[b]Median values.

the problems of inappropriate measurement of cross-reacting enzymes in smokers have remained, particularly where MAbs recognizing both PLAP and PLAP-like enzymes have formed the basis of the assay system. Such cross-reactivity is to be expected because the enzyme produced in smokers has been characterized by its reactivity with two MAbs (H317 and H17E2), of differing fine specificity, to be the PLAP-like, rather than the placental form of the enzyme (69,71). Thus the elevated PLAP levels observed in a proportion of the testicular tumor patients, who by other criteria are in clinical remission, are usually attributable to concomitant smoking. In patients on long-term follow-up after orchidectomy or combined orchidectomy and chemotherapy, the mean serum PLAP levels of smokers were between six- and 18-fold greater than those of nonsmokers (70). In addition, the fluctuations in PLAP profiles were consistently greater in smokers than in nonsmokers, and in one patient, who was persuaded to discontinue smoking, PLAP levels fell progressively to normal levels in a manner similar to that reported previously (33,66).

CONCLUSIONS

The development of murine MAbs specific for human PLAP, has seen a resurgence of interest in this highly polymorphic isoenzyme system as a tumor marker. The greater specificity of these MAbs not only eliminates the cross-reactivity with intestinal alkaline phosphatase that was formerly encountered with polyclonal xenoantisera, but it also allows discrimination within the placental and placentallike isoenzyme grouping. Predictably, several such MAbs have been substituted in previous polyclonal antibody-based immunoassays to improve both the specificity and sensitivity of PLAP detection. The MAb evaluations of tissue content and distribution and of the circulating levels of placental and placentallike isoenzymes found in various malignancies, have confirmed their clinical usefulness as a marker of testicular seminomas and certain ovarian tumors. Evidence is accumulating for coexpression of both placental and placentallike forms of enzyme in some instances of ovarian cancer. In seminomas, placentallike enzymes seem to be principally expressed and this complicates the monitoring of tumor activity because of the additional measurement of elevated placentallike enzyme levels induced by smoking.

This problem of falsely suspecting active disease in smokers could be obviated if patients gave up the habit. The alternative solution would be further development of MAbs capable of recognizing distinct epitope differences, if such exist, between the smoking-induced and disease-related forms of placentallike enzymes. An expansion of studies now appearing in the literature of molecular cloning and structural analysis of the placental and placental-related AP genes, may provide a rational basis for the production of such discriminant probes. Similarly produced MAbs also may be of value in further elucidating the interrelationships of PLAP and its placental-type counterparts expressed in clinically useful amounts in different malignancies. Finally, another area of high expectations, and one in which encouraging results are currently being obtained, is the application of MAbs to tumor imaging by immunoscintigraphy and their therapeutic potential in targeting drugs or toxins to tumor cells.

REFERENCES

1. R. B. McComb, G. N. Bowers, and S. Posen, *Alkaline Phosphatase*. Plenum Press, New York (1979).
2. K. B. Whitaker, P. G. H. Byfield, and D. W. Moss, *Clin. Chim. Acta 71*:285 (1976).
3. L. E. Seargeant and R. A. Stinson, *Nature 281*:152 (1979).
4. M. J. McKenna, T. A. Hamilton, and H. H. Sussman, *Biochem. J. 181*:67 (1979).
5. J. L. Millan and T. Stigbrand, *Eur. J. Biochem. 136*:1 (1983).
6 R. H. Kottle and W. H. Fishman, in *Biochemical Markers for Cancer* (T. Ming Chu, ed.), Marcel Dekker, Inc., New York (1982), p. 93.
7. T. S. Stigbrand, J. L. Millan, and W. H. Fishman, *Isozymes Curr. Top. Biol. Med. Res. 6*:93 (1982).
8. P. J. Greene and H. H. Sussman, *Proc. Natl. Acad. Sci. USA 70*:2936 (1973).
9. H. J. Cleeve and D. C. Tua, *Clin. Chem. 29*:715 (1983).
10. W. H. Fishman, N. R. Inglis, L. L. Stolbach, and M. J. Krant, *Cancer Res. 28*:150 (1968).
11. D. J. Goldstein, C. E. Rogers, and H. Harris, *Clin. Chim. Acta 125*:63 (1982).

12. P. J. McLaughlin, P. J. Travers, I. W. McDicken, and P. M. Johnson, *Clin. Chim. Acta 137*:341 (1984).
13. S. Nozawa, M. Ohta, S. Izumi, S. Kayashi, F. Tsutsni, S. Kurihara, and K. Watanabe, *Acta Histochem. Cytochem. 13*:521 (1980).
14. T. Nakayama, M. Yoshida, and M. Kitamura, *Clin. Chim. Acta 30*:546 (1970).
15. N. R. Inglis, S. Kirley, L. L. Stolbach, and W. H. Fishman, *Cancer Res. 33*:1657 (1973).
16. C. H. Chang, D. Angellis, and W. H. Fishman, *Cancer Res. 40*: 1506 (1980).
17. W. H. Fishman and L. L. Stolbach, in *Immunodiagnosis of Cancer* (R. B. Herberman and K. R. McIntire, eds.), Marcel Dekker, New York (1979), p. 442.
18. T. Stigbrand and E. Engvall, in *Human Cancer Markers* (S. Sell and B. Wahren, eds.), Humana Press, Clifton, N.J. (1982), p. 275.
19. S. Dass and K. D. Bagshawe, in *Human Alkaline Phosphatases, Progress in Clinical and Biological Research* (T. Stigbrand and W. H. Fishman, eds.), Vol. 166. Alan R. Liss, New York (1984), p. 49.
20. P. J. McLaughlin, H. M. Cheng, M. B. Slade, and P. M. Johnson, *Int. J. Cancer 30*:21 (1982).
21. C. A. Sunderland, C. W. G. Redman, and G. M. Stirrat, *Immunology 43*:541 (1981).
22. G. De Groote, P. De Waele, A. Van de Voorde, M. De Broe, and W. Fiers, *Clin. Chem. 29*:115 (1983).
23. P. Travers and W. Bodmer, *Int. J. Cancer 33*:633 (1984).
24. C.H. Self, *J. Immunol. Methods 76*:389 (1985).
25. J. L. Millan and T. Stigbrand, *Eur. J. Biochem. 136*:1 (1983).
26. L. J. Donald and E. B. Robson, *Ann. Hum. Genet. 37*:303 (1974).
27. P. J. McLaughlin, H. Gee, and P. M. Johnson, *Clin. Chim. Acta 130*:199 (1983).
28. J. O. Davies, E. R. Davies, K. Howe, P. Jackson, E. Pitcher, B. Randle, C. Sadowski, G. M. Stirrat, and C. A. Sunderland, *J. R. Soc. Med. 78*:899 (1985).
29. D. E. Pollet, E. J. Nouwen, and J. B. Schelstraete, *Clin. Chem. 31*:41 (1985).
30. D. F. Tucker, R. T. D. Oliver, P. Travers, and W. F. Bodmer, *Br. J. Cancer 51*:631 (1985).

31. E. H. Cooper, N. B. Pidcock, W. G. Jones, and A. Milford Ward, *Eur. J. Cancer Clin. Oncol. 21*:525 (1985).

32. J. L. Millan, K. Nustad, and B. Nørgaard-Pedersen, *Clin. Chem. 31*:54 (1985).

33. H. Muensch, W. Maslow, and F. Azama, in *Human Alkaline Phosphatases, Progress in Clinical and Biological Research* (T. Stigbrand and W. H. Fishman, eds.), Vol. 166. Alan R. Liss, New York (1984), p. 317.

34. J. A. Kellen, R. S. Bush, and A. Malkin, *Cancer Res. 36*:269 (1976).

35. H. G. Wada, J. G. Shindelman, A. E. Ortmeyer, and H. H. Sussman, *Int. J. Cancer 23*:781 (1979).

36. M. Usategui-Gomez, F. M. Yeager, and A. F. de Castro, *Cancer Res. 33*:1574 (1973).

37. L. Nathanson and W. H. Fishman, *Cancer 27*:1388 (1971).

38. I. W. McDicken, P. J. McLaughlin, P. M. Tromans, D. M. Luesley, and P. M. Johnson, *Br. J. Cancer 52*:59 (1985).

39. A. Van de Voorde, G. De Groote, P. De Waele, M. E. De Broe, D. Pollet, J. de Boever, D. Vandekerckhove, and W. Fiers, *Eur. J. Cancer Clin. Oncol. 21*:65 (1985).

40. M. W. Eerdekens, E. J. Nouwen, D. E. Pollet, T. W. Briers, and M. E. De Broe, *Clin. Chem. 31*:687 (1985).

41. A. Milford Ward and G. Bates, in *Advances in the Biosciences, Vol. 55, Germ Cell Tumours II* (W. G. Jones, A. Milford Ward, and C. K. Anderson, eds.), Pergamon Press, Oxford (1986), p. 149.

42. D. J. Goldstein, L. Blasco, and H. Harris, *Proc. Natl. Acad. Sci. USA 77*:4226 (1980).

43. P. J. McLaughlin, P. H. Warne, G. E. Hutchison, P. M. Johnson, and D. F. Tucker, *Br. J. Cancer 55*:197 (1987).

44. J. O. Davies, K. Howe, G. M. Stirrat, and C. A. Sunderland, *Histochem. J. 17*:605 (1985).

45. E. J. Nouwen, D. E. Pollet, J. B. Schelstraete, M. W. Eerdekens, C. Hansch, A. Van de Voorde, and M. E. De Broe, *Cancer Res. 45*:892 (1985).

46. C. A. Sunderland, J. O. Davies, and G. M. Stirrat, *Cancer Res. 44*:4496 (1984).

47. I. W. McDicken, G. H. Stamp, P. J. McLaughlin, and P. M. Johnson, *Int. J. Cancer, 32*:205 (1983).

48. A. A. Epenetos, P. Travers, K. C. Gatter, R. D. T. Oliver, D. Y. Mason, and W. F. Bodmer, *Br. J. Cancer 49*:11 (1984).

49. T. Uchida, T. Shimoda, H. Miyata, T. Shikata, S. Iino, H. Suzuki, T. Oda, K. Hirano, and M. Sugiura, *Cancer 48*:1455 (1981).

50. B. Wahren, P. A. Holmgren, and T. Stigbrand, *Int. J. Cancer 24*:749 (1979).

51. J. H. Beckstead, *Am. J.Surg. Pathol. 7*:341 (1983).

52. J. Paiva, I. Damjanov, P. H. Lange, and H. Harris, *Am. J. Pathol. 111*:156 (1983).

53. A. Horwich, D. F. Tucker, and M. J. Peckham, *Br. J. Cancer 51*:625 (1985).

54. A. A. Epenetos, A. J. Munro, D. F. Tucker, W. Gregory, W. Duncan, R. H. MacDougall, M. Faux, P. Travers, and W. F. Bodmer, *Br. J. Cancer 51*:641 (1985).

55. D. F. Tucker, Y. L. Pookim, and L. Bobrow (unpublished data).

56. B. G. Ward, D. J. Cruickshank, D. F. Tucker, and S. Love, *Br. J. Obstet. Gynaecol.* (in press).

57. M. Ellis and K. Sikora, in *Therapeutic Trials in Oncology* (G. Mathé, ed.), Bioscience, Geneva (1984).

58. W. G. Jones, in *Germ Cell Tumours* (C. K. Anderson, W. G. Jones, and A. Milford Ward, eds.), Taylor and Francis, London (1981), p. 3.

59. F. K. Mostofi, I. A. Sesterhenn, and C. J. Davis, in *Advances in the Biosciences, Vol. 55, Germ Cell Tumours II* (W. G. Jones, A. Milford Ward, and C. K. Anderson, eds.), Pergamon Press, Oxford (1986), p. 1.

60. F. Searle, in *Germ Cell Tumours* (C. K. Anderson, W. G. Jones, and A. Milford Ward, eds.), Taylor and Francis, London (1981), p. 233.

61. F. E. von Eyben, *Cancer 41*:648 (1978).

62. N. Javadpour, in *Advances in the Biosciences, Vol. 55, Germ Cell Tumours II* (W. G. Jones, A. Milford Ward, and C. K. Anderson, eds.), Pergamon Press, Oxford (1986), p. 209.

63. D. F. Tucker, R. T. D. Oliver, G. H. Ellard, D. Y. Wang, and Y. L. Pookim, in *Advances in the Biosciences, Vol. 55, Germ Cell Tumours II* (W. G. Jones, A. Milford Ward, and C. K. Anderson, eds.), Pergamon Press, Oxford (1986), p. 139.

64. A. Milford Ward and G. E. Bates, *Protides Biol. Fluids 27*: 356 (1979).

65. A. Milford Ward (unpublished data).

66. S. E. Tonik, A. E. Ortmeyer, J. E. Shindelman, and H. H. Sussman, *Int. J. Cancer 31*:51 (1983).

67. W. C. Maslow, H. A. Muensch, F. Azama, and A. S. Schneider, *Clin. Chem. 29*:260 (1983).

68. W. C. Maslow, H. Muensch, F. Carlson, and M. Betrand, *Am. J. Clin. Pathol. 81*:396 (1984) (abstr.).

69. P. J. McLaughlin, A. M. Twist, C. C. Evans, and P. M. Johnson, *J. Clin. Pathol. 37*:826 (1984).

70. D. F. Tucker, R. T. D. Oliver, and Y. L. Pookim (unpublished data).

71. G. H. Williams, P. J. McLaughlin, and P. M. Johnson, *Clin. Chim. Acta 155*:329 (1986).

12
Human Monoclonal Antibodies for Tumor Diagnosis

June Kan-Mitchell and Malcolm S. Mitchell / Kenneth Norris, Jr., Cancer Hospital and Research Institute, University of Southern California School of Medicine, Los Angeles, California

INTRODUCTION

The development by Köhler and Milstein (1975) of murine monoclonal antibodies (MAbs) by somatic cell hybridization techniques has revolutionized the histological analysis of human tumors and can provide the means for a far more detailed immunochemical and molecular analysis of tumor-associated antigens (TAAs) than was previously possible. This technology has been refined over the years to such a high degree that murine MAbs of known specificities are now available in large quantities for both therapeutic and diagnostic applications. Because of this success, a great deal of interest has recently been directed to the production of MAbs of human origin, particularly for therapy.

Human monoclonal antibodies (Hu-MAbs) offer several potential advantages over their murine counterparts. In therapeutic applications, Hu-MAbs should be much less immunogenic than those of mouse origin, inducing little or no neutralizing antibodies in patients, even after repeated administrations. The induction of a significant antimouse immunoglobulin (Ig) antibody response can severely limit the effectiveness of a therapeutic regimen that requires repeated administrations of murine MAbs. This has, in fact, been observed in clinical trials of murine MAbs for the therapy of lymphoma as well as solid tumors (1,2). In addition, the possibility exists that human antibodies to TAAs may have a different spectrum of reactivity than do mouse MAbs (3). An analogy might be found in tissue typing. Here, human antibodies are known to express a wider range of specificities against allotypic determinants of human leukocyte antigen (HLA) than do antibodies of xenogeneic origin (3). The production of Hu-MAbs with such specificities would provide a constant and well-defined source of specific human antibody to use in place of human immune sera for both therapeutic (such as Rh-immune globulin) and diagnostic purposes.

TECHNOLOGY FOR PRODUCTION OF HUMAN MONOCLONAL ANTIBODIES

The technology for the production of human MAbs is still in its developmental stages. Despite recent achievements, technical advances remain to be made, particularly in two aspects. These are the method(s) for the production of permanent antibody-producing cell lines and the generation of specifically sensitized human lymphocytes for immortalization by in vitro immunization.

Two basic approaches have been used to immortalize human B lymphocytes. First, cell lines derived from human B lymphocytes transformed in vitro by Epstein-Barr virus (EBV) can produce

human MAbs in tissue culture (5). Although many of these transformed lymphoblastoid cell lines (LCLs) lose their ability to secrete antibodies upon continuous cultivation (5), a very small
percentage have been isolated that remain stable for long periods
of time (6). The factors that are important for the stabilization
of antibody production are not known, although early cloning is
essential to prevent overgrowth by nonsecreting cells. In general,
the establishment of an antibody-producing line occurs at a very
low frequency, and the transformed cells are difficult to clone.
Furthermore, the cultures grow slowly, producing only small
amounts of Hu-MAbs. LCLs also do not grow in ascites form in
mice, thus making the production of larger quantities more difficult.

Human MAbs can also be produced by hybridoma technology.
However, an entirely satisfactory fusion partner of human origin
is not currently available. Of the most commonly used human
fusion partners, two are phenotypically myeloid and the majority
of the others are LCLs (7). Hybridomas, obtained by fusing
lymphocytes from patients with malignant diseases with an LCL,
secreted antibodies into the spent cultures that showed some
specificity of binding to tumor cells (8). As with LCLs, most of
these lines grew slowly in culture, were unstable, and produced
very small amounts of immunoglobulin (9). In addition, the
efficiency of antibody-producing hybrid cell formation was extremely low.

Interspecies hybrids obtained by fusing human lymphocytes
to mouse myeloma cells can produce human MAbs with specificity against a variety of antigens (10). With careful handling,
these heterohybridomas can stably produce Hu-MAbs for months,
and if a large number of early passages are preserved as frozen
stocks, it is possible to study the reactivities of these antibodies
over the course of several years. Nonetheless, these heterohybridomas are probably intrinsically impermanent, perhaps as a
result of the preferential segregation of the human chromosomes.

Considerable effort has been devoted to identifying better
fusion partners. Mouse × human hybrid myelomas (heteromye-
lomas) have been constructed (11,12) for this purpose. It was
hoped that the heterohybridomas would retain the superior fusion characteristics of the mouse myeloma cells, and, at the same
time, be more capable of supporting the production of Hu-MAbs

because of the presence of human chromosomes. Cell lines have
also been constructed by fusing a human myeloma line with peripheral blood mononuclear cells (13). Whether or not these prove
to be superior remains to be determined.

The largest obstacle for the production of Hu-MAbs is obtaining sufficient numbers of immune B lymphocytes. Despite
the identification of human B-cell growth and differentiation factors, human B cells have not been routinely maintained in long-
term culture. Human antibodies against infectious agents and
blood group antigens have been generated from lymphocytes of
immunized donors (10). However, the number of circulating
memory B cells in human peripheral blood appears to be fairly
low. In general, lymphocytes from lymph nodes and spleens give
better fusion frequency (14). Although primary human in vitro
immunization procedures have been established for isolated antigens, such as bombesin and tetanus toxoid (15) and bacterial
lipopolysaccharide and surface red cell antigens (10), a generally
applicable method is still not available.

RATIONALE FOR THE DEVELOPMENT OF HUMAN MONOCLONAL ANTIBODIES FOR DIAGNOSTIC APPLICATIONS

One observation, in particular, has spurred our interest in using
Hu-MAbs to study melanoma. Despite the use of a variety of immunization schedules and antigenic preparations of fresh, irradiated or cultured melanoma cells, many of the same melanoma
TAAs have been identified by several laboratories. This might
reflect the inability of mice to recognize certain human tumor
antigens (3) or more likely, their preference for the same "immunodominant" antigens. Although this limitation might be overcome with more ingenious immunization of the mouse (16),
Hu-MAbs may more directly identify TAAs. Moreover, unlike
the mouse when presented with an inoculum of xenoantigens,
human beings sensitized in vivo to their autologous tumor might
recognize exquisite differences between tumor and normal tissues.

Many of the melanoma-associated antigens identified by
mouse MAbs are *differentiation antigens* of cells of neural crest
origin (17), such as the core protein, p250, of a noncartilaginous
proteoglycan, which is found exclusively in cells of the melano-
cyte lineage and expressed as a cell surface macromolecule (18).

Other melanoma TAAs identified by mouse MAbs represent the abnormal presence of normal cellular antigens associated with cells of other lineages (such as the HLA-DR antigen) (19) or of rapidly proliferating cells (such as the transferrin receptor) (20). None of the TAAs yet identified appear to differentiate between normal and neoplastic cells, i.e., between skin melanocytes or benign nevus cells and melanoma cells. This also appears to be so in other tumor systems. A large battery of mouse MAbs with defined reactivities is available for the differential diagnosis of anaplastic tumors (21). However, their reactivities are directed to such antigens as the intermediate filaments of the cytokeratin type (22), and carcinoembryonic antigen (CEA) (23,24). Although the presence of these antigens can distinguish undifferentiated carcinomas from nonepithelial neoplasms, they are present in both normal and neoplastic epithelia and thus are not useful for the diagnosis of malignant changes in these tissues. In fact, most mouse MAbs do not identify antigens that differentiate tumors from their normal counterparts.

HUMAN MONOCLONAL ANTIBODIES WITH REACTIVITY AGAINST MELANOMA

Human MAbs have been generated in different laboratories from the lymphocytes of melanoma patients. Irie et al. (6) isolated a stable IgM-producing LCL by transforming peripheral blood lymphocytes by EBV. This antibody reacts against a melanoma cell surface glycolipid, GD2, which is a differentiation antigen of cells of neural crest origin. Houghton et al. (25,26) produced a large number of hybridomas from both human-human and human-mouse fusions from lymphocytes of melanoma patients. The Hu-MAbs secreted into the medium were found to react to intracellular antigens; less than 1% of the clones have cell surface reactivity. Some of their antibodies were subsequently shown to bind to cytoskeletal components, such as vimentin (14).

We have generated a series of Hu-MAbs by fusing lymphocytes from regional lymph nodes of melanoma patients with a nonsecreting mouse myeloma cell line. Regional lymph node cells generally, give better fusion efficiencies than peripheral blood lymphocytes, perhaps because they contain a higher number of memory B cells. One of our major objectives was to determine, by hybridoma technology, which TAAs might be antigenic to man to aid in the construction of antitumor vaccines. We therefore chose to use lymph node cells from patients not given previous immunotherapy. Thus, by definition, the TAAs identified by Hu-MAbs were spontaneously immunogenic to the autologous host. Whether or not antibodies with these reactivities are found circulating in the serum is another matter, to be determined.

Production of Human-Mouse Hybridomas: Generation of Large Quantities of Human Monoclonal Antibodies and Their Purification from Ascitic Fluids

Six stable hybridoma cell lines were cloned from different lymphocytes derived from three melanoma patients (27). We have maintained these human-mouse heterohybridomas for more than 4 years by the judicious recloning and the freezing of early passages. The three IgG antibody-producing hybridomas have been adapted to grow as ascites in nude mice, producing up to 20-25 mg of antibody from each mouse. A procedure was developed to purify Hu-MAbs from these ascites to greater than 80% homogeneity. An important step, termed *affinity depletion*, was included for the complete removal of mouse Ig from the ascites by an affinity column of sheep antimouse IgG with no cross-reactivity to Hu-IgG (28,29). After additional purification by a high-performance ligand chromatography (HPLC) hydroxyapatite column (HPHT), the human IgG MAbs migrate as a single sharp peak of 150 kd when examined by HPLC gel-permeation chromatography.

Altered Antigenicity of Human Monoclonal Antibody Molecules

Attempts to use enzyme immunoassays developed for mouse MAbs to quantitate IgG Hu-MAbs revealed rather unusual titration curves (28). This led to the discovery that the intact molecules of Hu-MAbs are antigenically distinct in both heavy and light chains from their polyclonal counterparts. A practical corollary is that different proportions of the antibodies in polyclonal goat antihuman Ig antisera recognize Hu-MAbs and polyclonal human Igs. Corrective measures must, therefore, be included when xeno-antibodies are used to study Hu-MAbs.

The reactivities of Hu-MAbs to melanoma antigens bound to a solid support can be demonstrated directly with biotin-conjugated Hu-MAbs or indirectly with a biotin-conjugated second (anti-Ig) antibody. Figure 1 shows the direct assay to be extremely sensitive, requiring only 25-100 ng of antibody protein. The binding was specific, since no binding by the biotin-conjugated human IgG was detected even at 20-fold greater concentrations. In contrast, the indirect assay was less sensitive, failing to detect binding at the same concentrations of antibody. Although not shown, no binding was detected using a class-matched nonreactive Hu-MAb. These results appear at first to disagree with the usual experience that a second antibody amplifies binding. This discrepancy is explained by the inability of many of the polyclonal goat antibody molecules to recognize the Hu-MAbs, resulting in a lower effective concentration of second antibody compared with that at the site of binding of the polyclonal first antibody.

In our screening procedure for reactivity, we have incorporated the use of the avidin-biotin-peroxidase complex both for detection and for amplification of binding (30). Hence, we have identified even those TAAs that appear to be present at lower concentrations in tumor cells than others defined by mouse and Hu-MAbs.

Immunoreactivities of Human Monoclonal Antibodies

Our Hu-MAbs appear to identify a new group of TAAs (Table 1). These Hu-MAb-defined antigens are found in the cytoplasm in all melanoma cells tested. On the other hand, they are not differentiation antigens of neuroectodermal lineage or obvious structural components of melanoma cells. Although they are present in tumors that are unrelated to melanoma embryologically, these antigens are preferentially expressed by tumor cells and not by their normal counterparts.

The reactivities of one IgG Hu-MAb have been studied most extensively and will be presented here. Antibody 2-139-1 was first analyzed by immunocytochemical methods against 88 cell lines. The cells were briefly fixed for 5 min with buffered formalin and their membrane permeabilized for 1 min with cold acetone. The antibody stained all 12 melanoma cell lines, including short-term ocular melanoma cultures and well-established lines from cutaneous metastases. In contrast to mouse MAbs, no reactivity was detected against all seven tumor cell lines of neuroectodermal origin. No reactivity was detected in any of the 45 lymphomas, leukemias and lymphoblastoid cell lines or in the six

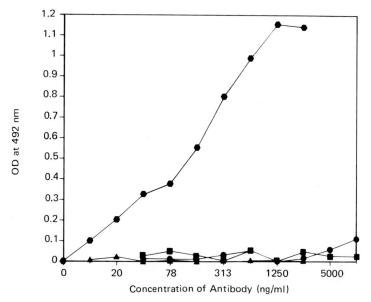

Figure 1   Comparison of sensitivity of the detection of binding by Hu-MAb
6-35-4 to its target antigen by direct versus indirect binding assays. A lysate
of melanoma cells was coated onto microtiter wells for 2 hr and washed.
Equal concentrations of purified Hu-MAb or polyclonal IgG antibodies were
added to the wells and incubated for an additional 2 hr. In the direct binding
assay, binding of 6-35-4 was visualized by the addition of the avidin-biotin-
peroxidase complex. In the indirect assay, a biotin-conjugated goat antibody
with reactivity against the gamma-chain of human immunoglobulin was added
for an hour and the binding was then visualized as before. ●, biotin-conjugated 6-35-4; ▲, biotin-conjugated polyclonal human IgG; ■, ●, indirect binding using a biotin-conjugated goat antihuman IgG to detect binding by 6-35-4
and polyclonal human IgG, respectively.

sarcoma cell lines. On the other hand, 2-139-1 reacted against 12
of the 16 carcinoma cell lines tested, staining all four lines of
colon origin rather strongly.

       We next tested the specificity of 2-139-1 against human tissue
sections. This allowed us to study the expression of the target
antigen not only in tumors, but also in nonneoplastic lesions and
normal tissues. To achieve this, special modifications of the immunohistochemical procedure were necessary. After purification

Table 1 Comparison of the Antigens Identified by Murine MAbs and Hu-MAbs

Biochemical nature of antigen	Name of antibody	Tissue distribution							Shed into			Detectable in fixed sections?
		Melanoma	Gliomas	Nevi	Melano-cytes	Fetal tissues	Other carcinomas	Lymphoid tissues	Super-natant	Serum	Vitreous	
Hu-MAbs												
protein	2-139-1	+(100%)[a]	−	−	−	−	+	−	Yes	?	Yes	Yes
protein	6-26-3	+(100%)	−	−	−	−	+	−	?	?	?	Yes
protein	10-3-44	+(100%)	−	−	−	−	+	−	Yes	?	Yes	Yes
Murine MAbs												
gangliosides												
GD2		+(100%)	+	+	+	+		+	Yes			No
GD3		+(95%)	+	+	+	+	+	+	Yes			No
o-Acetylated GD3		+(30%)	−	−	−	−	−	−				No
neuroectodermal differentiation antigens												
proteoglycan 105/130Kd(MAb		+(100%)	+	+	+	+	+		Yes	Yes		Yes
NU4B)		+(100%)	+	−	−	−	+	−	Yes	Yes		No
proliferation-related antigens												
transferrin receptor		+(100%)	+	+	+	+	+	+	Yes	Yes		
gp130		+(60%)	−	−	−	+	−	−	Yes	Yes		
melanocyte "differentiation antigen"												
HLA-DR		+(100%)[b]					+	+				

aPercent of melanomas positive.
bOnly a fraction of the tumor cells were positive.

by HPLC, the antibody was conjugated directly to biotin and its reactivities in tissue sections visualized by the avidin-biotin-peroxidase complex (ABC method) (27,31). This procedure has several advantages when MAbs of human origin are being tested. First, the variable amount of endogenous human immunoglobulin in human tissues would have no effect when a direct assay is used. Second, the binding is amplified by the ABC method. Finally, as mentioned before, our human IgG MAbs are poorly recognized by goat second antibody reagents.

No reactivity was detected against frozen sections of normal colon, stomach, breast, skin, and lung, although melanoma sections were stained with moderate or high intensity under these conditions. To test the specificity of 2-139-1 in detail against the broadest possible spectrum of tissues, we also examined the reactivity of 2-139-1 against formalin-fixed, paraffin-embedded sections of human tissues. The antibody recognized every melanoma tested, including both primary and metastatic lesions and ocular melanomas (27,31). Notably, it exhibited no reactivity against skin melanocytes and the cells in banal nevi. Also, no reactivity was detected in a variety of nonpigmented normal tissues, such as normal skin, liver, lung, and colon, or other benign tumors, such as mammary fibroadenoma and benign prostate hypertrophy.

As with our immunocytochemical results, the antibody exhibits strong cross-reactivity against adenocarcinomas of the colon, prostate, rectum, and pancreas. However, not all carcinomas were stained. Excluding the specimens of colon and prostate carcinomas, reactivity was observed against only 13 of 23 specimens of carcinoma studied, including only borderline reactivity against squamous cell carcinoma of the lung and transitional carcinoma of the bladder. No reactivity was detected with five specimens of sarcomas and miscellaneous tumors.

The most interesting and unique aspect of the reactivity of 2-139-1 is its ability to distinguish cutaneous malignant melanomas from benign nevi in fixed sections (31). It reacted with all 20 primary cutaneous malignant melanomas, 17 metastatic cutaneous melanomas, and 7 ocular melanomas. Reactivity was also noted against one of five specimens of lentigo mealigna. Two of five "dysplastic nevi" were also stained, although only 40% of the melanocytic cells in the sections were reactive. No reactivity was

found with 22 other banal nevi representing a spectrum of histologic types or with normal skin melanocytes.

We have begun a collaboration with Drs. Wain L. White and A.
Bernard Ackerman to further test the usefulness of this antibody in
patients in whom diagnosis is difficult. One particularly striking
result is shown in Figure 2, which depicts a melanoma in situ arising from a preexisting intradermal nevus. Antibody 2-139-1 reacted against all single and clusters (nests) of melanoma cells with
a staining intensity of 4+, without any reactivity against the morphologically well-defined nevus cells. The ability of 2-139-1 to
discriminate nonmalignant melanocytes from melanoma cells was
further illustrated in an unusual case of a benign congenital compound nevus. Diagnosis from this specmen was difficult on the
basis of morphological or cytological appearance because there were
several malignant characteristics: large nests of pagetoid melanocytes, some of which were detected above the epidermal-dermal
junction, and involvement of epithelial adnexae. No reactivity of
2-139-1 was found with these benign nevus cells.

HUMAN MONOCLONAL ANTIBODIES WITH REACTIVITY
TO OTHER TYPES OF TUMOR

Human MAbs with reactivity against glioma (32), breast carcinoma
(33), and colon carcinoma have been described. Many of these
antibodies remain to be characterized in greater detail. Haspel
et al. (34) generated Hu-MAbs from peripheral blood lymphocytes of patients with colon carcinoma after autologous immunization. Several of the LCLs appear to be stable and produced
large quantities of human IgM MAbs that react with surface antigens of colon carcinoma cells. Their specificities of binding and
their potential application in radioimaging is currently under investigation.

The striking cross-reactivity of 2-139-1 and the other melanoma MAbs to colon carcinomas suggests that perhaps Hu-MAbs
thus generated recognize only a limited number of target antigens. To test this hypothesis, we developed a series of Hu-MAbs
from regional lymph nodes of patients with colon cancer (30,35).
Immunohistochemical characterization against human tumor
xenografts revealed that some of the antibodies that reacted with

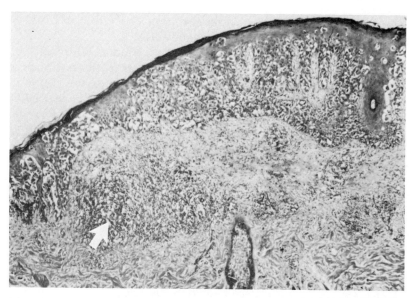

(a)

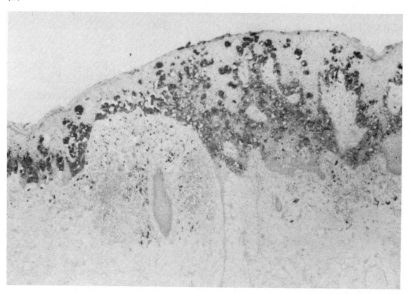

(b)

colon tumors also cross-reacted to melanomas and other adenocarcinomas. However, some of these MAbs did not cross-react
with melanoma.

One of the noncross-reacting IgG MAbs, 14-31-10, was selected for further characterization. The reactivity of 14-31-10
against human tissues was found to be rather restricted. The
MAb reacted against cytoplasmic antigens in all colon carcinomas
tested (30,35), although no binding was detected against normal
colon epithelium. No binding was detected against other normal
tissues, including skin, stomach, liver, pancreas, kidney, small
bowel, or lung. The lack of reactivity against melanoma was
more quantitatively confirmed by an enzyme immunoassay using
cell lysates.

In parallel studies of 2-139-1 in melanoma, MAb 14-31-10
was tested against inflammatory and preneoplastic lesions of the
colon. The antibody was not reactive against benign lesions such
as diverticulosis-diverticulitis, regional enteritis, or amebic colitis.
Staining was found in three of six specimens of villous adenomas
and one of three specimen of ulcerative colitis (35). In collaboration with Dr. George Mandarino, an enzyme immunoassay was
developed to detect the presence of this antigen in the sera of
cancer patients. Antibody 14-31-10 was used both as "trapper"
and an "indicator" antibody in this assay. The antigen, nonde-
tectable in normal sera, has been found in 30-50% of the sera of
patients with colon and breast carcinomas.

SUMMARY AND PERSPECTIVE

Our results illustrate that Hu-MAbs can add a new dimension to
identifying novel TAAs. Our Hu-MAbs derived from regional

Figure 2   Selective reactivity of Hu-MAb-2-139-1 against a melanoma in situ
and not against benign nevus cells in a subjacent intradermal nevus: (a) a
section stained with hematoxylin-eosin to illustrate the morphological features. The arrow indicates the location of the intradermal nevus; (b) same
section stained by the Hu-MAb 2-139-1. The melanoma in situ is clearly identified and is represented in this black and white photomicrograph by the dark
staining. (In the original section, the melanoma stained a deep red.) The
scattered dark granules in the dermis were brown melanin-containing nevus
cells, which were not stained by the MAb.

lymph node cells of melanoma patients defined a family of cytoplasmic TAAs. Extensive studies on the specificities of these antibodies using cell lines and tissue specimens revealed a high degree
of discrimination between tumor and normal tissues. While absolute discrimination may be impossible with any MAb, the spectra
of reactivity of these Hu-MAbs are sufficiently restricted to warrant further studies. Their target antigens are distinct from those
previously identified by mouse MAbs. Some of these, such as
those identified by 2-139-1 and 14-31-10, might have applications
in pathological and serological diagnosis.

We are in the process of biochemically identifying the TAA
defined by 2-139-1. Although the antigen is a protein, it cannot be
immunoprecipitated from detergent lysates of melanoma cells
after biosynthetic labeling with radioactive amino acids or phosphate. The possibility exists, therefore, that this TAA might have
a low turnover rate. The antigen eluted from an affinity column
of 2-139-1 consists of a homogeneous population of large detergent micelles when analyzed by HPLC molecular-sizing columns.
This hydrophobicity, perhaps, explains the antigen's stability, even
upon fixation of tissues and despite treatment with organic solvents.

In our studies, we have used only regional lymph node cells
as a source of sensitized lymphocytes. For in vitro diagnosis, cytoplasmic TAAs might even have advantages over surface antigens.
For the pathologist, it is preferable to see staining of the entire
cytoplasm. Because membrane proteins make up only a small
fraction of the total cellular proteins, cytoplasmic antigens may
be present at higher concentrations and, perhaps, may be more
easily detectable in sera. In fact, most of the TAAs identified by
our Hu-MAbs are shed into culture supernates. It is possible,
therefore, that these lymphocytes in the regional lymph nodes
may be especially sensitized to antigens that are shed by the
tumor.

With the development of better in vitro immunization procedures, it should be possible to generate Hu-MAbs with reactivity
to surface antigens of tumor cells. Such antibodies may have more
in vivo applications for tracing by scintigraphy for the treatment
of cancer by immunoconjugates. Although our human-mouse
heterohybridomas are most likely impermanent, sufficiently large
amounts of these Hu-MAbs can be produced for characterization

of the target antigens and perhaps to develop mouse MAbs with reactivity to the same antigen or epitope. However, it would be more desirable to develop better hybridoma technology, such as that involving directed in vitro immunization, for a less circuitous approach to this issue.

REFERENCES

1. R. A. Miller and R. L. Levy, *Lancet 2*:226 (1981).
2. R. L. Levy and R. A. Miller, *Ann. Rev. Med. 34*:107 (1983).
3. H. S. Kaplan and L. Olsson, in *Hybridomas in Cancer Diagnosis and Treatment* (M. S. Mitchell and H. F. Oettgen, eds.), Vol. 21, Raven Press, New York, (1982), p. 113.
4. M. Steinitz, G. Klein, S. Koskimies, and O. Makela, *Nature 269*:420 (1977).
5. D. Kozbor and J. C. Roder, *J. Immunol. 127*:1275 (1981).
6. R. F. Irie, L. L. Sze, and R. E. Saxton, *Proc. Natl. Acad. Sci. USA 79*:5666 (1982).
7. D. Kozbor, D. L. Dexter, and J. C. Roder, *Hybridoma 2*:7 (1983).
8. K. Sikora, T. Alderson, J. Ellis, J. Phillips, and J. Watson, *Br. J. Cancer 47*:135 (1983).
9. S. P. C. Cole, B. G. Campling, T. Atlaw, D. Kozbor and J. C. Roder, *Mol. Cell. Biochem. 62*:109 (1984).
10. J. W. Larrick and D. W. Buck, *BioTechniques 2*:6 (1982).
11. N. H. H. Teng, K. S. Lam, F. C. Riera, and H. S. Kaplan, *Proc. Natl. Acad. Sci. USA 80*:7308 (1983).
12. S. K. H. Foung, S. Perkins, A. Raubitschek, J. Larrick, G. Lizak, D. Fishwild, E. B. Engelman, and F. C. Grumet, *J. Immunol. Methods 70*:83 (1982).
13. M. R. Posner, S. F. Schlossman, and H. Lazarus, *Hybridoma 2*:369 (1983).
14. R. J. Cote, D. M. Morrissey, H. F. Oettgen, and L. J. Old, *Fed. Proc. 43*:2465 (1984).
15. M.-K. Ho, N. Rand, J. Murray, K. Kato, and H. Rabin, *J. Immunol. 135*:3831 (1985).
16. N. Hanai, K. Shitara, and H. Yoshida, *Cancer Res. 46*:4438 (1986).
17. R. A. Reisfeld, D. A. Cheresh, G. Schulz, J. R. Harper, and V. Quaranta, in *Immunity to Cancer* (A. Reif and M. S. Mitchell, eds.), Academic Press, New York (1985), p. 97.

18. R. A. Reisfeld, *Semin. Oncol. 13*:153 (1986).
19. B. S. Wilson, F. Indiveri, M. A. Pellegrino and S. Ferrone, *J. Exp. Med. 149*:658 (1979).
20. J. P. Brown, R. M. Hewick, I. Hellstrom, K. E. Hellstrom, R. F. Doolittle, and W. J. Dreyer, *Nature 296*:171 (1982).
21. F. C. S. Ramaekers, J. J. G. Puts, O. Moesker, A. Kant, A. Huysmans, D. Haag, P. H. K. Jap, C. J. Herman, and G. P. Vooijs, *Histochem. J. 15*:691 (1983).
22. K. C. Gatter, C. Alcock, A. Heryet, and D. Y. Mason, *Lancet 1*:1302 (1985).
23. C. Wagener, P. Petzold, W. Kohler, and V. Totovic, *Int. J. Cancer 33*:469 (1984).
24. K. Bosslet, G. Luben, A. Schwarz, E. Hundt, H. P. Harthus, F. R. Seiler, C. Muhrer, G. Klopperl, K. Kayser, and H. H. Sedlacek, *Int. J. Cancer 36*:75 (1985).
25. A. N. Houghton, H. Brooks, R. J. Cote, M. C. Taormina, H. F. Oettgen, and L. J. Old, *J. Exp. Med. 158*:53 (1983).
26. A. N. Houghton, *Transplant. Proc. 16*:351 (1984).
27. J. Kan-Mitchell, A. Imam, R. A. Kempf, C. R. Taylor, and M. S. Mitchell, *Cancer Res. 46*:2490 (1986).
28. J. Kan-Mitchell, K. L. Andrews, D. Gallardo, and M. S. Mitchell, *Hybridoma 6*:161 (1987).
29. J. Kan-Mitchell, D. M. Munoz, K. L. Andrews, and M. S. Mitchell, (submitted for publication).
30. S. C. Formenti, M. S. Mitchell, F. Rosen, R. A. Kempf, A. Imam, C. R. Taylor, and J. Kan-Mitchell, *Proc. Am. Assoc. Cancer Res. 26*:297 (1985).
31. A. Imam, M. S. Mitchell, R. L. Modlin, C. R. Taylor, R. A. Kempf, and J. Kan-Mitchell, *J. Invest. Dermatol. 86*:145 (1986).
32. K. Sikora, T. Alterton, J. Phillips, and J. V. Watson, *Lancet 1*:11 (1982).
33. J. Schlom, D. Wunderlich, and Y. A. Teramoto, *Proc. Natl. Acad. Sci. USA 77*:6841 (1980).
34. M. V. Haspel, R. P. McCabe, N. Pomato, N. J. Janesch, J. V. Knowlton, L. C. Peters, H. C. Hoover, Jr., and M. G. Hanna, Jr., *Cancer Res. 45*:3951 (1985).
35. S. C. Formenti, J. Kan-Mitchell, P. Jernstrom, C. R. Taylor, and M. S. Mitchell, *Proc. Am. Assoc. Cancer Res. 27*:337 (1986).

13
Monoclonal Antibody Assays for Human Cancer: Future Perspectives

Herbert Z. Kupchik / Boston University School of Medicine, and the Mallory Institute of Pathology, Boston, Massachusetts

INTRODUCTION

The preceding chapters have attempted to summarize the current diagnostic applicability of a number of monoclonal antibodies that recognize a variety of tumor-associated macromolecules. In most instances, the availability of virtually unlimited quantities of antibodies that react specifically with epitopes on human tumor markers has led to expectations of development of clinically useful diagnostic assays. Evaluations of these assays in clinical setting have demonstrated, for the most part, that the assays may be useful for monitoring response to therapy or for prognostic application. However, there are still no in vitro tumor-specific marker assays that can be relied upon for the diagnosis of solid human cancers. It may be that there are no macromolecules that are specific for human tumors or that those that are specific are not released in sufficient quantities to ever be measurable in body fluids. Those of us involved in this field would, however, prefer to assume a more optimistic view. That is, the advent of new technologies and innovative approaches to the problem of early diagnosis may lead to monoclonal antibodies (MAbs) and assay systems that will succeed where others have fallen short.

This chapter will identify and discuss three areas of investigation which may result in such improved in vitro assays. Namely (1) sources of new tumor markers, (2) production of more highly specific monoclonal antibodies, and (3) new assay designs.

SOURCES OF NEW TUMOR MARKERS

Over the years, investigators have sought to produce antibodies to markers identified in tumor tissue extracts, tumor cell extracts, purified putative markers, isolated tumor cells, etc. For the most part, these have met with limited success. In the search for new more highly specific tumor markers or markers that may appear at an earlier stage of tumor growth, innovative approaches must be used.

In 1969, Sela (1) coined the term *immunopotent* to describe those determinants that could provoke the production of specific antibodies in high concentration in the sera of immunized animals. It is possible that such immunopotent determinants may represent more common macromolecules, and the number of somatic cell fusion products responding to these determinants may be sufficiently large to swamp out fused cells responding to potentially more specific but less immunopotent determinants. In an effort to produce MAbs to less immunodominant macromolecules, which might prove to be more distinctive to human cancers, Morgan et al. (2) grew human colon adenocarcinomas as xenografts in nude mice. Peripheral protein extracts of these tumors were then combined with lectin and used as immunogens. Antibodies produced by the resulting cloned hybridomas were screened against cultured and xenografted colon, breast, lung, and lymphoid cells, and also extracts of colonic carcinoma membranes, glycolipids, and carcinoembryonic antigen (CEA), as well as paraffin and frozen sections of patient tumors and normal colonic mucosae. These MAbs, when compared with those obtained using whole cells or crude membrane extracts as immunogens, were produced in greater frequency, were more stable, were more frequently IgG (especially IgG3), and exhibited enhanced specificity for tumors.

Tong et al. (3) have used a different approach for the production of MAbs specific for small-cell lung carcinoma (SCLC). They postulated that immunization with multiple tumor cell lines that were histologically the same would enhance the generation of cells producing antibody to SCLC common tumor-associated antigens. Following simultaneous immunization with two distinct SCLC cell lines, two MAbs were produced that recognized the original cell lines as well as a substantial number of SCLC and other lung carcinoma tissue specimens, but that did not react with numerous other (normal and tumor) cell lines and tissues.

It is widely accepted that one of the problems inherent in identifying human carcinomas is the noticable heterogeneity among tumors of the same type as well as within a given tumor. Using membrane-enriched fractions of human metastatic mammary carcinoma lesions, Schlom et al. (4) developed MAbs that could be divided into five major groups based on differences in reactivity with different carcinomas and carcinoma cell line surfaces and with the molecular size of the reactive antigens. Their data demonstrated a diversity of antigen expression among various mammary carcinomas as well as within a given tumor mass. Our laboratory is attempting to reduce such heterogeneity in human colonic carcinoma cell lines by separating invasive and noninvasive cells from the parental populations (5). Whether based on invasiveness, degree of differentiation, or a particular phenotypic trait, the use of such selected cells as immunizing agents may enhance our ability to develop MAbs that recognize a marker associated with a specific characteristic of tumors.

In 1972, Halliday and Miller (6) developed an assay of cell-mediated antitumor immunity called leukocyte adherence inhibition (LAI). The assay was based on the presence of factors in the serum of cancer patients that could inhibit the normal adherence of nonsensitized leukocytes to glass. Numerous laboratories have demonstrated a high degree of "tumor-type" specificity over the past decade. The tumor factor(s) recognized by the leukocytes have been the subject of several investigative efforts and a polypeptide with a relative molecular weight of 40,000 has been identified by Artigas et al. (7). They used an MAb (anti-p40) to monitor the isolation of the polypeptide which exhibited organ specificity and appeared to be immunogenic and antigenic in the patient. This group has also presented data to suggest that the

T8$^+$ (Lai-2a$^+$) subset of T cells that are reactive in the LAI system
is triggered by tumor antigen to generate leukotrienelike mediators
(8). Thus, in addition to the identification of putative tumor
specific antigens, the LAI phenomenon may provide host-syn-
thesized markers (mediators) to which MAbs may be generated.
Such mediators, because they are produced by the host in response to tumors, may be generated sufficiently early and in
sufficiently high concentrations to be useful diagnostically. Hadas
et al. (9) have recently been able to produce an MAb against an
organ-specific neoantigen (OSN) defined by LAI assay of colon
carcinoma. Although they were unable to use the antibody to
clearly distinguish between the OSNs of different tumor patients
and normal cross-reactive proteins, they suggested that MAbs can
be produced against affinity-purified OSNs and these may be useful in immunoassays for the detection of colon cancer.

Oncogenes are cellular genes that are thought to be responsible
for the acquisition of the malignant phenotype by normal cells
(10). Amplification of several oncogenes, including c-myc, c-myb,
c-ras^{ki}, c-ras^{Ha}, c-abl, c-erb B and N-myc have been described for
human cancers (11). These oncogenes appear to code for protein
products that may play a role in cell growth or behavior. Investigators have begun making antibodies to such oncogene products
directly (12,13) or by using NIH 3T3 fibroblast cells that have
been transfected with human tumor DNAs as immunizing agents
(14). The latter provides an ideal situation for immunizing mice
because transfected cells can be selected and cloned based on a
specific phenotypic property, and the lymphocytes of the immunized mice will respond to the human gene products, even though
they may be relatively minor components of the cell. Such procedures may go a long way in producing MAbs capable of identifying gene products responsible for a specific aspect of malignancy.

PRODUCTION OF MONOCLONAL ANTIBODIES

Although the basic format designed by Köhler and Milstein in
1975 (15) is used widely for somatic cell fusion, cloning, and MAb
production, a number of investigators have sought to make modifications that might result in increased opportunities to obtain
more clinically useful antibodies. Grant et al. (16,17) have investi-

gated and compared a number of different immunization protocols in their attempts to produce MAbs to human pancreatic cancer. In the earlier study, they found that fusion of splenic lymphocytes, from immunocompetent mice immunized with serum
from nude mice bearing human pancreatic tumor xenografts,
yielded fewer hybrids, but proportionally more of these produced
antibodies selective for the pancreatic tumor cell used (16). Their
more recent studies showed that immunization of the nude
mouse's hairy litter mates with extracts of the pancreatic tumor
xenografts plus the cultured tumor cells resulted in the highest
proportion of antibody (selective for the tumor cell line)-produc-
ing hybrids. These studies suggest that immunogenic markers
comparable with those in the original tumor may be expressed
during in vivo growth, although they may be absent or present in
only low amounts in in vitro culture. In addition, the putative
markers are "prescreened" by the syngeneic tumor bearer.

The development of human MAbs is another approach that
may lead to the generation of more useful diagnostic reagents.
Haspel et al. (18) have generated tumor cell-reactive human MAbs
from peripheral blood lymphocytes of cancer patients who were
actively immunized with autologous tumor cells. Although they
sought to fuse such cells with mouse myeloma cells, they also generated diploid human B cells that were stable producers of human
MAbs. Their findings suggested that the specificity of these antibodies was restricted to those macromolecules recognized as immunogenic in the autologous host. In spite of a number of technical problems in generating such human antibodies, this is an
extremely important field of study and has been summarized in
more detail in Chapter 12.

Perhaps the most critical step in the production of MAbs is
the availability of a sensitive assay with which one can screen a
multitude of potential antibody-producing hybridomas. In the
search for antibodies to new tumor markers, the problem is com-
pounded by the anonymity of small quantities of markers that may
be present in the sera of cancer patients. In an attempt to resolve
these problems, Katz et al. (19) have developed a microenzyme-
linked immunosorbent assay (ELISA) based on the inhibition, between suspected antibody and tumor membranes, brought about
by cancer patient sera. The assay required only 0.003 ml of hybridoma culture supernatant per test. Using sera from over 100

patients, they screened 100 fusions and identified four antibodies that reacted with the determinant(s) found in sera from cancer patients but not found in sera from control patients or normal donors. These and other innovative assay systems will be helpful for future screening of hybridomas.

ASSAY DESIGNS

In addition to searching for new tumor markers that may be more representative or specific for selected tumors, or for tumors in general, it is anticipated that redesign of assays that use existing reagents (or that will use the new reagents) will improve the in vitro diagnostic usefulness of MAbs. Improved sensitivity does not appear to be the problem because existing radioimmunoassays, enzymoimmunoassays, and fluorometric methods can detect 1 ng or less of marker per milliliter of body fluid, and the tumor markers that have been now identified have been associated with nonmalignant diseases or with normal individuals at such levels.

One approach, which has been investigated with polyclonal antisera and merits additional consideration with MAbs, is the coordinated use of multiple assays for existing markers associated with a common tumor type. For example, several groups have shown that the combined use of CEA and CA 19-9 assays was superior to either assay alone when evaluating patients with pancreatic carcinoma (20,21). Mercer and Talamo (22) came to similar conclusions with a "colon panel" of markers for colorectal carcinoma and Kuriyama et al. (23) suggested that a multiple marker test of tissue-specific antigens would be of value in the diagnosis of prostatic cancer.

The exquisite specificity of an MAb for a single epitope on a macromolecule can also be the cause of gross nonselectivity if that epitope is common to one or more other macromolecules expressed by normal or by other cells that are not of interest. On the other hand, this "problem" can be used to great advantage if one has several MAbs against the same macromolecule but reacting with different epitopes on that molecule. The totality of the specificity of the antibodies would greatly enhance the selectivity if the macromolecule in question was exclusive to the cell sought (i.e., cells within the tumor being examined).

Ehrlich et al. (24,25) have demonstrated how the use of multiple MAbs to different epitopes on human chorionic gonadotropin can result in enhanced affinity and increased sensitivity when appropriately combined in an assay system. Several investigators have used this approach in their studies of CEA and related assay system. Neumaier et al. (26) developed five MAbs to CEA that recognized different epitopes on different preparations of CEA and related macromolecules. Their data suggested that, of the sources of CEA and CEA-like material examined, only CEA from colorectal carcinoma tissues was recognized by all five antibodies. Buchegger et al. (27) produced three MAbs that reacted with three different epitopes of CEA and successfully incorporated them into a sensitive sandwich enzyme immunoassay, as did David et al. (28) with two antibodies. Although neither group has shown significant enhancement of specificity for carcinoma, similar studies with other markers may yet succeed.

In addition to the potential for tumor specificity that is afforded by MAbs directed against tumor markers, methodology now exists for the production of chimeric antibodies that can simultaneously bind the marker and offer an effector function (29). Newberger et al. (30) have shown that in vitro mutagenesis and DNA transfection techniques can be used to produce recombinant MAbs and have successfully produced a chimeric antibody in which the antigen-binding portion of the immunoglobulin was fused to an enzymatic moiety. Such chimeric antitumor marker antibodies would simplify ELISA-type assays by reduction of the number of steps required.

For several years now, a number of investigators have been evaluating a heterogeneous category of chemicals, generally termed *biologic response modifiers*, as differentiation agents for clinical application. These studies are based on the thesis that differentiated functions are more highly expressed in nonproliferating cells. In the course of such studies, alterations in the expression of various tumor-associated markers have correlated with increased differentiation. Hager et al. (31) noted that in addition to alterations in the degree of differentiation brought about by N,N-dimethylformamide, treated colon cancer cells showed increased cell surface-associated CEA and colonic mucoprotein antigen. Similarly, Tsao et al. (32) noted that butyrate-treated colon cancer cells not only presented characteristics of increased differentiation but also expressed more CEA. Theophylline-treated melanoma cells showed morphological changes associated with increased differentiation and concomitant enhanced surface expression of HLA-A,B,C antigens and β_2-microglobulin (33). Greiner et al. (34) have demonstrated that treatment of breast and colon carcinoma cells with interferon also resulted in increased surface expression of tumor-associated macromolecules which were recognized by their MAbs. Thus, biological modifiers that may find their way into the clinical armament as antiproliferative agents, may also enhance the sensitivity of tumor marker assay systems designed to evaluate therapy. In addition, studies such as those cited above may result in the identification of new markers associated with nonproliferative states of tumors. Monoclonal antibodies to these new markers might be extremely useful in identifying patients with early stage malignancy.

CONCLUSION

It is unrealistic to expect that screening assays to detect the presence of tumor markers in body fluids will be forthcoming regardless of the development of MAb technology. This, in a large measure, is due to the heterogeneous and complex nature of human cancer. In addition, although it is commonly suggested that a test that is 90% accurate (10% false-positive, 10% false-negative) would be clinically useful if the appropriate reagents could be developed, one has to question whether this would be economically and logistically practical. For example, the average annual age-adjusted incidence rate for all forms of malignant neoplasms during 1973-1977 was approximately 3.3:1000 population (35). For each 1000 individuals screened, 100 false-positive (10%) could be anticipated while only 3.3 true-positives (a 30:1 ratio). All of these would have to undergo thorough, expensive, and psychologically traumatic clinical examination.

It would, therefore, seem more appropriate to attempt to develop assays that will be clinically useful for the diagnosis of cancer in individuals at risk, for prognostic application, and for monitoring response to surgery or to therapy. The plethora of new technology being developed for the production of new and more relevant MAbs and the innovative use of such techniques, either individually or in combination, may meet this challenge within this century for a significant number of tumor types.

REFERENCES

1. M. Sela, *Science 166*:1365 (1969).
2. A. C. Morgan, Jr., C. S. Woodhouse, J. A. Knost, K. A. Foon, and R. K. Oldham, *Hybridoma 3*:64 (1984).
3. A. W. Tong, J. Lee, and M. J. Stone, *Hybridoma 3*:82 (1984).
4. J. Schlom, D. Colcher, P. H. Hand, D. Wunderlich, M. Nuti, and Y. A. Teramoto, in *Understanding Breast Cancer: Clinical and Laboratory Concepts* (M. A. Rich, J. C. Hager, and P. Furmanski, eds), Marcel Dekker, New York (1983). p. 169.
5. H. Z. Kupchik and S. Aznavoorian, *Proc. Am. Assoc. Cancer Res. 27*:57 (1986).
6. W. J. Halliday and S. Miller, *Int. J. Cancer 9*:477 (1972).
7. C. Artigas, D. M. P. Thomson, M. Durko, M. Sutherland, R. Scanzano, G. Shenouda, and A. E. J. Dubois, *Cancer Res. 46*:1874 (1986).
8. N. Labateya and D. M. P. Thomson, *J. Natl. Cancer Inst. 75*:987 (1985).
9. E. Hadas, A. Fink, E. Gembom, N. Harpaz, A. Shani, Z. Bentwich, and Z. Eshhar, *Cancer Res. 46*:5210 (1986).
10. R. A. Weinberg, *Adv. Cancer Res. 36*:149 (1982).
11. J. Yokota, Y. Tsunetsugu-Yokota, H. Battifora, C. Le Fevre, and M. J. Cline, *Science 231*:261 (1986).
12. A. Thor, P. Horan Hand, D. Wunderlich, A. Caruso, R. Muraro, and J. Schlom, *Nature 311*:562 (1984).
13. W. P. Carney, D. Petit, P. Hamer, C. J. Der, T. Finkel, G. M. Cooper, M. Lefebore, H. Mobtaker, R. DeLellis, A. S. Tischler, Y. Dayal, H. Wolfe, and H. Rabin, *Proc. Natl. Acad. Sci. USA 83*:7485 (1986).
14. M. A. Hollingsworth, L. M. Rebellato, J. W. Moore, O. J. Finn, and R. S. Metzgard, *Cancer Res. 46*:2482 (1986).
15. G. Köhler and C. Milstein, *Nature 256*:495 (1975).
16. A. Grant, P. Harris, B. Pym, and J. Hermon-Taylor, *Br. J. Cancer 50*:278 (1984).
17. A. G. Grant, P. M. Harris, E. Heyderman, S. E. Larkin, B. Pym, and J. Hermon-Taylor, *Br. J. Cancer 52*:543 (1985).
18. M. V. Haspel, R. P. McCabe, N. Pomato, N. J. Janesch, J. V. Knowlton, L. C. Peters, H. C. Hoover, Jr., and M. G. Hanna, Jr., *Cancer Res. 45*:3951 (1985).
19. D. V. Katz, D. Chia, M. Hermes, J. Galton, M. Hirota, and P. I. Terasaki, *J. Natl. Cancer Inst. 74*:335 (1985).

20. W. H. Schmiegel, W. Eberl, C. Kreiker, H. Kalthoff, G. H. But-
    zow, K. Jessen, R. Klapdor, N. Soehendra, N. Wargenau, and
    M. Classen, *Hepatogastroenterology 32*:141 (1985).
21. W. M. Steinberg, R. Gelfand, K. K. Anderson, J. Glen, S. H.
    Kurtzman, W. F. Sindlar, and P. P. Toskes, *Gastroenterology
    90*:343 (1986).
22. D. W. Mercer and T. S. Talamo, *Clin. Chem. 31*:1824 (1985).
23. M. Kuriyama, M. C. Wang, C. L. Lee, C. S. Killian, L. D. Pap-
    sidero, H. Inaji, R. M. Loor, M. F. Lin, T. Nishiura, N. H.
    Slack, G. P. Murphy, and T. M. Chu, *J. Natl. Cancer Inst. 68*:
    99 (1982).
24. P. H. Ehrlich, W. R. Moyle, Z. A. Moustafa, and R. E. Can-
    field, *J. Immunol. 128*:2709 (1982).
25. P. H. Ehrlich and W. R. Moyle, *Science 221*:279 (1983).
26. M. Neumaier, U. Fenger, and C. Wagener, *J. Immunol. 135*:
    3604 (1985).
27. F. Buchegger, C. Mettraux, R. S. Accolla, S. Carrel, and J.-P.
    Mach, *Immunol. Lett. 5*:85 (1982).
28. G. S. David, R. Wang, R. Bartholomew, E. D. Sevier, T. H.
    Adams, and H. E. Greene, *Clin. Chem. 27*:1580 (1981).
29. S. L. Morrison, *Science 229*:1202 (1985).
30. M. S. Neuberger, G. T. Williams, and R. O. Fox, *Nature 312*:
    604 (1984).
31. J. C. Hager, D. V. Gold, J. A. Barbosa, Z. Fligiel, F. Miller,
    and D. L. Dexter, *J. Natl. Cancer Inst. 64*:439 (1980).
32. D. Tsao, A. Mouta, A. Bella, Jr., P. Luu, and Y. S. Kim,
    Cancer Res. 42:1052 (1982).
33. S.-K. Liao, P. C. Kwong, J. W. Smith, P. B. Dent, and D. A.
    Clark, *J. Biol. Resp. Mod. 2*:280 (1983).
34. J. W. Greiner, P. H. Hand, P. Noguchi, P. B. Fisher, S. Petska,
    and J. Schlom, *Cancer Res. 44*:3208 (1984).
35. J. L. Young, C. L. Percy, A. J. Asire, J. W. Berg, M. M. Cusano,
    L. A. Gloeckler, J. W. Horn, W. I. Lourie, E. S. Pollack, and
    E. M. Shambaugh, in *Surveillance, Epidemiology, and End
    Results: Incidence and Mortality Data, 1973-77* (J. L. Young,
    C. L. Percy and A. J. Asire, eds.), NIH Publication No. 81-
    2330, Bethesda, Maryland (1981), p. 3.

Index